Social Development and Social Work Perspectives on Social Protection

Social protection is now considered a development milestone and an important tool in combating poverty. Interventions can include, for example, health insurance, public works programs, guaranteed employment schemes, or cash transfers targeting vulnerable populations groups.

This innovative volume is designed to develop understanding about the role and contribution of social protection globally and to share innovative practices and policies from around the world. It explores how to cover an entire population effectively, especially those who are at risk or who are already in a situation of deprivation, and in a sustainable manner. Divided into two parts, the book begins by exploring the theoretical underpinnings of social protection, discussing the social work and social development perspectives and concepts that currently shape it. The second part is comprised of case studies from countries implementing successful social protection initiatives, including Brazil, India, South Africa, Ghana, Nigeria and Indonesia, and reveals how the impact of a successful social protection intervention on poverty, vulnerability and inequality can be dramatic.

This volume is an important reference for students and researchers from a range of disciplines including social policy, social work, development studies, geography, planning, economics, sociology, population health and political science.

Julie Drolet is Associate Professor in the Faculty of Social Work, University of Calgary, Canada.

Routledge advances in health and social policy

Social Development and Social Work Perspectives on Social Protection

Edited by Julie Drolet

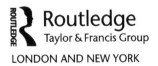

Routledge
Taylor & Francis Group

LONDON AND NEW YORK

First published 2016
by Routledge

2 Park Square, Milton Park, Abingdon, Oxfordshire OX14 4RN
711 Third Avenue, New York, NY 10017

Routledge is an imprint of the Taylor & Francis Group, an informa business

First issued in paperback 2018

British Library Cataloguing-in-Publication Data
A catalogue record for this book is available from the British Library

Library of Congress Cataloging in Publication Data
Names: Drolet, Julie, 1971- editor.
Title: Social development and social work perspectives on social
protection / edited by Julie L. Drolet.
Description: Abingdon, Oxon ; New York, NY : Routledge, 2016.
Identifiers: LCCN 2015042907| ISBN 9781138780392 (hardback) |
ISBN 9781315770796 (ebook)
Subjects: LCSH: Social service. | Public welfare. | Social security. | Social
policy.
Classification: LCC HV40 .S6163 2016 | DDC 361–dc23
LC record available at http://lccn.loc.gov/2015042907

ISBN: 978-1-138-78039-2 (hbk)
ISBN: 978-1-138-34587-4 (pbk)

Typeset in Times New Roman
by Wearset Ltd, Boldon, Tyne and Wear

Contents

Illustrations

Figures

Tables

Contributors

Ziblim Abukari received a bachelor's degree in social work and sociology from the University of Ghana, Legon. He began his social work career as a community organizer and facilitator for the non-profit, Opportunities Industrialization Centers International (OICI) Ghana where he taught low-income women and farmer groups about food security initiatives including microcredit, water and sanitation, and agribusiness development. He obtained an MSW from the University of Denver, Colorado as a Ford Foundation scholar from 2004 to 2006. He conducted his doctoral dissertation research in Ghana on academic outcomes of Ghanaian youth. Dr. Abukari presently teaches as an Assistant Professor at Westfield State University in Westfield, Massachusetts, and has published journal articles on human security, academic achievement, and international social work with a primary focus on Ghana and Sub-Saharan Africa.

Chidimma Aham-Chiabuotu teaches Public Health in Babcock University, Nigeria. She is also a nurse/midwife and specialized in mixed-methods research on women and adolescents. She co-authored *ABC of Women's Health, Financing Higher Education without Tears* and two articles on collaborative social work practice. Chidimma is a recipient of several academic and service awards including the Babcock University Presidents' Award as the student with the best overall performance in leadership, academic, community and spiritual services in 2011.

Vivienne Bozalek is a professor of Social Work and the Director of Teaching and Learning at the University of the Western Cape (UWC), South Africa. She holds a PhD from Utrecht University. Her areas of research, publications and expertise include the use of post-structural, feminist materialist, social justice and the political ethics of care perspectives, critical family studies, innovative pedagogical approaches in higher education, and feminist and participatory research methodologies. She has co-edited three books – one entitled *Community, Self and Identity: Educating South African Students for Citizenship* with Brenda Leibowitz, Ronelle Carolissen and other colleagues (2013), *Discerning Hope in Educational Practices* with Brenda Leibowitz, Ronelle Carolissen and Megan Boler (2014) and *Activity Theory, Authentic*

Learning and Emerging Technologies: Towards a Transformative Higher Education Pedagogy with Dick Ng'ambi, Denise Wood, Jan Herrington, Joanne Hardman and Alan Amory (2015).

Julie Drolet is an associate professor in the Central and Northern Alberta Region of the Faculty of Social Work, University of Calgary. She holds a PhD from McGill University. She is principal investigator of a study titled *Rebuilding Lives Post-Disaster: Innovative Community Practices for Sustainable Development* funded by a SSHRC partnership development grant (2012–2015), and is currently leading the *Alberta Resilient Community (ARC) Research Project* funded by Alberta Innovates Health Solutions (2015–2018). Her research program is supported by infrastructure awarded by the Canadian Foundation for Innovation (CFI). She has published extensively in international social work and social development with a particular focus on climate change and disasters, international social protection initiatives, gender and development, social work field education, qualitative research, and international migration and Canadian immigration.

Tessa Hochfeld is a senior researcher at the Centre for Social Development in Africa, University of Johannesburg. Her work includes research on social justice, social welfare, social policy, transformative social protection and gender and development, with a focus on the social impacts of the Child Support Grant. Tessa has a BA in social work from the University of the Witwatersrand, an MSc in gender and development from the University of London, and will have a PhD in development studies conferred on her during 2016 from the University of the Witwatersrand.

Malakkaran Johny Jino is a researcher in organizational behavior and human resource management in the Department of Management Studies at Indian Institute of Technology, Madras (IIT-M), India. His research considers how contextual factors impact an individual's internal moral capacity that provide motivation for ethical action. He graduated in philosophy (1999–2002) from Mahatma Gandhi University, Kerala, India. After which he spent a year in various social work activities such as tribal development programs, self-help group formation, and also served for the rehabilitation of prisoners, orphans, alcoholics and sex workers. He completed his bachelor's course in theology (2003–2006), in affiliation with Katholieke Universiteit Leuven, Belgium. He is an ordained Catholic priest. He completed a master's in Human Resource Mangement (2008–2010) from Rajagiri Centre for Business Studies (RCBS), Kerala, India.

Linda Kreitzer is presently teaching at the University of Calgary, Faculty of Social Work, in the Central and Northern Region office in Edmonton. She began her career in the USA and moved to the UK in 1981 where she worked as a social worker in London and Oxford. From 1994–1996, she taught social work at the University of Ghana, Legon-Accra. She completed her MSW at the University of Calgary, conducting research at a Liberian refugee camp in

Ghana. After working in Armenia, she started a PhD, looking at culturally relevant social work in Ghana. Linda continues to engage with social workers concerning social issues and social work education in Africa.

Klaus Kuehne worked as a professor at the University of Applied Sciences, Social Work in Bern, Switzerland and lectured in psychology and social psychology. His main topics were: prejudice, racism, poverty, migration and social welfare. For 20 years he was responsible for international student and staff exchange, international cooperation and study trips. He is now retired and lectures in international social work on global social policy and social development. Since 2010 he is the main IFSW representative at the UN in Geneva where he has organized World Social Work Day at the UN since 2012.

Crystal Kwan is a PhD candidate in Social Work at the University of Calgary. Her research interests and experiences include a variety of topics/areas within social work, specifically: community and international development, gerontological social work, social and public policy, climate change and social work. Her proposed PhD study is focused on disaster resilience and older adults. She has a keen interest in integrating creative media techniques with social work research and promotes dissemination through non-traditional networks to reach a broader audience.

Valter Martins holds a bachelor's degree in Social Work and doctorate from the Graduate Studies Program in Social Work at the Pontifical Catholic University of São Paulo, Brazil. He is a professor in the Department of Social Work of the Federal University at Santa Catarina, Brazil. He is also a researcher in the Center for Studies and Research on Labor and Employment. His resesarch interests include labor and social work, social policy, social protection and poverty.

Vickie Ogunlade is Assistant Director of Counseling and Disability Services of Spelman College, with over 30 years of clinical and administrative professional social work experience. Her professional experiences have included presentations and facilitation of workshops, within the USA and Nigeria. With a respect of cross-cultural perspectives, Vickie has participated in on-site support of village projects from a family system perspective, as well as lecturing as an adjunct at Babcock University in Nigeria. Dr. Ogunlade received the Chieftaincy Title of YeYe Otunba Gbasaga of Osogboland in 2007.

Augusta Y. Olaore is a social work practitioner and educator. She has obtained a doctoral degree from the University of South Africa and master's degree in Social Welfare from the University of California, Los Angeles. Her areas of interest are transformative social work, indigenous social care, and child and family services. She is a social services entrepreneur and has developed several programs and services for youth and their families in higher education.

She is the pioneer Chair for the Department of Social Work and Human Services and Director for Student Support Services at Babcock University in Nigeria.

Alpian A. Pratama is a researcher at Resilience Development Initiative (RDI), Bandung, Indonesia. Alpian has conducted a number of research studies on climate change adaptation, children, social capital, tourism development, community institution, and remittances of migrant workers in several areas of Indonesia. Moreover, he also serves as a volunteer of Bandung Disaster Study Group that actively arranges disaster education for children and youth in West Java and Jakarta, Indonesia. He also actively writes articles for international and national journals and presents conference papers, at both international and national conferences.

Elisabeth Rianawati is a Director of Resilience Disaster Initiative (RDI), Indonesia, an Indonesian think tank initiative that focuses on environmental change and sustainable development. She has published in a number of international journals, among others: *Physics and Chemistry of the Earth*, *Environ. Sci. Technol.* She also likes to disseminate and build networks with other researchers through attending national and international conferences. While her background is in environmental engineering, she has developed her passions on social aspects of environmental and risk management. Her main interest is social-ecological resilience, climate change adaptation, resilience and adaptive capacity, water management.

Saut Sagala is an assistant professor at the School of Architecture, Planning and Policy Development, Institute of Technology Bandung (ITB), Bandung, Indonesia. He has conducted intensive research and consultancy on disaster risk management, climate change adaptation and community participation and works as an Editorial Board Member of *ASEAN Engineering Journal*. He also serves as a senior research fellow at the Resilience Development Initiative and an adviser for Bandung Disaster Study Group, empowering university students to conduct disaster education. Most recently, he has been selected as a PARR (Pan Asia Risk Reduction) Fellow (July 2014–January 2015) by START Washington.

Tiffany Sampson received her Bachelor of Social Work degree in 2012 at Thompson Rivers University in Kamloops, British Columbia, Canada. Before pursuing a degree in social work, Tiffany obtained a Bachelor of Arts degree in Intercultural Religious Studies in 2002 from Trinity Western University as well as a Graduate Diploma in International Development Studies in 2008 from Saint Mary's University. Tiffany is presently working as a Community Social Worker at the University of Alberta. Current research interests include: community development, social development, social protection, and disaster vulnerability and resilience.

Miriam Samuel is Associate Professor and Head of the Department of Social Work at Madras Christian College in Chennai, India. Her specialization is in the field of medical and psychiatric social work and gender. She has served as Dean of Humanities and the Coordinator of the Internal Quality Assurance Cell of the College. She is particularly interested in research and projects on gender, women's empowerment, mental health and research. She is President of the Centre for International Social Work. Her research interests have centered on gender, mental health, natural disasters, community engagement and sexual minorities.

Maria Ozanira da Silva e Silva is Professor in the Graduate Program in Public Policies at Universidade Federal do Maranhão. She is coordinator of the Group for the Evaluation and Study of Poverty and Policies Focused on Poverty (GAEPP: www.gaepp.ufma.br) at Universidade Federal do Maranhão. She serves as IA level researcher of CNPq – Conselho Nacional de Desenvolvimento Científico e Tecnológico (CNPq), a Brazilian government agency that promotes research.

Edakkat Subhakaran Sriji is UGC-JRF scholar of Department of Management Studies, IIT Madras. She completed her MBA in 2009 at Jansons School of Business, Coimbatore, India and received a master's degree in Applied Psychology in 2011 from Bharathiar University, Tamilnadu. She was a teaching faculty at Gnanam School of Business, Tamilnadu, India (2010–2012). She conducted a study on "attrition of sales managers in an insurance company, Kerala, India" as part of her master's thesis. Her research interests include employee voice and organizational behavior. She has industry experience as a Human Resource Professional.

Sekar Srinivasan is currently a PhD research scholar at Department of Management Studies, Indian Institute of Technology Madras (IIT-M), Chennai, India. His present research is on "Motivators for Corporate Social Responsibility (CSR)." Previously, he was engaged in "Alternative water system project," a collaborative research project between the Department of Environmental and Water Resources Engineering, IIT-Madras and University of Guelph, Canada funded by IDRC, Canada during 2010–2012. He was also worked as a research coordinator on a "Post Tsunami Reconstruction" collaborative research project between Thompson Rivers University, Canada and Department of Social Work, Madras Christian College, Chennai, India funded by SSHRC, Canada during 2008–2009. He was involved in socio-economic assessment research work for National Thermal Power Corporation (NTPC) – Govt. of India enterprises in the year 2010.

Haorui Wu is a postdoctoral fellow in the Faculty of Social Work at the University of Calgary in Alberta, Canada. With a background of architecture and urban design, he focuses on applying interdisciplinary knowledge and methods into built environment field, to address global post-disaster recovery, reconstruction and rehabilitation, by examining the interplay between the built environment and local residents' social capacity. His research dwells on how the renewal or redevelopment of the built environment could fulfill its residents' social requirements.

Dodon Yamin is a researcher at Resilience Development Initiative (RDI), Bandung, Indonesia. Dodon has conducted research studies on climate change adaptation, social protection, disaster risk reduction, micro-finance for disaster and micro-insurance. He writes articles for international and national journals and presents papers at international and national conferences.

Foreword

Klaus Kuehne, IFSW UN Representative accredited at the ECOSOC in Geneva

As the International Federation of Social Work's representative at the United Nations in Geneva I warmly welcome the publication of the book *Social Development and Social Work Perspectives on Social Protection* and wish it a wide distribution. The editor, Dr. Julie Drolet, has conceived and realized a valuable and useful publication, which will promote knowledge and understanding among social workers about concepts of social protection systems worldwide.

Decades ago the right for social protection was enshrined in the Universal Declaration of Human Rights (1948) and in the Covenant of Economic, Social and Cultural Rights (1966). Nonetheless the International Labour Organization (ILO) World Social Protection Report 2014/2015 "Building economic recovery, inclusive development and social justice" shows that about 73% of world population have no or a very restricted access to social protection systems meaning that three out of four people in the world live in social insecurity if not in extreme poverty and have no access to comprehensive social protection, when they lose income due to personal, economic or environmental crisis. If there is no accessible and affordable health service for all, falling sick is a great risk for losing one's job or livelihood, habitation and schooling. The World Health Organisation (WHO) estimates that yearly 100 million persons fall into poverty due to unaffordable health costs.

The ILO Declaration on Social Justice for a Fair Globalisation (2008) calls for the need for a strong social dimension to counter the negative social impacts of economic globalization, which had become even more obvious in the financial and economic crises in 2008. The ILO and the WHO were the lead agencies in the social protection floor initiative which found a broad support among UN organizations, governments and NGO as cooperating agencies. With this initiative the discussion and the implementation of social protection systems, especially in the global south, have gained momentum. In many countries there is a renewed and growing importance given to social protection as a human right and as a precondition for social coherence and economic stability and development. This is contrasting with the recent development in rich countries where the attained level of social security is under attack as result of financial crisis and austerity policy.

The ILO Recommendation No. 202 on the implementation of National Floors of Social Protection (SPF) was adopted in 2012 by 185 ILO member states.

SPFs guarantee universal access to health services and income security through the life cycle: for children, unemployed and poor, older and disabled persons. Rights-based national social protection floors or parts of it have been successfully implemented in many countries. There is growing evidence, also documented in the case studies in this book, that they are ambitious but feasible, affordable and effective in the reduction of extreme poverty and of excessive inequality. SPFs contribute to wellbeing, to gender equality and improve educational and health status in underprivileged and vulnerable groups and enforce resilience in reaction to hardship of life in the broad population. SPFs have contributed to achievements reaching Millennium Developmental Goals and are an essential element to realize social rights. The Sustainable Developmental Goals 2016–2020 adopted by the UN Summit in September 2015 include three targets aiming for social protection and explicitly for SPFs as a contribution to end poverty and to reduce inequality for the Post-2015 Development Agenda.

The ILO Recommendation No. 202 on the national implementation of SPFs is the most important and promising initiative in global social policy and has found a broad support among development agencies. It marks an innovative change in global social and development policy away from the primacy of financial issues (Washington Consensus), away from a targeted protection of vulnerable population to an inclusive social policy postulating and implementing social protection for all. In this context the concept note of the World Bank Group and the ILO from April 2015 for a shared mission and action plan for universal social protection is remarkable.

The International Federation of Social Workers (IFSW) strongly supports the implementation of SPFs as they stand for an integrated approach addressing multidimensional vulnerabilities. SPFs, with the guarantees for health services and basic income through the life cycle, will stabilize and better the life of many clients of social work. SPFs will eliminate extreme poverty but will not result in the disappearance of poverty altogether, as the experiences of rich countries with well-developed social protection systems show. SPFs will not make social work superfluous; on the contrary the IFSW is convinced that social protection systems without the services of social workers are incomplete.

IFSW support of SPF is stated explicitly in the Global Agenda for Social Work and Social Development, a joint commitment to action of the three global organizations of professionals (IFSW) and educators (IASSW) in social work and social development activists (ICSW) adopted in 2012 (www.ifsw.org/globalagenda). The IFSW welcomes that with the implementation of SPFs governments are assuming their responsibility for the welfare of people living within their geographical boundaries and for the provision of appropriate social services. And the IFSW is willing to assume its role to contribute to the implementation and functioning of SPFs. So the IFSW Delegate Meeting 2014 in Melbourne adopted a motion requesting the elaboration of an IFSW policy paper on the "Role of Social Work in Social Protection Floors." This IFSW statement is still in development and will be presented at the next General Assembly in Seoul in 2016. This text presents a first sketch for such a statement.

The basic concept of SPFs is convincing and promising, but there is no guarantee that states will follow the recommendation they adopted with their signature and will implement SPFs. It is too important to wait until governments and politicians in power will introduce it. Social workers and their organizations can and should engage to promote SPFs in two different roles: as members of civil society and as professionals in public or private social services.

Civil society has to intervene, to engage and to participate in the decision process, in the conception and development, in the implementation and in the monitoring of SPF adapted to national, economic, social and cultural realities. Social workers and their organizations cannot do this alone and have to unite with other civil society organizations to have a voice. On the international level the IFSW is member of the Global Coalition for Social Protection Floors, together with many international and national civil society organizations lobbying with some success for SPFs in the United Nations, especially for the integration of SPFs in Post 2015 Sustainable Developmental Goals (www.socialprotectionfloorscoalition.org). The IFSW encourages its members in 120 countries worldwide to engage in national coalition for the implementation of SPFs. A helpful guideline for this engagement is the *Civil Society Guide for National Social Protection Floors*, launched in April 2015. The *Guide*, published by the Friedrich-Ebert-Stiftung, member of the Global Coalition, aims at supporting civil society organizations to take over the concept of SPFs, to get a better understanding of their role and to give orientation for getting engaged in SPF advocacy and monitoring work. And I can only recommend the guide to social workers and social workers' organizations as part of civil society to get engaged in the process of realizing the right of social protection for all. Social workers have the knowledge and the experience to make substantial contributions to the development of SPFs adapted to the needs, the values and cultural traditions of the vulnerable people they work with. They have to make the voice of their clients heard, advocate for them and empower them to claim their rights.

But even the implementation of a SPF is no guarantee that it will work, that it will meet the demands of the potential beneficiaries and that they will accept it. Many good governmental reform projects had poor results or failed completely due to incompetence, inefficiency, ideology, fraud, corruption, discrimination or lack of adequate means, information or acceptance on any political or administrative level. Social services are the place where civil servants, administrative and professional personnel, among them professional social workers, are meeting the beneficiaries on a day-to-day basis. This "street level bureaucracy" is decisive for a successful and accepted implementation of such fundamental reforms. With the expected proliferation of social protection systems and especially of SPFs it is important that social workers prepare themselves for this task and understand the active role they can play in the conception, implementation, managing, delivering and monitoring of SPFs.

An IFSW statement must give clear orientation and it will be based on fundamental values and principles laid down in the powerful framework set by the IASSW and IFSW:

- The "International definition of social work" (2014) and elaborated code of ethics in all 120 IFSW member national associations.
- "Statement of principles: Ethics of social work" (2004).
- "Global standards for the education and training of social work profession" (2004).
- Furthermore there are guidelines and orientations for conceiving the role of social workers in the specific field of social protection (e.g., in health, disability).
- In addition there are several pertinent IFSW policy papers, e.g., "Effective and ethical working environments for social work: The responsibilities of employers of social workers", to name only one.

The other important point of reference for the IFSW policy paper is the ILO-Recommendation No. 202 on Social Protection Floors, as it provides guidance to establish and maintain national SPFs and details the principles that states should apply (Article 3). These principles are highly relevant for social services and social workers and merit a thorough study and consideration and they will guide in our task to produce an IFSW policy paper. I name only a few examples of those principles:

- social inclusion also for persons in the informal economy (3.e);
- non-discrimination, gender equality and responsiveness to special needs (3.d);
- respect for the rights and dignity of people (3.f);
- coherence across institutions responsible for delivery of social protection (3.m);
- high quality public services (3.n);
- with efficient and accessible, impartial and transparent, simple, rapid and inexpensive complaint and appeal procedures (3.o + 7).

The communalities between the principles named in the ILO document and in the Statement on Ethics in Social Work are striking, reflecting the fact that both are based on human rights.

Besides giving clear orientation and guidance an IFSW statement must be open for national peculiarities and this is a big challenge as social protection is conceived differently in different countries according to historical development, laws, values and traditions. Social welfare benefits may include a variety of benefits in cash or in kind such as child and family, sickness and health care, maternity, disability, old age and unemployment benefits and others (ILO Rec. 202, 9.2). The schemes providing such benefits may also vary, including, among others, schemes of social insurances, of negative income tax, public employment, employment support, universal benefit or social assistance schemes. Accordingly the role of social work varies in relation to different benefits and provision schemes depending on the organizational and administrative structures, on division of labor, on the acquired status of the profession, and on traditional and ways of support for and by families and communities. Neither social protection systems nor social work's role and methods can just be copied on existing models. The transfer to other countries needs an adaptation to existing national and local values and traditions, laws and administrative structures.

The IFSW policy statement is still in discussion. But I already can name some postulates that will be part of the IFSW recommendations concerning the role of social work in social protection:

Need for integrated social services: Social services are the entry point for users into sometimes complicated structures of social protection systems. For high quality of services a one-window approach is recommended as it enhances the accessibility and citizen outreach; it promotes good coordination between administrators and professionals, and it facilitates referral to adequate specialised services.

SPF inclusion for all:
- Special attention must be given to the outreach to persons living in remote rural areas, where travel to social services is time-consuming and unaffordable.
- Birth registration for all children is essential for an inclusive social protection and easy possibility for late registration must be provided.
- Persons without legal status (*sans papiers*) shall not be excluded from health services and other basic need provision.

Inclusion of social workers: In social services there is a need for the specific knowledge and skills of social workers. With their holistic approach social workers have a core position handling multidimensional problems of users. A SPF without the inclusion of social workers in social services is incomplete and will not fulfill its mission at its best.

Tasks of social workers: Social workers are trained to work with disempowered clients. Many clients of social workers are living in poverty, are excluded and discriminated and are so disempowered that they neither have the knowledge nor the capability, neither the self-confidence nor the means to claim for their rights and benefits. On a daily basis social workers are dealing with those who cannot access social protection or whose rights are denied.

The task of social workers is informing and counseling their clients about their rights and the benefits they are entitled to claim. Often social workers have to support the clients to receive what they have the right to. Social workers have to support beneficiaries, individuals, families and communities to gain control over their own lives. Sometimes they have to advocate for the clients. They have to educate and possibly to organize communities to campaign for their rights and for adequate services. Social workers have to provide all their services with as much participation of the clients as possible, to empower them to decide and to advocate for themselves instead of making them dependent on helpers and welfare benefits.

Adequate training for social workers: In many countries social work is a new profession and there are not enough qualified social workers to work in social services. Often a social service workforce without adequate training in social work is nonetheless employed and called "social workers." Possibilities for in-service training and part-time studies for experienced and mature students in social work must be provided.

Decent work conditions: Employers of social workers have the responsibility to provide effective working environments, which allow effective work in respect of the ethical principles of social work.

Too often social protection has been conceived as an "end-of-the-pipe" solution. It comes into play only when a problem occurs, when people get sick or injured, when people lose their job or livelihood, when they are getting old or disabled. You have to be poor before you are eligible for social assistance. Social protection means not only that in such situations benefits are available but also that these benefits are predictable. But this is not enough. Besides giving guarantees for health services and basic income, social assistance benefits should aim as much as possible at prevention of those problems, their effects and repetition. But this is not enough. Social protection must also be transformative and be coordinated and integrated in strategies of social development. And recent developments brought forward a new and distinctive approach to social work practice, explicitly called developmental social work. This can contribute a great deal to social development mainly by facilitating the full inclusion of their clients in social and economic life, by capacity building, and by promotion of small-scale enterprises in the formal but also in the informal economy.

The IFSW invites all social workers to participate in the realization of the Sustainable Development Goals and especially in the promotion of SPFs. With these remarks we wish all social workers, students and professionals, readers of this book, perseverance in their studies and professional life, and success in the common engagement for social justice and for the realization of social protection for all, leaving no one behind.

August 31, 2015
Klaus Kuehne
IFSW UN Representative
accredited at the ECOSOC
Geneva

1   Introduction

Julie Drolet

Social protection, or social security as it is also known, is a key social develop-ment strategy that has been increasingly recognized by the international com-munity (Midgley, 2014). Social protection systems aim to protect individual women, men and children against the risks of impoverishment in situations of sickness, disability, maternity, employment injury, unemployment, old age, death of a family member, high health care or child care costs, and general poverty and social exclusion (Hautala, 2012). With increasing inequalities in and between countries, there is a need for social protection policies grounded in social justice and human rights with a strong state commitment toward universal programs (Dimmel, 2014). This is a unique time in the history of social protec-tion and of the social work profession, both in terms of the challenges we face as well as the solutions that we can develop (Hoffler & Clark, 2014). Social workers have historically advocated on behalf of vulnerable and oppressed groups and have acquired resources for clients, organized communities for causes, and coordinated grassroots advocacy campaigns, and have played signi-ficant roles in enacting important legislation into law such as social security, civil and women's rights, health insurance, among others (Hoffler & Clark, 2014). Social workers as human service professionals guide people to critical resources, counsel them on important life decisions, and help them reach their full potential (Hoffler & Clark, 2014). The eradication of poverty in all its forms is the ultimate goal of social work and social development (Dimmel, 2014). One important aspect of the social work profession, and probably the most well-known and understood, is that of a social safety net (Hoffler & Clark, 2014). New initiatives and innovative social protection programs introduced in many developed and developing countries deserve our attention. The emergence of new forms of social protection is a "recent global development [that offers] inspiration and renewed hope for the possibility of social change and for a better world" (Smith, 2014, p. 57). This book is about social work and social develop-ment perspectives on social protection.

This introductory chapter examines the social protection floor initiative, and the post-2015 development agenda including the Sustainable Development Goals (SDGs). As will be shown, the Global Agenda for Social Work and Social Development is a platform for social workers around the world to lend their support. This chapter presents the perspectives of social work and social development and how this relates to social protection. It concludes by reviewing the mandates, principles, practice and roles of social workers and discusses how social work involvement can be enhanced.

Social protection floor initiative

The ILO Recommendation concerning National Floors of Social Protection (No. 202) was adopted in June 2012. This Recommendation reflects a commitment to building nationally defined social protection floors which guarantee at least a basic level of social security to all, with access to health care and income security throughout people's lives and ensuring their dignity and human rights (ILO, 2014). It is a legal instrument that explicitly recognizes the triple role of social security as a universal human right and an economic and social necessity (ILO, 2014, p. 5). "For the purpose of this Recommendation, social protection floors are nationally defined sets of basic social security guarantees which secure protection aimed at preventing or alleviating poverty, vulnerability and social exclusion" (ILO, 2012, para. 2). These guarantees can be materialized through transfers in cash and in kind such as child benefits, income support benefits combined with employment guarantees for the working-age poor, tax-financed university pensions for older persons, and benefits for persons with disabilities and persons who have lost the main breadwinner in the family (United Nations, 2015). The overall and primary responsibility of meeting these guarantees lies with the state.

"Social protection is both a human right and sound economic policy" (ILO, 2015, p. 1). It strongly contributes to reducing poverty, exclusion, vulnerability and inequality, and contributes to political stability and social cohesion (ILO, 2015). Implementation of the Social Protection Floors Recommendation, 2012 (No. 202) is an indispensable tool to accelerate poverty reduction and promote sustainable development (ILO, 2015). Expanding social protection coverage to the informal economy, rural areas and vulnerable populations is a critical priority for our times (ILO, 2015). Social protection is recognized for delivering positive results and making a real difference in peoples' lives (ILO, 2015, p. 1).

Social protection was not included in the Millennium Development Goals Agenda, but emerged in the response to the global financial crisis of 2008. The social protection floor concept was formally adopted in April 2009 as one of nine joint initiatives. With the ongoing economic repercussions of the global financial crisis, the world is faced with a deep social crisis that is also a crisis of social justice, with fiscal austerity measures that threaten living standards in many countries (ILO, 2014).

Social protection and Sustainable Development Goals (SDGs)

The United Nations' new post-2015 global development agenda includes social protection as a practical action that governments can take to effectively reduce inequalities, eradicate extreme poverty, and promote gender equality, decent work, climate adaptation and universal health coverage. The Open Working Group on Sustainable Development Goals recognized the need to strengthen social protection floors as part of the SDGs in the post-2015 development agenda. Social protection is represented in the SDGs and targets as follows:

> Social protection and SPFs feature prominently in Goal 1 – Ending poverty in all its forms everywhere. Target 1.3 proposes that countries implement nationally appropriate social protection systems and measures for all, including floors, and by 2030 achieve substantial coverage of the poor and the vulnerable.
>
> Goal 3 is on achieving universal health coverage. Target 3.8 includes financial risk protection, access to quality essential health care services, and access to safe, effective, quality, and affordable essential medicines and vaccines for all.
>
> Goal 5 is dedicated to achieving gender equality and empowerment for all women and girls, and social protection features as a strategy. Target 5.4 calls on countries to recognize and value unpaid care and domestic work through the provision of social services, infrastructure and social protection policies, and the promotion of shared responsibility within the household and the family as nationally appropriate.
>
> Goal 10 aims to reduce inequality within and among countries. Target 10.4 proposes that countries adopt fiscal, wage, and social protection policies and progressively achieve greater equality.
>
> (Social Protection Floor, n.d.b, para. 3)

The importance of social protection in the SDGs and targets is significant, and the case for social protection floors is compelling (ILO, 2015). The implementation of the SDGs will require policy coherence, coordination and integration among multi-stakeholder partners. The SDG goals are universally applicable to all countries including both developed and developing countries.

International context

Despite the importance of social protection as a policy tool to ensure that individuals and families are able to realize their full potential, it is estimated that "73% of the world's population do not enjoy access to comprehensive or adequate social protection coverage" (ILO, 2014, p. v).

> For example, 39% of the people around the world are not affiliated to a health system or insurance scheme. The lack of social protection affects people throughout the life cycle. 50% of the world's children live in poverty, 300 million elderly do not have income security to live in dignity, and only 12% of unemployed individuals have access to unemployment benefits.
>
> (Social Protection Floor, n.d.a, para. 2)

Building social protection floors worldwide is required to help guarantee income and food security, and access to essential services such as health, education, housing, water and sanitation. Social protection benefits and services are recognized as powerful tools for combatting poverty and inequality by investing in social and economic development in the short and long term (ILO, 2014). According to the United Nations Research Institute for Social Development (UNRISD, 2010), "economic growth is important, but alone does not necessarily reduce poverty and inequality" (p. 2). The 1995 World Summit for Social Development outlined a vision of an inclusive society as a "society for all" in which every individual, each with rights and responsibilities, has an active role to play. Social policy continues to play "an integral part of the development strategies of countries that have transformed their economies and reduced poverty relatively quickly" (UNRISD, 2010, p. 2).

> In the past, access to social security was the privilege of formal sector workers. Being a salaried worker protected by labour law would guarantee access to existing mandatory social security coverage. It was assumed that by formalizing the economy, more and more people would have access to social security. The Social Protection Floor reaffirms that all residents regardless of their work contract types or occupations are entitled to social security, it is universal and delinks access to social security from the condition of being formally employed.
>
> (ILO, 2013, p. 16)

The social protection floors approach calls for universal coverage of all residents and children, and recognizes that special support may be needed for disadvantaged groups and people with special needs (ILO & UNDG, 2014). The Asia-Pacific region has experienced some of the most damaging disasters in recent decades, with alarming consequences for human development, and this reinforced the need to continue to build nationally defined social protection floors (ILO & UNDG, 2014). "Many countries have significantly extended their social security coverage during recent years and have stepped up their efforts to ensure that all in need benefit from at least basic protection, while continuing to develop their social security systems" (ILO, 2014, p. 2).

Access to basic income security and equal access to essential services are a basic right of all people, and governments are duty bearers to ensure that all people can realize these rights (National Institute for Health and Welfare, 2015). Social protection floors do not define new rights, but they contribute to the realization of the human right to social security and to social services, established in Articles 22, 25 and 26 of the Universal Declaration of Human Rights and Articles 26 and 27 of the Convention on the Rights of the Child, and other international legal instruments. Greater efforts are necessary to work toward the goal of establishing social protection floors, and there is a need to better understand the role of social workers in this process.

The Global Agenda for Social Work and Social Development

A program for strengthening social work's role in setting an agenda for global action was developed in 2012 in a document titled "Global Agenda for Social Work and Social Development – Commitment to Action" by the International Association of Schools of Social Work (IASSW), International Federation of Social Workers (IFSW) and International Council on Social Welfare (ICSW). The Agenda calls for international, regional and national commitment to advocate for a new world order, which makes a reality of respect for human rights and dignity (Staub-Bernasconi, 2014). During the period 2012–2016 international social work efforts are focused in four areas:

1   promoting social and economic equalities;
2   promoting the dignity and worth of peoples;
3   working toward environmental sustainability; and
4   strengthening recognition of the importance of human relationships (Global Agenda for Social Work and Social Development, 2012).

The social protection floor initiative is identified as a major focus in the post-2015 development agenda in order to promote social and economic equalities, and is bringing together the profession of social work to support the realization of the right to social protection.

Global definition of the social work profession

According to the IFSW the global definition of the social work profession is the following:

> Social work is a practice-based profession and an academic discipline that promotes social change and development, social cohesion, and the empowerment and liberation of people. Principles of social justice, human rights, collective responsibility and respect for diversities are central to social work. Underpinned by theories of social work, social sciences, humanities and indigenous knowledge, social work engages people and structures to address life challenges and enhance wellbeing. The above definition may be amplified at national and/or regional levels.
>
> (IFSW, 2014)

The social work profession's core mandates include promoting social change, social development, social cohesion and the empowerment and liberation of people (IFSW, 2014). Social work recognizes the connections between historical, socio-economic, cultural, spatial, political and personal factors that serve as opportunities and/or barriers to human well-being and development (IFSW, 2014). Structural barriers contribute to the perpetuation of oppression and discrimination (Mullaly, 2007). The social work profession strives to alleviate poverty, liberate the vulnerable and oppressed, and promote social inclusion and social cohesion (IFSW, 2014). A social change perspective is realized when a social work intervention at the level of the person, family, small group, community or society is deemed to be in need of change and development. It is driven by the need to challenge and change those structural conditions that contribute to marginalization and oppression. Social change initiatives recognize the place of human agency in advancing human rights and economic, social and environmental justice.

The principles of social work include respect for the inherent worth and dignity of human beings, doing no harm, respect for diversity and upholding human rights and social justice (IFSW, 2014). Advocating and upholding human rights and social justice is the motivation and justification for social work (IFSW, 2014). Social workers advocate for the rights of people at all levels, and work to facilitate outcomes where people take responsibility for each other's well-being, realize and respect the interdependence among people and between people and the environment.

Social work embraces first, second and third generation rights. First generation rights refer to civil and political rights such as free speech and conscience and freedom from torture and arbitrary detention; second generation to socio-economic and cultural rights that include the rights to reasonable levels of education, healthcare, and housing and minority language rights; and third generation rights focus on the natural world and the right to species biodiversity and inter-generational equity (IFSW, 2014). These rights are mutually reinforcing and interdependent, and accommodate both individual and collective rights.

Social work knowledge

Social work is both interdisciplinary and transdisciplinary, and draws on a wide array of scientific theories and research from other human sciences, including but not limited to community development, administration, anthropology, ecology, economics, education, management, nursing, psychiatry, psychology, public health and sociology. The uniqueness of social work research and theories is that they are applied and emancipatory, and largely co-constructed with service users in an interactive, dialogic process and informed by specific practice environments (IFSW, 2014).

Social work is informed not only by specific practice environments and Western theories, but also by indigenous knowledge. Part of the legacy of colonialism is that Western theories and knowledge have been exclusively valorized, and indigenous knowledge has been devalued, discounted and hegemonized by Western theories and knowledge (IFSW, 2014). Social work seeks to redress historic Western scientific colonialism and hegemony by listening to and learning from indigenous peoples around the world.

Social work's legitimacy and mandate lie in its intervention at the points where people interact with their environment (IFSW, 2014). The environment includes the various social systems that people are embedded in and the natural, geographic environment, which has a profound influence on the lives of people. Consistent with the social development paradigm, social workers utilize a range of skills, techniques, strategies, principles and activities at various system levels, directed at system maintenance and/or system change efforts (IFSW, 2014). Social work practice spans a range of activities including various forms of therapy and counseling, group work and community work; policy formulation and analysis; and advocacy and political interventions (IFSW, 2014). Social work strategies are aimed at increasing people's hope, self-esteem and creative potential to confront and challenge oppressive power dynamics and structural sources of injustices (IFSW, 2014). A proactive, inclusive and empowering approach to community development as well as to essential societal services helps people to (re)gain and improve their own control over their livelihoods, living conditions, opportunities and social relations (National Institute for Health and Welfare, 2013). The holistic focus of social work is universal, but the priorities of social work practice will vary from one country to the next, and from time to time depending on historical, cultural, political and socio-economic conditions (IFSW, 2014).

Social work and social development perspectives

Social work is widely recognized across the globe as a "formal helping system to improve the well-being of individuals, families, groups, communities, and societies" (Osei-Hwedie & Rankopo, 2012, p. 723). The social work profession is engaged in social and political action to advance development, alleviate poverty and secure justice for all, especially vulnerable and oppressed people (Desai & Solas, 2012). "Poverty on a local or national level and its consequences has been present at the historical beginning of social work" (Staub-Bernasconi, 2014, p. 37). It is important to note that social work is a profession that has taken a keen interest in matters of justice, and it can be said to be one of its most distinguishing features (Desai & Solas, 2012). Professional social work began in Europe, with important developments occurring in the UK and the Netherlands toward the end of the 19th century on issues of poverty, unemployment and housing (Dominelli, 2014). Social work education and practice was exported from Western contexts to other parts of the world, and has often ignored and displaced developing nations' indigenous knowledge systems (Osei-Hwedie & Rankopo, 2012; Gray & Coates, 2008). Social work expanded rapidly over the 20th century due to improved international relations across the globe, and many developing countries put in place formal social welfare systems in their effort to address social and economic debt (Osei-Hwedie & Rankopo, 2012).

Social work is one of a minority of professions dedicated to anti-oppressive practice and remains a driving force for global partnership, regional cooperation and local engagement (Desai & Solas, 2012, p. 96). Social workers have been actively involved in promoting social development since the 1970s when a group of social work educators founded the International Consortium for Social Development (Midgley, 2012). Social development is primarily focused on the tasks of alleviating poverty, meeting social needs and addressing social problems (Midgley, 2012).

Critical social workers are committed to achieving social justice through social work practice, which is not surprising since social justice is a core value of social work practice and reflected in the ethical codes of many social work associations throughout the world (Healy, 2012; Banks, 2006). Conventional social work focuses on casework and assisting clients in conforming to any oppressive system by helping them learn to accept responsibility for their plight (Mullaly, 2007). Progressive social work values are consistent with a social change model such as feminist, anti-racist, postmodern and structural social work paradigms that focus on social problems as an outgrowth of oppressive social constructions (Mullaly, 2007).

Social development is conceptualized to refer to strategies for intervention, desired end states and a policy framework, the latter in addition to the more popular residual and institutional frameworks. It is based on holistic assessments and interventions that transcend the micro–mezzo–macro divide by incorporating multiple system levels and inter-sectorial and inter-professional collaboration. It prioritizes socio-structural and economic development, and does not subscribe to conventional wisdom that economic growth is a prerequisite for social development.

Social workers are active in the delivery of social protection programs. For example, social work practice can include facilitating access to health services, unemployment benefits, social insurance programs, assistance for older people (pensions and basic allowances), child protection, family allowances, welfare and social services, cash and in-kind transfers, temporary subsidies for utilities and staple foods, employment programs and skills development (Winther-Schmidt, n.d.). Social workers as professionals of care are needed to meet poor, vulnerable and disadvantaged families, understand their diverse life situations in their real contexts, and be inclusive and offer high quality services (Voipio, 2011). It is important to recognize and respect the role of social workers and community development workers at the local level in social protection.

Social work and human service professionals also play a role in increasing awareness of people's needs, and facilitating referrals to services and programs. There is a potentially important role for social workers to play in advocacy and raising awareness to inform the public about the Social Protection Floor Recommendation No. 202, to share country experiences, and to include social protection in training courses and curriculum materials. Building and strengthening partnerships to ensure that social protection is featured in the national policy agenda is also a feature in the social work profession. Finally, there is a need to build capacity within the social work profession to better contribute to the design, implementation, monitoring and evaluation of social protection policies and social security strategies, particularly in relation to vulnerable groups. In the next section the role of social workers in social policy and social protection will be further discussed.

Social workers and policy practice

The idea that social workers should seek to influence the policies that affect the societies in which they work has existed for nearly as long as the profession itself (Weiss-Gal & Gal, 2014). Social policies are interventions by governments that affect the welfare of individuals and communities (UNRISD, 2014). This tradition of social worker involvement in social policy formulation reflects values and assumptions that lie at the very foundation of social work (Weiss-Gal & Gal, 2014).

> Social workers are ethically bound to understand the applicable laws, policies, and regulations affecting the profession and the clients they serve because they have the knowledge and expertise to improve social systems and institutions that have caused inequality and despair.
>
> (Hoffler & Clark, 2014, p. 46)

Yet despite the profession's tradition of involvement in social change and social work's formal commitment to engage in the policy process, until recent decades the social work discourse in most national settings tended to delegate the role of involvement in social policy to a small group of social policy experts and to community social workers (Weiss-Gal & Gal, 2014). There is a general agreement that all social workers should and can be involved in policy practice regardless of the focus of their professional activities or field of practice (Weiss-Gal & Gal, 2014).

In a study conducted by Weiss-Gal and Gal (2014) it was found that social workers seek to affect social policies through social work organizations by lobbying efforts or participation in the policy discourse. Social workers also seek to influence policy by participating directly in activities initiated and organized by social work organizations. For example, the ICSW has adopted the Social Protection Floor Initiative as its major policy agenda at an international level (ICSW, 2015). The ICSW is comprised of member organizations that represent tens of thousands of community organizations, and the ICSW supports a life course approach in development strategies with anti-poverty measures and social protection schemes to promote gender equality and social inclusion (ICSW, n.d). The Global Coalition for Social Protection Floors brings together the ICSW and the International Association of Schools of Social Work (IASSW) with over 80 non-government organizations (NGOs) that strive to raise awareness and promote a more people-oriented and humane economic order (Social Protection Floor Coalition, 2015).

Civil society organizations such as advocacy organizations, social movements and social welfare provider organizations play a major role in the policy formulation process in different countries. Social workers as members or employees of these civil society organizations, or in conjunction with them, appear to be a more viable option than direct engagement on the part of social workers who are civil servants (Weiss-Gal & Gal, 2014). Social work academics use their professional status and access to policy makers and the media to influence policy, and contribute through research and the publication of findings that have implications for policy (Weiss-Gal & Gal, 2014). Social workers who are civil servants engage in policy directly within the context of their workplace in various forms (Weiss-Gal & Gal, 2014).

Structure of the book

This book brings together a growing number of scholars and practitioners who are engaged internationally in social protection aimed at addressing poverty, promoting human rights, reducing inequality and other important social issues. This book offers current social work and social development perspectives that shape social protection and provides case studies grounded in country experiences. The strengthening of civil society and the role of NGOs and governments both internationally and nationally is covered. The book aims to stimulate interest and discussion on successful social protection initiatives across the world, including the new Social Protection Floor Initiative.

The Social Protection Floor Initiative promotes universal access to essential social transfers and services. Presently 80% of the global population does not enjoy a set of social guarantees that allows them to deal with life's risks. Ensuring basic social protection for these people, many of whom are struggling to survive, is a necessity. This book is needed to develop understanding about the role and contribution of social protection. Investing in social protection supports a range of Millennium Development Goals, and the new SDGs, and has the potential to reduce poor people's vulnerabilities to global challenges such as economic shocks, instability in food prices and other essential commodities, and the impacts of climate change and related natural disasters. In today's protracted economic and financial crisis, social protection strategies are receiving increasing attention as a crucial element in effective policy responses in support of sustainable social and economic development.

During the past few years a number of low income and middle income countries have launched innovative social protection pilot initiatives, and many countries are seeking to integrate fragmented social protection projects into coherent national systems (National Institute for Health and Welfare, 2015). Many developing countries have already successfully taken measures to build their nationally defined social protection floors or to introduce elements thereof. Governments and UN agencies have developed a range of interventions to strengthen social protection for all and particularly the most vulnerable. These include, for example, health insurance, school feeding programs, public works programs or guaranteed employment schemes, or cash transfers targeting different populations groups including older people, children, pregnant women, people with disability, people with HIV/AIDS and the poor. There is an important gender dimension in social protection because women are often not entitled to social security benefits and pensions for their work in the informal economy or unpaid work that is not recognized as an economic contribution to their communities (United Nations, 2015). The challenge is how to cover the entire population effectively, especially those who are at risk or who are already in a situation of deprivation, and in a sustainable long-term manner. The results of these programs show that the impact of the social protection floor on poverty, vulnerability and inequality can be dramatic.

The book is divided into two main sections. The first part of the book features key concepts, definitions and theoretical perspectives drawn from the field of social work, social development as well as the international development literature. The introductory chapters will discuss the social protection floor initiative and ground the role of social work in supporting social protection and social development in policy and practice. The book is intended to provoke further reflection and analysis, and stimulate action among stakeholders to better realize human rights and face challenges.

Chapter 2 by Julie Drolet and Crystal Kwan situates the context of social protection in a historical context and traces the development of the Social Protection Floor Initiative. The post-2015 development context and SDGs are reviewed, and the role of social protection in addressing new and enduring global challenges.

Chapter 3 by Crystal Kwan and Julie Drolet discusses the impacts of the global economic crisis of 2008 and recovery measures due to fiscal stimulus and countercyclical policies. A critical social work lens is used to understand a "recovery for all" policy approach. The impacts of the global crisis are traced such as rising unemployment and vulnerability, loss of access to healthcare and health insurance, gendered dimensions, youth unemployment, and the situation of migrant workers, indigenous groups, older workers and ethnic and religious minorities. Stimulus measures adopted in developed and developing countries are presented, and the impacts of more recent austerity, and the role of social protection in reducing poverty and vulnerability.

Chapter 4 by Sekar Srinivasan et al. considers the right to social protection and social security enshrined in international treaties, national legislations and constitutional provisions. A rights-based approach is proposed in order to promote social justice and equity. The contributors explain key concepts and principles related to human rights, justice and equity with respect to social protection.

Julie Drolet and Tiffany Sampson define key terms and concepts such as social protection, social development, sustainable development, livelihoods, gender and poverty in Chapter 5. Social development as a theory and an approach is presented in a developmental perspective that concerns people's well-being and progressive social change. The concept of sustainable development is traced since its origin in the 1960s, and later adoption in 1987 with the Brundtland Commission. The concept of livelihood is discussed as well as sustainable livelihoods and poverty reduction. The importance of gender roles and gender relations are situated in the context of gender equality and the need for an integrated approach in the post-2015 development framework.

Chapter 6 by Haorui Wu and Julie Drolet presents adaptive social protection, or social protection in the context of climate change and disasters. Adaptive social protection aims to reduce vulnerability, enhance resilience and achieve sustainable development. This chapter traces sustainable development concepts of importance in order to advance the global development framework. The Sendai Framework for Disaster Risk Reduction 2015–2030 identified priorities for action such as the protection of human rights in disaster mitigation. As social workers are being called upon to help rebuild lives due to devastating disasters and climate-related events, the importance of adaptive social protection is shared in several brief country examples such as the Wenchuan earthquake in China.

Chapter 7 by Valter Martins presents the role of social protection in the fight against poverty. While there is no single definition of poverty, Martins explores income poverty, inequality and the complex, relative and multidimensional nature of poverty. The role of social workers in anti-poverty initiatives is discussed with respect to social rights. Industrialization and urbanization processes are considered, and the labor and worker movements in liberal democracies for greater protections. The development of social protection and the impacts of economic recessions on the mechanisms of social protection are reviewed, and examples of social protection and income transfer programs from Latin America and the Caribbean are discussed in the context of inequalities.

The second part of the book presents a number of case studies. The purpose of the case studies is not to objectively compare them, given the diverse realities in each country, but to highlight promising practices, and the actual and potential roles of social work and social development. While the field of international development has contributed to debates on political economy perspectives and gendered access to labor markets, the case studies consider the role of social work and social development in promoting and strengthening social protection, in policy and practice, from anti-oppressive and critical perspectives. The knowledge, expertise and experience that countries have gained in their own efforts at establishing a social protection floor represent a valuable source of information for other countries interested in planning, expanding, extending or reorienting their social protection systems.

Chapter 8 by Maria Ozanira da Silva e Silva presents the first case study in the book on the Bolsa Família program in Brazil. This conditional income transfer program is the main and largest social protection national initiative in Brazil. Silva considers the characteristics of the program, and its beneficiary families using socio-economic and National Household Survey data. The impact of the Bolsa Família on the reduction of extreme poverty and social inequality is discussed, and the role of social work practice.

The Mahatma Gandhi National Rural Employment Guarantee Act (MGNREGA) in India is presented by Miriam Samuel and Sekar Srinivasan in Chapter 9. This social protection initiative aims to reduce poverty in rural areas by providing a minimum of 100 days of employment to any rural household. Samuel and Srinivasan review the features and provisions of MGNREGA in the context of a number of important social, economic and environmental issues and priorities. The role of social workers adopting a community development and rights-based approach is discussed for the realization of social protection in rural areas.

Chapter 10 by Vivienne Bozalek and Tessa Hochfeld examines the Child Support Grant (CSG) in South Africa through a social justice perspective. A trivalent view of social justice considers social protection and the following dimensions: the redistribution of resources, recognition of work and representation of people's voice or social inclusion. The research results of a study are provided that investigated the social impacts of the CSG using a narrative inquiry framework, and the women participants' experiences are presented as a case study. The chapter finds that more is needed to counter existing severe inequalities in South Africa, and the role of social workers in the pursuit of social justice is discussed.

Ziblim Abukari and Linda Kreitzer examine social protection initiatives in Ghana in Chapter 11. Ghana has developed a national strategic framework for social protection with a focus on vulnerable populations. The Livelihood Empowerment Against Poverty (LEAP) cash transfer program, the National Health Insurance Scheme and the Education Capitation Grant and School Feeding program are reviewed. Challenges in the implementation of social protection programs are reviewed and suggestions for the future are offered.

Chapter 12 by Augusta Y. Olaore et al. focuses on child-sensitive social protection initiatives in Nigeria, Africa. The role and importance of indigenous social care practices in traditional and community settings is discussed in the absence of comprehensive social protection systems. Social work is an emerging profession in Nigeria. Contemporary social protection initiatives are presented including the In Care of the People Cash Transfer Program (COPE CCT) and the Family Nutritional Support Program (FNSP). Children face vulnerabilities including extreme poverty, HIV/AIDS, among others, and depend on others for the provision of their survival needs, education and healthcare, as well as protection from emotional and physical harm. In the absence of social protection children become victims of child trafficking, child labor, and experience child abuse. The chapter argues for a child-sensitive social protection system to build a protective environment to meet the needs of children. Complementary indigenous social care practices and the role of developing community partnerships is discussed to strengthen social protection of children and persons affected by HIV/AIDS in Nigeria.

Chapter 13 by Saut Sagala et al. discusses social protection in Indonesia in the context of disaster risk reduction and community resilience. Rural areas in Indonesia are prone to climate and disaster risks, and there is a role for social protection to contribute to disaster risk reduction. Adaptive social protection measures are discussed in the context of the National Program on Community Empowerment (PNPM). Results of field research are presented, drawing from two regions affected by the impacts of climate change and volcanic eruption disasters. The role of social workers as facilitators is presented to demonstrate their role and involvement in adaptive social protection and community resilience. Many countries are now designing social policy initiatives that also incorporate environmental concerns, also known as eco-social policies, in order to strengthen the resilience or adaptive capacities of individuals and communities while also achieving social goals (UNRISD, 2014, p. 3).

This is the first book on social work and social development perspectives on social protection. The book is unique, and contributes to debates on social protection initiatives and aims to build capacity on the actual and potential role of social workers in contributing to social protection in diverse settings. It is important to consider how social workers and departments of social work are engaging with broader social protection programs and schemes. Social work perspectives present an opportunity to strengthen what is often a very narrow economic focus in many of the large-scale social protection initiatives, especially among public works programs.

The chapters aim to improve understanding of social protection, and share successful and emerging experiences among stakeholders on promising practices. Building critical knowledge and innovative practices in social protection is of interest to social workers and students who are seeking to develop a new understanding and to implement actions in support of the right to social protection. The book will be of interest to academics, researchers, practitioners, government officials, policy makers, social planners, program officers, activists and students in social work, and many disciplines in the social sciences, humanities and health fields, such as international development, geography, planning, economics, sociology, engineering, population health, nursing, anthropology, social policy, political science and international collaboration.

References

Banks, S. (2006). *Ethics and values in social work* (3rd ed.). Basingstoke: Palgrave.

Desai, M., & Solas, J. (2012). Poverty, development and social justice. In K. Lyons, T. Hokenstad, M. Pawar, N. Huegler, & N. Hall (Eds.), *The Sage handbook of international social work* (pp. 85–99). London: Sage Publications Ltd.

Dimmel, N. (2014). Fighting poverty and social protection. In S. Hessle (Ed.), *Global social transformation and social action: The role of social workers* (pp. 31–56). Surrey: Ashgate.

Dominelli, L. (2014). Learning from our past: Climate change and disaster interventions in practice. In C. Noble, H. Strauss, & B. Littlechild (Eds.), *Global social work: Crossing borders, blurring boundaries* (pp. 341–351). Sydney: Sydney University Press.

Global Agenda for Social Work and Social Development – Commitment to Action. (2012). Retrieved on September 22, 2015, from http://cdn.ifsw.org/assets/globalagenda 2012.pdf.

Gray, M., & Coates, J. (2008). From "indigenization" to cultural relevance. In M. Gray, J. Coates, & M. Yellow Bird (Eds.), *Indigenous social work around the world: Towards culturally relevant education and practice* (pp. 1–12). Aldershot: Ashgate.

Hautala, H. (2012). Foreward. In M. Sepulveda & C. Nyst, *The human rights approach to social protection* (pp. 6–8). Ministry of Foreign Affairs of Finland. Retrieved on October 6, 2015 from www.ohchr.org/Documents/Issues/EPoverty/HumanRights ApproachToSocialProtection.pdf.

Healy, K. (2012). Critical perspectives. In M. Gray, J. Midgley, & S.A. Webb (Eds.), *The Sage handbook of social work* (pp. 191–205). London: Sage Publications Ltd.

Hoffler, E.F., & Clark, E.J. (2014). The congressional social work caucus: A renewed focus on the social safety net. In S. Hessle (Ed.), *Global social transformation and social action: The role of social workers* (pp. 43–47). Surrey: Ashgate.

International Council on Social Welfare (ICSW). (n.d.). *ICSW statement to the 59th session of the commission on the status of women.* Retrieved on September 30, 2015, from www.icsw.org/index.php/activities/social-protection-floor-initiative.

International Council on Social Welfare (ICSW). (2015). *Social protection floor initiative.* Retrieved on September 30, 2015, from www.icsw.org/index.php/activities/social-protection-floor-initiative.

International Federation of Social Workers (IFSW). (2014). *Review global definition of social work.* Retrieved on February 17, 2014, from http://ifsw.org/get-involved/global-definition-of-social-work/.

International Labour Organization (ILO). (2012, June 14). *R202 – social protection floors recommendation, 2012 (No. 202).* Retrieved on September 20, 2015, from www.ilo.org/dyn/normlex/en/f?p=NORMLEXPUB:12100:0::NO::P12100_INSTUMENTID:3065524.

International Labour Organization (ILO). (2013). *Social protection: Assessment based national dialogue: A good practices guide.* Retrieved on September 20, 2015, from www.socialprotectionfloorgateway.org/files/ABND_guide.pdf.

International Labour Organization (ILO). (2014). *World social protection report: Building economic recovery, inclusive development and social justice.* Retrieved on September 20, 2015, from www.socialprotectionfloor-gateway.org/files/WSPR.pdf.

International Labour Organization (ILO). (2015, February 23). *Area of critical importance: Creating and extending social protection floors.* Retrieved on September 22, 2015, from www.ilo.org/wcmsp5/groups/public/--ednorm/- relconf/documents/meetingdocument/wcms_346516.pdf.

International Labour Organization and United Nations Development Group. (2014). *UNDG Asia-Pacific: Social protection issues brief.* Retrieved on September 20, 2015, from www.socialprotectionfloor-gateway.org/files/UNDG_Asia_Issues_Brief.pdf.

Midgley, J. (2012) Welfare and social development. In M. Gray, J. Midgley, & S.A. Webb (Eds.), *The Sage handbook of social work* (pp. 94–107). London: Sage Publications Ltd.

Midgley, J. (2014). *Social development: Theory & practice.* Thousand Oaks: Sage Publications Ltd.

Mullaly, R.P. (2007). *The new structural social work: Ideology, theory, practice* (3rd ed.). Oxford: Oxford University Press.

National Institute for Health and Welfare. (2013, January 4). *Comprehensive social policies.* Retrieved on September 20, 2015, from www.thl.fi/en/web/thlfi-en/topics/information-packages/globalsocial-policy/comprehensive-social-policies.

National Institute for Health and Welfare. (2015, September 3). *New: EU social protection systems programme.* Retrieved on September 15, 2015, from www.thl.fi/fi/web/thlfien/topics/information-packages/global-social-policy/in-focus-2015-1.

Osei-Hwedie, K., & Rankopo, M.J. (2012). Social work in "developing" countries. In M. Gray, J. Midgley, & S.A. Webb (Eds.), *The Sage handbook of social work* (pp. 723–739). London: Sage Publications Ltd.

Smith, L. (2014). Amandia, Ngawethu (the Power is with us): Finding new social work discourse in movements for change. In S. Hessle (Ed.), *Global social transformation and social action: The role of social workers* (pp. 57–64). Surrey: Ashgate.

Social Protection Floor. (n.d.a). *Why the SPF?* Retrieved on September 20, 2015, from www.socialprotectionfloorgateway.org/55.htm.

Social Protection Floor. (n.d.b). *Global initiatives.* Retrieved on September 20, 2015, from www.socialprotectionfloor-gateway.org/216.htm.

Social Protection Floor Coalition. (2015). *Members of the core team.* Retrieved on September 30, 2015, from www.socialprotectionfloorscoalition.org/members/members-core-team/.

Staub-Bernasconi, S. (2014). Transcending disciplinary, professional and national borders in social work education. In C. Noble, H. Strauss, & B. Littlechild (Eds.), *Global social work: Crossing borders, blurring boundaries* (pp. 27–40). Sydney: Sydney University Press.

United Nations. (2015, March 6). *Statement on social protection floors: An essential element of the right to social security and of the sustainable development goals.* Retrieved on September 22, 2015, from www.socialprotection.org/gimi/gess/Ressource PDF.action?ressource.ressourceId=50857.

United Nations Research Institute for Social Development (UNRISD). (2010, May). *UNRISD research and policy brief 210: Combating poverty and inequality.* Retrieved on September 20, 2015, from www.unrisd.org/80256B3C005BCCF9/httpNetITFrame PDF?ReadForm&parentunid=82BBE4A03F504AD9C1257734002E9735&parentdoctype =brief&netitpath=80256B3C005BCCF9/%28httpAuxPages%29/82BBE4A03F504AD 9C1257734002E9735/$file/Policy-Brief-10.pdf.

United Nations Research Institute for Social Development (UNRISD). (2014). *Social inclusion and the post-2015 sustainable development agenda.* Retrieved on September 20, 2015, from www.unrisd.org/unitar-social-inclusion.

Voipio, T. (2011, January). *Social protection for all: An agenda for pro-child growth and child rights.* Retrieved on September 20, 2015, from www.unicef.org/socialpolicy/files/ Jan2011_ChildPovertyInsisghts_ENG%284%29.pdf.

Weiss-Gal, I., & Gal, J. (2014). Social workers and policy practice: A cross-national perspective. In S. Hessle (Ed.), *Global social transformation and social action: The role of social workers* (pp. 190–195). Surrey: Ashgate.

Winther-Schmidt, T. (n.d.). *Evolution of ODA for social protection.* Retrieved on September 20, 2015, from www.oecd.org/dac/povertyreduction/Evolution%20of%20 ODA%20for%20Social%20Protection.pdf.

2 The historical and current context of social protection

The development of the Social Protection Floor Initiative

Julie Drolet and Crystal Kwan

Historical context

The 20th century witnessed a major restructuring of the global economy with profound implications for the lives, livelihoods and life chances of people across the world (Kabeer, 2008). Historically, colonial governments and interests shaped trade and the economy, with poorer countries producing and exporting primary commodities to the richer countries while the latter specialized in the production and export of manufactured goods (Kabeer, 2008). After World War II there were high rates of economic growth and full employment in advanced industrialized countries, which strengthened state-provided social protection for the majority of workers in the formal sector of these countries, contributing to different forms of the welfare state (e.g., liberal, conservative, social democratic). Many systems of social protection were based on a "family model" or "male breadwinner model," with the idea of a male "primary breadwinner" in full-time employment, and with access to insurance benefits secured through the relationship of family members to the working person (Lund, 2006). The OECD model of welfare state regimes relied upon a legitimate state and a pervasive, formal sector labor market (Wood, 2004). Poorer regions of the world did not conform to these two key assumptions (Wood, 2004). Many developing countries lacked comprehensive social protection systems:

> Developing countries had inherited weak and highly restricted systems of social protection from the colonial era that were intended for a small proportion of workers in the formal sector. While efforts were made to expand these measures to the wider population, the results were very uneven. In most countries, social security measures remained restricted to the small, male-dominated section of the workforce employed in the formal state and private sector.
>
> (Kabeer, 2008, p. 1)

Social protection was long regarded as being unaffordable in developing countries or being detrimental to economic growth, whereas, in recent years, many policy-makers consider social protection as an instrument for poverty reduction, fostering social cohesion or even for promoting economic growth (Bender, Kaltenborn, & Pfeiderer, 2013). Social cohesion is understood as a cohesive society where citizens feel they can trust their neighbors and state institutions, seize opportunities for improving well-being, and feel protected when facing illness, unemployment or old age (Jutting & Prizzon, 2013). In the 1990s, social protection underwent a significant transformation in developing countries to define an agenda for social policy that focuses on poverty reduction and providing support to the poorest (Barrientos & Hulme, 2008). There is a renewed interest in social policies, and some governments have increased social spending to soften the impacts of economic reform as well as the realization of the failure of neo-liberal economic models to generate economic growth and reduce poverty (Hassim & Razavi, 2006). The neo-liberal policy agenda of stabilization, structural adjustment and public sector retrenchment led to cutbacks in social spending and resulted in devastating human costs (Cook, 2013). Social movements in many parts of the developing world have successfully opened spaces to demand more effective social policies that mitigate the effects of market failures and reduce inequalities (Hassim & Razavi, 2006). Social workers face many contemporary challenges, and alongside the difficulties of upholding human rights, social justice and active citizenship, are those of affirming environmental justice in and through social work practice (Dominelli, 2013). This chapter provides a historical context of social protection and social policy. Indigenous and informal types of social protection in developing countries are discussed. Then, it traces the development of the Social Protection Floor Initiative. Finally, the chapter will end with a discussion about social protection in light of a post-2015 context and the new challenges that ensue.

Indigenous and informal forms of social protection

Indigenous informal or semi-formal systems of social protection have existed alongside formal social protection systems in developing countries (Patel & Triegaardt, 2008). While some remnants of traditional systems have survived modernization and colonialism, other traditional practices have evolved due to the lack of access to formal systems of social provision (Patel & Triegaardt, 2008). For example, traditional and informal systems of social security are evident in the form of credit and savings schemes, burial societies, cooperative arrangements, and remittances of migrant workers to relatives in rural areas, in-kind support, social networks of family and friends, volunteerism, and mutual aid and self-help groups (Patel & Triegaardt, 2008).

Informal safety nets are informal mechanisms for coping with difficulties such as borrowing, drawing down savings, selling assets, mutual support from family and friends, and seeking additional income-generating activities. Family systems of support and private transfers continue to play an important role in social protection. Community and family provide important social solidarity, kinship and friendship ties as a form of informal social protection, with informal transfers in the form of remittances from family members working abroad.

Mupedziswa and Ntseane (2014) report on the contribution of non-formal social protection to social development in Botswana, and explain that "non-formal social protection consists of self-organized safety nets based on membership of a particular social group or community that includes family, kinship, age group, neighbourhood or ethnic group" (p. 85). These measures are predicated on people's cultural beliefs, norms and values, and deliver a variety of benefits, including income and psychosocial and emotional support (Mupedziswa & Ntseane, 2014). With the majority of populations falling outside formal systems, those with most limited access to social protection tend to be those marginalized on the basis of a number of factors such as ethnicity (and caste in India), gender, age, migrant status, and by economic status (Cook, Kabeer, & Suwannarat, 2003).

Many people employed in the informal sector, as well as the working poor, the self-employed and the unemployed have no social protection or social security coverage and no access to safety nets. Many workers are trapped in informality by chronic poverty, social exclusion and lack of voice (Kabeer, 2008). Women from low-income households are over-represented in precarious and poorly paid jobs and experience a variety of gender-related constraints that limit their ability to overcome labor market disadvantages through their own efforts (Kabeer, 2008). There is a need for a gender perspective in the design of social protection measures given the different barriers faced by women and men (Kabeer, 2008), and this will be further discussed later in this chapter. The next section will discuss social policy and social protection.

Social policy and social protection

According to Ortiz (2007):

> Modern government is based on a social contract between citizens and the state in which rights and duties are agreed to by all to further the common interest. Citizens lend their support to a government through taxes and efforts to a country's good; in return, governments acquire legitimacy by protecting the people's rights and through public policies that benefit all.
>
> (p. 7)

This is particularly evident in social policy and social protection systems. The objective of social protection activities is to enhance livelihood security, reduce risk and enable households to cope better with shocks (Cook, Kabeer, & Suwannarat, 2003). A significant body of evidence points to the importance to households of human and social capital both in protecting against shocks and in enabling coping with or recovery from economic shock. The principal role of government in social protection is generally through sectoral policies (including health, education and welfare) and through direct provision of relief or social assistance (Cook, Kabeer, & Suwannarat, 2003). Basic support in the form of health and education has been eroded in recent years with the introduction of user fees; this affects access to basic services by the poor (Cook, Kabeer, & Suwannarat, 2003).

As a policy approach, social protection is relatively new in the field of international development. It reflects attempts to integrate concerns about social security and poverty reduction within a unified conceptual and policy framework in response to the perceived increase in vulnerability of populations across the world and reflects a greater appreciation of the need to have protection measures in place before a crisis occurs rather than in its aftermath (Kabeer, 2008; 2010). Social policy scholars in different parts of the world use the term social policy in different ways. According to Mkandawire (2004):

> Social policy is collective interventions in the economy to influence the access to and the incidence of adequate and secure livelihoods and income. As such, social policy has always played redistributive, protective and transformative or developmental roles ... the weight given to each of these elements of social policies has varied widely across countries and, within countries, over time. In the context of development, there can be no doubt that the transformative role of social policy needs to receive greater attention than it is usually accorded in developed countries and much more than it does in the current focus on "safety nets."
>
> (p. 1)

Some definitions of social policy are broad and include income programs, health insurance, and the provision of social work services, and governments in many parts of the world recognize social protection as an effective policy instrument for both poverty prevention and poverty alleviation (Tang & Midgley, 2008). Redistribution is a primary legitimate objective of social policies (Ortiz, 2011). Equity enhancing policies are needed to balance the unequal distribution of the benefits from economic growth resulting from unregulated market forces (Ortiz, 2007). Public policies can mitigate or exacerbate social differences; the design of any social policy should carefully evaluate its distributive impacts to ensure coverage to excluded groups such as the poor, and above all, avoid regressive redistribution (e.g., building systems with public resources that mostly benefit upper income groups) (Ortiz, 2011). Financing social policies implies some transfer of resources, either from taxed citizens to those outside the formal sector, or, as in the case of social insurance, from the working population to the unemployed and older people. There is national capacity to fund economic and social development even in the poorer countries (Ortiz, 2011). Improved taxation, reprioritization of expenditures, external financing and debt relief, domestic borrowing, more accommodating macroeconomic framework (e.g., tolerance to some inflation, fiscal deficit), fighting illicit financial flows, and use of reserves for national development are measures available to finance social protection in developing countries (Ortiz, 2011). The implementation of social protection occurs through the public sector's central ministries and local governments, which is normally best to achieve expansion of coverage and to reduce poverty and social exclusion nationwide, as well as market-based, NGOs and charitable institutions, and a combination of these measures (Ortiz, 2011). Given the scarcity of resources for social policies in developing countries, Ortiz (2011) claims that the best solution may be a mixed delivery system, and it is important to ensure that any proposed social protection measure or social policy can be effectively implemented; often social policies may be good on paper but fail because of the lack of implementation capacity (e.g., legal restrictions on child labor but no labor inspectors).

The origins of social assistance can be traced to the charitable works and activities mandated by religious institutions and cultural beliefs (Tang & Midgley, 2008). The Elizabethan Poor Law of 1601 created the first centralized, nationwide system of public poor relief in England, and recognized that traditional forms of familial and community support were not always able to cope and that religious charity needed to be augmented by public provision (Tang & Midgley, 2008). Many social policy scholars acknowledge the importance of the Elizabethan Poor Law in the history of social security by shaping its subsequent evolution and served as a model for many social assistance programs created in the United States and many parts of the developing world (Tang & Midgley, 2008).

"Extending social security is a necessary condition for achieving broad-based and inclusive development" (van Ginneken, 2008, p. 288). Access to basic social services, such as health care and education, play a crucial role in processes toward inclusion and empowerment (van Ginneken, 2008). Safety nets are most effective if they are integrated into the overall development strategy of the country rather than one-off, stand-alone programs. "Millions of people work all their lives yet remain poor, and cohorts are entering their elderly years with no savings for retirement … this crisis will not be solved by patchwork responses" (Lund, 2006, p. 231). Social policies are necessary because the benefits of economic growth do not automatically reach all people (Ortiz, 2007). In the early 21st century, a consensus has emerged that social policy is a primary function of the state, and that social policy is more than a limited set of safety nets and services to cover market failure (Ortiz, 2007). The next section will discuss the development of the Social Protection Floor Initiative.

The development of the Social Protection Floor Initiative

On April 5, 2009, the United Nations (UN) Systems Chief Executives Board for Coordination (CEB) reached an inter-agency agreement of nine joint initiatives as a response to the Global Financial Crisis (ILO, 2010). The Social Protection Floor Initiative (SPF-I) is one of the nine, and it is co-led by the International Labour Organization (ILO) and the World Health Organization (WHO) (ILO, 2010). The social protection floors approach has gained widespread recognition and discussion among international bodies and in the global development fora (ILO, 2012). For instance, in September 2010 the SPF-I was endorsed by the UN General Assembly during the Millennium Development Goals summit (ILO, 2012). The role and potentials of SPFs were recognized and discussed in the G20

Meeting of Labour and Employment Ministers (in November 2011) and in the resolutions adopted by the UN Commission for Social Development in February 2012 (ILO, 2012).

Civil society has played an integral role in supporting the SPF-I. Civil society refers to a range of non-governmental, community and religious organizations, family and other informal networks that contribute to social protection (Cook, Kabeer, & Suwannarat, 2003). For instance, many non-governmental organizations (NGOs) stress a rights-based approach grounded in international conventions to protect jobs and wages, assets of the poor (land titles, rights to housing) and protection of worker rights in the informal sector. In efforts to support the SPF-I, on March 2012, 17 NGOs came together in a workshop to write a joint statement to support the ILO's SPF recommendations (Global Coalition for Social Protection Floors, 2012). From this workshop, the interest in continuing to support the SPF approach, through joint initiatives, was so great that the NGOs decided to create the Global Coalition for Social Protection Floors (Global Coalition for Social Protection Floors, 2013). In the end, 59 NGOs signed the joint statement and the NGO coalition grew in members (Global Coalition for Social Protection Floors, 2013).

NGOs within the Coalition each have their various focus areas and population groups, however what bonds them together is the desire to "achieve real social protection based on human rights for all people in all parts of the world" (Global Coalition for Social Protection Floors, 2013, p. 1). The Coalition has four key aims:

1   to raise awareness of the ILO's SPF recommendations and influence international discourse on social protection;
2   to promote forums for knowledge exchange among civil society organizations;
3   to enhance collaboration and coordination with other social protection platforms and/or coalitions (at national and regional levels); and
4   to promote the creation of "inclusive coalitions, where these do not exist, aimed at promoting the design, implementation, monitoring and evaluation of social protection floors" (Global Coalition for Social Protection Floors, 2013, p. 1).

ILO's Social Protection Floors Recommendation No. 202

Part of the ILO's two-dimensional strategy. On June 2012, the ILO launched the Social Protection Floors Recommendation No. 202, which are the new international standards for national protection floors (ILO, 2012). Recommendation No. 202 completes the ILO's two-dimensional social security strategy for countries at all levels of development (ILO, 2012). The strategy includes:

1   a horizontal dimension of "establishing and maintaining of social protection floors as a fundamental element of national social security systems"; and

2   a vertical dimension of "pursuing strategies for the extension of social security that progressively ensure higher levels of social security to as many people as possible" (ILO, 2012, p. 3).

Efforts, toward establishing and maintaining social protection floors, are guided by Recommendation No. 202 (ILO, 2012), while efforts toward the vertical dimensions of the strategy are guided by the ILO's Convention No. 102 and other more advanced social security standards (ILO, 2012). The strategy also implicates the state as the overall and primary-responsibility holder in initiating, developing and maintaining social security strategies (ILO, 2012).

Key messages. There are several key messages within the Recommendation No. 202 (ILO, 2012). First, the notion that social security is a human right is reconfirmed. Second, social security is socially and economically necessary, as it is a mechanism to:

1   reduce poverty and social exclusion; and
2   bolster development and equality (ILO, 2012).

Third, SPFs are economically affordable to introduce, complete and maintain within all societies, at all development levels (ILO, 2012). Fourth and finally, as societies' economies and fiscal space widens, continued efforts need to be made to promote more advanced social security levels guided by the ILO's social security standards (e.g., Convention No. 102) (ILO, 2012). The ILO states that:

> at the heart of these messages is this: there is no excuse for any society to put off building social security for its members, and it can be done at any stage of development, even if gradually. All societies can grow with equity.
>
> (ILO, 2012, p. vi)

In this way, the Recommendation No. 202 demystifies the belief that only societies with advanced economies can afford social security systems, and facilitates a new understanding of social security – "as a condition for growth rather than a burden to society" (ILO, 2010, para. 5).

What are National SPFs? National SPFs are "nationally-defined sets of basic social security guarantees which secure protection aimed at preventing or alleviating poverty, vulnerability and social exclusion" (ILO, 2012, p. 5). At minimum these guarantees should ensure that all people, throughout the life cycle, have access to basic income security and essential health care (ILO, 2012). There should be at least four social security guarantees (defined at national levels) in any national SPFs (ILO, 2012). First, access to essential health care (including maternity care) should be guaranteed (ILO, 2012). Second, children should be guaranteed basic income security that provides access to "nutrition, education, care and any other necessary goods and services" (ILO, 2012, p. 5). Third, persons who are in active age but are unable to earn sufficient income (e.g., due to sickness, unemployment, maternity and disability) should be guaranteed basic income security (ILO, 2012). Fourth and finally, basic income security should be guaranteed to older persons (ILO, 2012). The goal of SPFs is toward improved coordination and impact of social protection policies and programs (ILO, 2012). SPFs are not meant to disregard existing efforts and start from scratch but rather a key strength of SPFs is facilitating "the prioritization and sequencing of the different elements of the floor" (UNDP & ILO, 2011, p. 14). Thus, a "careful analysis of capacities, needs and existing schemes already in place will enable a rationalization of the policy making process for a gradual building up of the social protection floor" (UNDP & ILO, 2011, p. 14).

Resolutions 2012. The "Resolution concerning efforts to make social protection floors a national reality worldwide" was adopted at the same time as the Recommendation 202, on June 2012 at ILO's 101st Session (ILO, 2012, p. 41). These efforts include:

1   awareness-raising initiatives to promote the "widespread implementation of the Recommendation";
2   capacity-building with government, employers' and workers' organizations "to enable them to design, implement, monitor and evaluate national social protection floor policies and programmes";
3   providing technical support and forums for shared knowledge, information and good practices on social protection among members;
4   "supporting national dialogue processes on the design and implementation of national social protection floors"; and
5   enhancing cooperation and coordination among members and other stakeholders/organizations to further develop national social protection strategies (ILO, 2012, p. 41).

The Global SPF Advisory Network is an example of efforts that contribute to the Resolutions 2012. The Network provides technical support and advice to countries that intend to build, expand or re-orient their social protection systems (ILO, 2010). The support provided includes: "policy design, awareness raising, fiscal space analysis, legislation and evaluation" – which covers the entire process of establishing and maintaining a national SPF (ILO, 2010, para. 8).

Social protection and the post-2015 development agenda

Post-2015: new context and challenges

The current and post-2015 context for development is fundamentally different due to new challenges and risks societies are facing worldwide. First, since the Global Economic Crisis (that started in 2008), widespread inequality (both between and within countries) and unemployment ensued, which has generated social instability and set back the economic progress many countries had achieved (Camfield, Crabtree, & Roelen, 2013). Further, within a neo-liberal global context, governments are pressured to adopt austerity measures, which entail the reduction of public spending on social protection programs (Cook & Dugarova, 2014). Parallel to the global economic crisis, are shortfalls to global food production and increasing volatility in food and energy prices (Camfield, Crabtree, & Roelen, 2013). Second, the ecological threats associated with climate change are increasing (Cook & Dugarova, 2014). For instance, climate-related disasters are increasing in frequency and intensity (UN, 2015). The UN (2015) states that in the last decade:

> Over 700 thousand people have lost their lives, over 1.4 million have been injured and approximately 23 million have been made homeless as a result of disasters. Overall, more than 1.5 billion people have been affected by disasters in various ways, with women, children and people in vulnerable situations disproportionately affected. The total economic loss was more than $1.3 trillion. In addition, between 2008 and 2012, 144 million people were displaced by disasters.
>
> (p. 10)

Ecological threats pose serious social and economic consequences. Countries are now pressed to reduce greenhouse gas emissions, which conflicts with the traditional carbon-led growth/development model that continues to dominate (Camfield, Crabtree, & Roelen, 2013). Such a model is no longer sustainable and new sustainable development pathways are necessary in a post-2015 world (Cook & Dugarova, 2014). Third and finally, demographics are shifting worldwide, whereby all societies are (or will be) experiencing rapidly aging populations (Cook & Dugarova, 2014). For instance, in 2000, the global number of adults aged 60 years or older exceeded the number of children aged 14 or younger (UNFPA & HelpAge International (HAI), 2012). This demographic trend is unprecedented in human history and projected to continue, whereby in 2050 one in five people will be 60 years of age or older (tripling the global number of older adults) (UNFPA & HAI, 2012). Rapidly aging populations pose various challenges to social protection schemes and designs (e.g., pensions), as they raise the age-dependency ratios of a country (Cook & Dugarova, 2014). Age-dependency ratio is the ratio of dependents (e.g., those younger than 15 years of age or older than 64 years of age) to the working age population (e.g., those between 15 and 64 years of age) (World Bank, 2015).

The new global context and inter-related challenges requires contemporary social policies to diverge from the classic welfare state and neo-liberal approaches (Cook & Dugarova, 2014). Within the classic welfare state and neo-liberal approaches, social policies are primarily focused on addressing the symptoms – social issues (e.g., poverty) while neglecting the underlying structural/systemic causes (e.g., patterns of social stratification) (Cook & Dugarova, 2014). Social policies, within this framework, often act "as residual in the sequencing of policy decisions, [whereby] social, environmental or other consequence (or 'externalities') of growth-focused economic policies are addressed through compensatory measures such as social assistance or target poverty alleviation" (Cook

& Dugarova, 2014, p. 32). Targeted social protection measures are not ideal in a context of widespread poverty, inequality and deprivation (Cook & Dugarova, 2014). Cook and Dugarova (2014) insightfully state:

> A new approach to social development needs to move from a primary focus on particular problems and groups towards addressing the structures of opportunity or constraint that generate better social outcomes and to focus on the drivers of social transformation rather than only on symptoms and consequences.
>
> (p. 32)

Role of social protection in addressing the challenges

The global economic crisis, global food shortages, volatile food and energy prices and continued ecological threats, among others, highlight an increasingly volatile world. Yet, currently, 80% of the global population are without access to comprehensive social protection to help cope with the potential implications of such threats (UN, 2012). In a post-2015 context, social protection can play various critical roles, including among others:

1   acting as an effective automatic stabilizer in times of economic crisis;
2   building the adaptive capacities and resilience of households to climate change threats; and
3   supporting the well-being and quality of life of aging populations.

Social protection – an automatic economic stabilizer. Euzeby (2010) posits that "among the lessons from the economic crisis, it would be remiss to overlook the fact that it could put an end, once and for all, to the widespread belief that social protection constitutes as an economic handicap" (p. 71). Stiglitz (2009) argues, "when the economy gets weaker, spending on social protection and unemployment schemes should automatically go up, helping to stabilize the economy" (p. 4). The Global Economic Crisis has shown that social protection act as a social buffer and as an automatic economic stabilizer (Euzeby, 2010). Countries with well-developed social protection systems faired (and continue to do) better than their counterparts during the recession (Euzeby, 2010). For instance, member countries of the European Union who had least developed social protection systems (e.g., Latvia, Lithuania and Estonia in Eastern Europe, and Ireland in Western Europe) experienced the greatest decline in GDP and increases in unemployment due to the crisis (Euzeby, 2010).

Social protection – building adaptive capacities and resilience to climate change. Climate change is one of the most pressing challenges of the 21st century, and "is now recognized to be an (increasing) source of hazard and vulnerability for populations in both developed and developing countries" (Béné, 2011, p. 67). Rarely discussed within the literature are the relationships between social protection and climate change (Béné, 2011). Social protection plays a critical role:

1   in the short-term by, acting as a buffer against climate-related shocks; and
2   in the long-term, by strengthening the adaptive capacities and building the resilience of households to future shocks (Wood, 2011).

For instance, climate-related shocks can pressure individuals and households to adopt damaging coping strategies (which also affect their long-term adaptive capacities to future shocks) (Wood, 2011). Social protection, in the form of cash transfers, for example, can lighten the pressures to adopt such strategies (Wood, 2011). Further, climate change can also gradually decrease the viability of livelihood options available (Wood, 2011). Social protection systems that guarantee employment and decent work can help to facilitate livelihood transitions (Wood, 2011).

The increased complexity and changing nature of disasters and emergencies has underlined the need to identify linkages between humanitarian action and social protection. In other words, work is needed to assess the potential role of social protection contributing to strengthening households' resilience and preparedness and risk management; supporting the accumulation of human capital and assets prior to crises in relief; secure a transition from relief to recovery; and address key elements of peace-building such as social cohesion and access to services. Social workers engaged in disaster response and recovery efforts are acutely aware of the challenges involved in transitioning from the short-term emergency response phase to the longer-term sustainable development phase. Although there is considerable evidence on cash-based interventions in humanitarian contexts, there is limited evidence on linkages with medium and/or long-term social protection interventions.

Gender and social protection

Poverty and deprivation are not static conditions (Ortiz, 2007). Populations, households, and individuals may be in a good condition at one point, but may face various risks that can plunge them into poverty over time (Ortiz, 2007). Men and women face specific risks over the life cycle, and specific groups are excluded from access to social protection in specific ways (Lund, 2006). Vulnerability is generally correlated with poor education and health status, limited fluency in the national language, undocumented civil status, and low levels of political empowerment and organization. Marginalized groups are vulnerable to serious violations of their basic rights – for example in the trafficking of women and children, labor exploitation of undocumented migrants and children – and are thus in greatest need of protection from society and state. Social workers recognize the interaction of multiple forms of disadvantage due to structural barriers such as poverty, social location, age, gender, and caste that can lead to the most severe forms of vulnerability and exclusion.

Domestic workers, who are mainly women and girls, are amongst the least recognized and least protected workers. Worldwide they share common characteristics, most notably their isolation, invisibility and lack of recognition and of workers' rights (OECD, 2012). Tens of millions of women and girls around the world are employed as domestic workers in private households where they clean, cook, care for children, look after elderly family members, and perform other essential tasks for their employers (Human Rights Watch, 2012). Despite their important role, they are among the most exploited and abused workers in the world (Human Rights Watch, 2012). For example, domestic work is the largest source of employment for women in Latin America, and although significant steps have been taken to improve the situation, it is a sector where informality prevails (ILO, 2014). Remittances from the incomes of domestic workers account for as much as 10% of the Gross Domestic Product (GDP) in some countries (OECD, 2012). These monetary investments – used for food, housing, education and medical services – along with the newly acquired skills of return-ees, can potentially contribute significantly to poverty reduction and provide safety nets that sustain communities in their home countries (OECD, 2012). Yet, while migration can bring new employment and opportunities, it also bears great risks for women, many positioned at the lower end of the job market. Migrant populations have less access to basic social services and social protection than resident populations, and face discrimination in accessing employment, housing and services. There is a need to consider social protection measures for all.

Resilience

An increasing number of women and men, girls and boys are finding their lives and rights disrupted and threatened by a range of interconnected shocks and stresses caused by various and often interlocking factors such as climate change, increasing inequality, globalization and unsustainable resource use (Smyth & Sweetnam, 2015). Over the past decade, resilience has become a significant new area of development, policy and debate, and programs and services are evolving in response. According to Ungar (2013):

> resilience is both the capacity of individuals to navigate their way to the psychological, social, cultural and physical resources that build and sustain their well-being, and their individual and collective capacity to negotiate for these resources to be provided in culturally meaningful ways.
>
> (p. 17)

This understanding of resilience goes beyond an individual notion, to a more relational and holistic approach (Drolet et al., 2015). Social protection can assist in fostering resilience at the individual and community levels. Women are often assumed to be inherently more vulnerable – and hence less resilient – than men. While this may be true of some women in some contexts, a more nuanced under-standing is needed (Smyth & Sweetnam, 2015). Holmes and Jones (2013) advocate for a transformative social protection approach that will empower women and ensure more gender-equitable outcomes, as well as address the root causes of poverty and vulnerability, driven by gendered inequities at the societal level. Gender inequality and gendered norms create and intensify vulnerability by constraining women's responses to sudden shocks, and placing longer-term strain on livelihoods, stability and well-being.

> Women perform 66 percent of the world's work, and produce 50 percent of the food, yet earn only 10 percent of the income and own 1 percent of the property. Whether the issue is improving education in the developing world, or fighting global climate change, or addressing nearly any other challenge we face, empowering women is a critical part of the equation.
>
> (Former President Bill Clinton addressing the annual meeting of the Clinton Global initiative (September 2009), cited in OECD, 2012)

Resilience is greatly enhanced by policies that ensure women's equal rights, and active participation and leadership in social protection, livelihood and disaster management. This means working in partnership with women as individuals, and with feminist movements and women's organizations, and many social workers are engaged in such solidarity practices. Drolet et al. (2015) present two case studies from Pakistan and the United States to demonstrate how women contribute to building resilience and promoting sustainable development in diverse post-disaster contexts. Resilience requires more than reducing vulnerability – it calls for empowering responses to disasters, which aim to support and foster people's resilience, enhancing their ability to respond to disasters, against a backdrop of the longer-term challenges of building sustainable livelihoods (Drolet et al., 2015). "Differentiated vulnerabilities require differentiated interventions, so gender-specific and gender-intensified vulnerabilities and inequalities require gender-sensitive social protection" (Devereux, 2013, p. xi). Vulnerability and capacity vary throughout the life cycle, with the young and old being particularly affected.

Children and social protection

More than 200 million children younger than five years old from low-income and middle-income countries do not attain their developmental potential, primarily because of poverty, nutritional deficiencies and inadequate learning opportunities; economic recession and climate change will probably increase the number of children affected (Walker et al., 2011). Biological and psychosocial risk factors associated with poverty lead to inequalities in early child development, which undermine educational attainment and adult productivity, thereby perpetuating the poverty cycle (Walker et al., 2011). Social protection is a response to fulfill children's rights, including the right to access services and an adequate standard of living. At the same time, social protection contributes to an equity-focused approach to development, as it ensures equal access to services and is conducive to equitable human development outcomes for children. For example, UNICEF has recently launched its Social Protection Strategic Framework, which lays out its approach to social protection and articulates the underlying key principles that guide the organization's work, including national integrated systems and the progressive realization of universal coverage (UNICEF, 2014). The development and strengthening of integrated social protection systems is a promising approach to address the multiple and compounding vulnerabilities of children, families and communities. Children have developmental needs with nutritional, emotional and psychological needs, as well as education and health care. Social workers play a key role in child protection and in meeting children's rights across the world. Addressing the needs of children requires specific measures to support universal access to basic social services, health and education. A child-sensitive and transformative approach to social protection is required.

Aging and social protection

Worldwide, societies are experiencing unprecedented shifts in their age compositions and population demographics (Kwan & Drolet, 2015). For the first time in human history the number of older people will surpass the number of children under the age of 14, representing one of the "biggest social transformations" societies will experience in recent decades (WHO, 2014, para. 2). The great shift in demographics demand that sustainable development efforts are age-inclusive and support the well being of people throughout their life course – including the later life years (Kwan & Drolet, 2015). The challenge of aging populations raises a number of social protection concerns related to illness, disability, widowhood and old age, that may not be best addressed by measures to increase their rates of economic activity (Kabeer, 2008). There is a need to extend social protection to formerly excluded categories of people irrespective of their working or labor-protection status. The lack of basic and universal social protection systems for older adults further create challenges to eradicate old age poverty (Dhemba, 2013).

The well-being and quality of life of the older adult population are linked to their capacity to address risks and opportunities in the rapidly changing and complex context of the post-2015 era (Llyod-Sherlock, 2004). Social protection plays a key role in building the capacity and resilience of older adults to manage such risks and opportunities. For instance, the risks of old age poverty can be reduced by pension systems that recognize that as one ages, income potentials may decline (Dhemba, 2013). Strong public social protection systems are essential to addressing old age poverty. Bolivia, for example, launched in 2008 a universal (non-contributory) pension scheme, called the Dignity Pension (Renta Dignidad) (UNDP & ILO, 2011). This pension scheme covered 800,000 beneficiaries, which is 97% of the total eligible beneficiaries, and the impact was a 5.8% decline in extreme poverty between 2007 and 2009 (particularly in rural areas) (UNDP & ILO, 2011).

Conclusion

In an increasingly volatile world with heightened economic, social and demographic challenges and risks, there is a greater need for an integrated social protection system that addresses such complexity. ILO's Recommendation No. 202 is an example of a new approach to social development that Cook and Dugarova (2014) argue is necessary in the post-2015 era. The strategy is a movement away from a piecemeal approach to social protection and toward an integrated system of social protection predicated on universality and social justice (ILO, 2012).

It is now widely recognized that the objective of sustainable and inclusive development can hardly be achieved without the extension of social security to larger groups of the population (Behrendt, 2013). The role of social protection for economic and social development has been emphasized in a number of international policy documents and initiatives (Behrendt, 2013). This major paradigm shift is evident in recent policy reforms in developing countries with the implementation of social protection programs (Behrendt, 2013). Identifying and targeting vulnerable groups, reducing inequality and addressing structural vulnerability are essential to sustaining development over an individual's lifetime and across generations (UNDP, 2014, p. 131). The most successful countries in achieving long-term sustainable growth and poverty reduction have put in place extensive systems of social security (Behrendt et al., 2009).

National Development Strategies are often designed by economists and specialists with inadequate attention to people's perceptions and claims (Ortiz, 2007). There is a need to ground social policies and social protection initiatives in the lived experiences of those most affected by these social and economic development interventions. Social workers represent the "voices" of the marginalized and oppressed in society, and work to build alliances across borders and build bridges across similarities and differences (Sewpaul, 2015). This chapter traced the history of social protection in developed and developing countries, and considered the important role of indigenous and non-formal social protection supports in the absence of formal social protection measures. With the recent international initiatives to further support and develop social protection in developing countries the Social Protection Floor Initiative and the ILO's Social Protection Floors Recommendation No. 202 was discussed. Finally, the post-2015 development context and the role of social protection in addressing the historical and current challenges were considered. Social workers across the globe are called upon to further realize the right to social protection in their national plans, and provide support at the national and international level to achieve these goals.

References

Barrientos, A., & Hulme, D. (2008). Social protection for the poor and poorest: An introduction. In A. Barrientos & D. Hulme (Eds.), *Social protection for the poor and poorest: Concepts, policies and politics* (pp. 1–24). New York: Palgrave Macmillan.

Behrendt, C. (2013). Building national social protection floors and social security systems: The ILO's two-dimensional social security strategy. In K. Bender, M. Kaltenborn, & C. Pfleiderer (Eds.), *Social protection in developing countries: Reforming systems* (pp. 207–218). London: Routledge.

Behrendt, C., Cichon, M., Hagemejer, K., Kidd, S., Krech, R., & Townsend, P. (2009). Rethinking the role of social security in development. In P. Townsend (Ed.), *Building decent societies: Rethinking the role of social security in development* (pp. 325–337). New York: Palgrave Macmillan.

Bender, K., Kaltenborn, M., & Pfeiderer, C. (2013). Introduction. In K. Bender, M. Kaltenborn, & C. Pfleiderer (Eds.), *Social protection in developing countries: Reforming systems* (pp. 1–9). London: Routledge.

Béné, C. (2011). Social protection and climate change. *IDS Bulletin, 42*(6), 67–70.

Camfield, L., Crabtree, A., & Roelen, K. (2013). Editorial: Poverty, vulnerability and resilience in a post-2015 world. *Social Indicators Research, 113*(2), 599–608.

Cook, S. (2013). Rescuing social protection from the poverty trap: New programmes and historical lessons. In K. Bender, M. Kaltenborn, & C. Pfleiderer (Eds.), *Social protection in developing countries: Reforming systems* (pp. 13–23). London: Routledge.

Cook, S., & Dugarova, E. (2014). Rethinking social development for a post-2015 world. *Development, 57*(1), 30–35.

Cook, S., Kabeer, N., & Suwannarat, G. (2003). *Social protection in Asia*. New Delhi: Har-Anand Publications.

Devereux, S. (2013). Foreword. In R. Holmes & N. Jones, *Gender and social protection in the developing world* (pp. x–xiii). London: Zed Books.

Dhemba, J. (2013). Overcoming poverty in old age: Social security provision in Lesotho, South Africa and Zimbabwe revisited. *International Social Work, 56*(6), 816–827.

Dominelli, L. (2013). Environmental justice at the heart of social work practice: Greening the profession. *International Journal of Social Welfare, 22*, 431–439.

Drolet, J., Dominelli, L., Alston, M., Ersing, R., Mathbor, G., & Wu, H. (2015). Women rebuilding lives post-disaster: Innovative community practices for building resilience and promoting sustainable development. *Gender & Development, 23*(3), 433–448.

Euzeby, A. (2010). Economic crisis and social protection in the European Union: Moving beyond immediate responses. *International Social Security Review, 63*(2), 71–86.

Global Coalition for Social Protection Floors. (2012). *Autonomous recommendation on the social protection floor (joint statement by a group of NGOs)*. Retrieved on June 12, 2015, from www.socialprotectionfloorscoalition.org/wp-content/uploads/2014/09/LOGO_2012_EN_NGO-SPF-statement-ILC2012_FINAL_version.pdf.

Global Coalition for Social Protection Floors. (2013). *Terms of reference*. Retrieved on June 12, 2015, from www.fes-globalization.org/geneva/documents/2013_04_08-09_SPF-NGO_Terms%20of%20References_revised.pdf.

Hassim, S., & Razavi, S. (2006). Gender and social policy in a global context: Uncovering the gendered structure of "the Social." In S. Razavi & S. Hassim (Eds.), *Gender and social policy in a global context: Uncovering the gendered structure of "the Social"* (pp. 1–39). New York: Palgrave Macmillan.

Holmes, R., & Jones, N. (2013). *Gender and social protection in the developing world*. London: Zed Books.

Human Rights Watch. (2012). Domestic workers. Retrieved on October 18, 2015, from www.hrw.org/topic/womens-rights/domestic-workers.

International Labour Organization (ILO). (2010, June 16). *ILO-UN Social Protection Floor Initiative: The role of social security in crisis response and recovery, and beyond*. Retrieved on June 15, 2015, from www.ilo.org/global/about-the-ilo/newsroom/features/WCMS_141818/lang-en/index.htm.

ILO. (2012). *The strategy of the International Labour Organization: Social security for all*. Retrieved on June 15, 2015, from www.socialprotectionfloor-gateway.org/files/social_security_for_all.pdf.

ILO. (2014, March 8). 100 million women in Latin America's labour force. Retrieved on October 18, 2015, from www.ilo.org/global/about-the-ilo/newsroom/comment-analysis/WCMS_237488/lang-en/index.htm.

Jutting, J., & Prizzon, A. (2013). Social cohesion: Does it matter for growth and development? In K. Bender, M. Kaltenborn, & C. Pfleiderer (Eds.), *Social protection in developing countries: Reforming systems* (pp. 43–50). London: Routledge.

Kabeer, N. (2008). *Mainstreaming gender in social protection for the informal economy*. London: Commonwealth Secretariat.

Kabeer, N. (2010). *Gender and social protection strategies in the informal economy*. New Delhi: Routledge.

Kwan, C., & Drolet, J. (2015). Toward age-inclusive sustainable development goals: Exploring the potential role and contributions of community development. *Community Development Journal, 50*(4), 589–607.

Llyod-Sherlock, P. (2004). *Living longer: Ageing, development & social protection*. London: Zed Books.

Lund, F. (2006). Working people and access to social protection. In S. Razavi & S. Hassim (Eds.), *Gender and social policy in a global context: Uncovering the gendered structure of "the Social"* (pp. 217–233). New York: Palgrave Macmillan.

Mkandawire, T. (2004). Social policy in a development context: Introduction. In T. Mkandawire (Ed.), *Social policy in a development context* (pp. 1–33). New York: Palgrave Macmillan.

Mupedziswa, R., & Ntseane, D. (2014). The contribution of non-formal social protection to social development in Botswana. In L. Patel, J. Midgley, & M. Ulriksen (Eds.), *Social protection in Southern Africa: New opportunities for social development* (pp. 84–97). London: Routledge.

OECD. (2012). *Women's economic empowerment*. Retrieved on October 15, 2015, from www.oecd.org/dac/povertyreduction/50157530.pdf.

Ortiz, I. (2007). *Social policy*. Retrieved on October 18, 2015, from http://esa.un.org/tech-coop/documents/PN_SocialPolicyNote.pdf.

Ortiz, I. (2011). *Social policy in national development strategies*. UNICEF Bangkok, June 13–17, 2011. PowerPoint presentation. Retrieved on October 20, 2015, from www.slideserve.com/tarik-hoffman/social-policy-in-national-development-strategies.

Patel, L., & Triegaardt, J. (2008). South Africa: Social security, poverty alleviation and development. In J. Midgley & K.-L. Tang (Eds.), *Social security, the economy and development* (pp. 85–109). New York: Palgrave Macmillan.

Sewpaul, V. (2015, October 16). Hokenstad International Lecture. Council on Social Work Education (CSWE) 61st Annual Program Meeting. Denver, Colorado.

Smyth, I., & Sweetnam, C. (2015). Introduction: Gender and resilience. *Gender & Development, 23*(3), 405–414.

Stiglitz, J. (2009). The global crisis, social protection and jobs. *International Labour Review, 148*(1/2), 1–13.

Tang, K.-L., & Midgley, J. (2008). The origins and features of social security. In J. Midgley & K.-L. Tang (Eds.), *Social security, the economy and development* (pp. 17–50). New York: Palgrave Macmillan.

UNDP. (2014). *Human development report 2014: Sustaining human progress: Reducing vulnerabilities and building resilience*. Retrieved on October 18, 2015, from www.undp.org/content/dam/undp/library/corporate/HDR/2014HDR/HDR-2014-English.pdf.

UNDP & ILO. (2011). *Sharing innovative experiences: Successful social protection floor experiences.* Retrieved on June 12, 2015, from www.ilo.org/gimi/gess/ShowRessource. do?ressource.ressourceId=20840.

Ungar, M. (2013). *The social ecology of resilience: A handbook of theory and practice.* New York: Springer.

UNICEF. (2014). *Social protection strategic framework.* Retrieved on October 18, 2015, from www.unicef.org/socialprotection/framework/.

United Nations. (2012). Social protection: A development priority in the post-2015 UN development agenda. Retrieved on October 18, 2015, from www.un.org/millennium-goals/pdf/Think%20Pieces/16_social_protection.pdf.

United Nations. (2015). *Sendai Framework for Disaster Risk Reduction.* Retrieved on June 12, 2015, from www.preventionweb.net/files/43291_sendaiframeworkfordrren. pdf.

United Nations Population Fund (UNFPA) & HelpAge International (HAI). (2012). *Ageing in the twenty-first century: A celebration and a challenge.* Retrieved on June 15, 2015, from www.unfpa.org/public/home/publications/pid/11584.

Van Ginneken, W. (2008). India: Inclusive development through the extension of social security. In J. Midgley & K.-L. Tang (Eds.), *Social security, the economy and development* (pp. 287–304). New York: Palgrave Macmillan.

Walker, S.P., Wachs, T.D., Grantham-McGregor, S., Black, M.M., Nelson, C.A., Huffman, S.L., Baker-Henningham, H., Chang, S.M., Hamadani, J.D., Lozoff, B., Gardner, J.M., Powell. C.A., Rahman, A., & Richter, L. (2011). Inequality in early childhood: Risk and protective factors for early child development. *Lancet, 378,* 1325–1338.

Wood, G. (2004). Informal security regimes: The strength of relationships. In I. Gough & G. Wood with A. Barrientos, P. Bevan, P. David, & G. Room (Eds.), *Insecurity and welfare regimes in Asia, Africa and Latin America* (pp. 49–87). Cambridge: Cambridge University Press.

Wood, R.G. (2011). Is there a role for cash transfer in climate change adaptation? *IDS Bulletin, 42*(6), 79–85.

World Bank. (2015). *Age dependency ratio.* Retrieved on June 15, 2015, from http://data. worldbank.org/indicator/SP.POP.DPND.OL.

World Health Organization (WHO). (2014). *Are you ready? What you need to know about ageing.* Retrieved on June 15, 2015, from www.who.int/world-health-day/2012/ toolkit/background/en/.

3 "Recovery for all" and reducing inequality

Austerity and poverty elimination

Crystal Kwan and Julie Drolet

Introduction

What began as a crisis within the real estate and financial markets in the United States, spread quickly into a global financial crisis in 2008 (Shrivastava & Statler, 2012). The financial crisis impacted labor markets worldwide, creating massive job loss and unprecedented unemployment levels; it was deemed as the worst financial crisis since the Great Depression (Shrivastava & Statler, 2012).

Governments worldwide were facing failing economies which also brought along with it social and political consequences. The default response for recovery by many governments was to adopt austerity measures (Dymski, 2013). Austerity refers to economic policies that are aimed to reduce a government's budget deficit through a combination of decreasing public expenditures and increasing taxes (Atkinson, 2014). Austerity programs may entail various combinations of decreasing public expenditures and increasing taxes, however the majority of programs adopted in response to the crisis are dominated by a focus on cutting public programs, which are considered essential services and basic rights (e.g., social welfare benefits, unemployment benefits, pensions, education and health care services, amongst others) (Atkinson, 2014).

The promises of austerity are that such fiscal adjustments would restore economic growth and reduce unemployment (Dymski, 2013). The mounting evidence and literature since the crisis has shown that austerity policies have not only failed to achieve its economic promises but have high human and development costs (Dymski, 2013). Yet, austerity programs continue to persist and often presented as the only option (Atkinson, 2014). Strong advocates of austerity measures are powerful international institutions, such as the International Monetary Fund (IMF) and the European Union (EU), who due to the rise of neo-liberal economic globalization have developed strong influences in the social and economic policy development processes of various nation states (Atkinson, 2014). The aim of this chapter is to employ a critical social work lens to:

1 delineate implications of the global crisis and subsequent austerity measures adopted, with a focus on vulnerable populations; and
2 suggest alternative policies to austerity that support a "recovery for all."

The chapter is organized around five sections. First, a description of a Critical Social Work lens is provided. Second, a brief review of the global economic crisis is given, and some key contributing causes identified. Third, we trace the development of the current neo-liberal economic global system, and outline its inability to address long-standing development challenges and its contributions to new forms of insecurities. Fourth, the negative impacts of the global crisis and the austerity measures adopted are examined, which include increasing unemployment and vulnerability, loss of access to health care and health insurance, impacts on public health and education, social unrest and instability, and setbacks to global development goals (e.g., progress made by the Millennium Development Goals). Such impacts are considered in light of vulnerable populations (e.g., women, youth, migrant workers, older adults, indigenous groups, and religious and ethnic minorities). Fifth and finally, the chapter concludes with a discussion about the role of social protection in building a recovery for all – one that is equitable and just.

A Critical Social Work lens

A theoretical lens can be a useful tool for policy analysis and development (Dannefer, 2011). Each theoretical lens offers a specific explanatory focus, and highlights issues and possibilities that may not have been thought of previously (Dannefer, 2011). By imploring a particular lens, policy-makers are encouraged to look at a situation, issue, problem/challenge, process and opportunity in a different way (Dannefer, 2011). Marshall (2009) states: "put simply, to invoke a theoretical perspective is to say, 'look at it this way'" (Marshall, 2009, p. 573). Policy-makers have approached the crisis and recovery largely through various macroeconomic theoretical lenses and as such policy analysis and development are censured by the myopia of such theoretical assumptions and explanatory focuses (Atkinson, 2014). As the crisis continues to impact individuals, families, communities and public institutions, and the macroeconomic interventions adopted fail to provide a "recovery for all," it is important that policy-makers look to alternative disciplines and theoretical lens to support policy analysis and development. Critical Social Work offers potential insights to the implications of the global economic crisis and alternative measures for recovery.

What then does it mean to employ a Critical Social Work lens? First, a Critical Social Work lens encourages one to see how the daily lives of individuals are linked to wider (political, social, cultural and/or economic) structures and systems (Allan, 2003). Second, there is a focus on social injustices (e.g., poverty, social exclusion, inequalities, discrimination, oppression, abuse and exploitation, amongst others) and how these structures and systems may create and/or exacerbate such injustices (Fook, 2002). Third, analyses of power relations (at all levels: micro, mezzo and macro) are integral when employing a Critical Social Work lens (Fook, 2002). Fourth, employing such a lens moves beyond critiquing and pointing at issues/problems, to offering insights into possibilities (which are empowerment and emancipatory based) for transformation (Dominelli, 2010). Fifth and final, employing a Critical Social Work lens entails

> ideology-critique [which] aims to expose how ideologies function to conceal the forms of oppression from which they emanate. Thus a proper analysis of how an ideology leads agents astray should reveal important facts about the non-ideational aspects of society in question, and may even provide some insights into how we might overcome their most undesirable features.
>
> (Shelby, 2003, p. 188)

The global economic crisis

In September of 2008, the bankruptcy and failures of major investment banks (such as Lehman Brothers and Merrill Lynch) was a clear indicator that the United States and its interdependent economies were in a financial crisis (Shrivastava & Statler, 2012). Within 10 months the crisis had spread, derailing financial systems and markets worldwide, whereby an estimated wealth of US$10 trillion (approximately 40% of the global wealth) was lost in financial markets within 10 months (Shrivastava & Statler, 2012). Greed, reckless risk-taking and inadequate banking regulations are argued as the causes of the crisis (Naude, 2010). While these factors may have contributed to the crisis, the "fundamental inequities in the structure and governance of the global economic and financial systems" are probable causes of the crisis as well (Naude, 2010, p. 225). Policy-makers need to look beyond issues, problems and solutions within the system, and take a step back to critically question/challenge the equity and sustainability of the system in itself (McBride & Merolli, 2013). Preceding a discussion of the implications of the crisis, the background context of the current global economic system (its emergence and ideological basis) is provided.

A neo-liberal global economic system

Since the 1970s, a combination of factors have set in train processes of growing integration of the world's economies and the intensified flow of goods, services, people and ideas across national boundaries (Kabeer, 2010). These factors include the rising costs of labor in advanced industrialized countries together with rapid advances in information technology and transportation systems that have allowed production processes to be broken down and their labor-intensive stages relocated to different regions of the world (Kabeer, 2010). Politics have also played a major role in driving the pace of globalization.

The ascendance of neo-liberal ideologies in some of the world's most powerful countries spearheaded the liberalization of their economies and the downsizing of welfare regimes (Kabeer, 2010). These factors have given rise to a global economic system guided by the neo-liberal paradigm, which is "premised on the goal of market-led economic growth" that is largely left unregulated (McBride &

Merolli, 2013, p. 302). In order to achieve this goal, economic policies that promote:

1   privatization;
2   capital mobility;
3   free trade;
4   deregulation and the reduced role of the state;
5   balanced budgets and reduced public expenditures;
6   "acceptance of market-driven inequality"; and
7   "flexibilization of labour markets"

are most favourable (McBride & Merolli, 2013, p. 302). With the aim of propelling economic growth through market forces alone and prioritizing economic policies identified above, this new economic paradigm has failed to address (and even exacerbated) long-standing forms of development challenges. The persistence of chronic poverty and inequality are examples.

Long-standing development challenges

Chronic poverty. While the past decades have witnessed a decline in overall global poverty rates, to date the situation of the chronically poor has not improved (Chronic Poverty Research Centre, 2014). Chronic poverty describes people who live in extreme poverty (living on US$1.25/day) "for many years, or for their entire lives, and who often pass their poverty down to their children" (Chronic Poverty Research Centre, 2014, p. 3). In its 2008–2009 report, the Chronic Poverty Research Centre found that while the last five years witnessed unprecedented wealth creation and growth, chronic poverty had increased (Chronic Poverty Research Centre, 2008). The chronically poor are often "effectively locked out of national growth process and globalization" benefits because of the poverty traps they experience, including: social discrimination/exclusion, "poor working opportunities," "spatial disadvantage" (e.g., living away from main national markets and/or natural resource bases), "limited citizenship" and "insecurity" (e.g., having few assets and/or entitlements) (Chronic Poverty Research Centre, 2008, p. 4). The chronically poor are not only economically marginalized, but are also the most socially and politically excluded within a society (Addison, 2009). Addressing chronic poverty requires more than a blind reliance on economic growth, led by free market principles and mechanisms, to trickle down to benefit the situation of the poor (Addison, 2009). "Social protection and public services for the hard to reach" are key policy priorities to address this long-standing development challenge (Chronic Poverty Research Centre, 2008, p. 2).

Inequality. A premise of the neo-liberal ideology is that a globalized economic system based on free-market principles and mechanisms has a positive effect on inequalities (Schuerkens, 2010). The rise in inequality since the 1980s (the beginning of the era of the neo-liberal economic system) challenges such a premise (Schuerkens, 2010). In particular some global trends regarding inequality highlight a different relationship between neo-liberal economic globalization and inequality. First, while various countries may have experienced overall economic growth, within-country inequality (or domestic inequality) has increased significantly in almost all countries (Schuerkens, 2010). Second, the gap between poor and rich countries has widened since economic globalization. Third and final, the focus on increasing capital mobility has fueled global competition for foreign investments whereby governments are encouraged to prioritize global competitiveness and in doing so may refrain from redistributive interventions to address inequality (ILO, 2005). The persistence of the situation of the chronically poor and rising inequalities (both within-country and between countries) questions whether globalization based on the neo-liberal model represents "a globalization for all people" (ILO, 2005, p. 54).

New forms of insecurities

Chronic poverty and inequality are long-standing forms of development changes, which precede the neo-liberal economic global system. However, the system has contributed to new forms of insecurities for individuals, families, communities and the public sector/institutions. The United Nations Development Programme (UNDP), in its 1999 report, focused on globalization and human development, and stated:

> The markets in today's global system are creating wonderful opportunities, but distributing them unevenly – and the volatility of markets is creating new vulnerabilities. What's worse, the success of global markets has marginalized many non-market activities for human development, making human well being even more vulnerable.
>
> (UNDP, 1999, p. 4)

Economic security, defined as having "an assured basic income – usually from productive and renumerative work or in the last resort from some publicly financed safety net," is a critical component to human well-being and security (UNDP, 1999, p. 25). Within the neo-liberal economic global system, employment patterns and trends have shifted and achieving economic security has become much harder for many people around the globe (Shari, 2003). For instance, full-time and longer (or lifetime) employment opportunities are increasingly replaced with part-time, contract and/or temporary employment (Shari, 2003). The latter types of employment opportunities also tend to involve "lower wages, less representation and fewer social entitlements" (Shari, 2003, p. 254).

Neo-liberal economic globalization has also given rise to powerful multinational corporations (who are bound by the bottom-line of profit in decision-making), global competitiveness and foreign direct investment (FDI) as the main engines of economic growth, which have serious social and economic implications for the laborer. For instance, economic policies geared toward increasing labor flexibility promote "social dumping, that is, moving or threatening to move operations to locations with lower wages and poorer working conditions" (Shari, 2003, p. 252). In order to stay competitive and attract FDI, governments are encouraged to have lax labor protection rights (Shari, 2003). Within such an environment, laborers become more vulnerable to insecure, unsafe and irregular employment (Shari, 2003).

The new forms of economic insecurities brought about by the neo-liberal system also have a gendered dimension leaving women, in particular women living in developing countries, more vulnerable and at risk. For instance, many governments in developing countries have been strongly encouraged, by the International Monetary Fund (IMF) and the World Bank, to adopt an export-led economic growth strategy (ILO, 2012). As part of this strategy, export-processing zones (EPZs) are promoted and established. EPZs are "industrial zones with special incentives set up to attract foreign investors, in which imported materials undergo some degree of processing before being exported again" (ILO, 1998). Due to the liberal regulatory and anti-trade union environments of EPZs, laborers working within such zones face even greater insecurities. The ILO states there is an "urgent need for decent work (defined as work that is productive and provides a fair income, security and social protection for individuals and their families) in EPZs" (ILO, 2012, p. 3). There are an estimated 3,500 EPZs globally across 130 countries, which employ approximately 66 million people. The large majority (90%) of those employed in EPZs are women, and in some cases close to 100% of EPZ workers are women. While the ILO notes some progress has been made in regards to decent work within such zones, the problems women face remain relatively unchanged whereby they continue to experience "workplace discrimination, sexual harassment, and concerns related to maternity leave and childcare" (ILO, 2012, p. 2).

Neo-liberal globalization has created an global economy that continues to exclude various social groups (e.g., the chronically poor) and create new forms of insecurities that have left many individuals, families, communities and the public sector vulnerable and unable to cope with and recover from the global financial crisis. In the next section, the human and development costs associated with the crisis and the subsequent austerity measures are considered.

Impacts of the global crisis

Rising unemployment and vulnerability

The *2011 Report on the World Social Situation* reviews the adverse social consequences of the economic crisis and resulting economic slowdown that reduced social spending in most developing countries and precipitated a turn to fiscal austerity undermining social spending in developed countries. A rapid rise in unemployment and vulnerability, particularly in countries without comprehensive social protection, is estimated to have affected tens of millions more people who fell into, or were trapped in, extreme poverty due to the global crisis.

Vulnerable employment is associated with workers who are less likely to have formal work arrangements and lack decent employment such as social security, health benefits and effective collective bargaining mechanisms. "In 2009, half of the world's workers of nearly 1.53 billion people were in vulnerable employment" (UN, 2011, p. 33).

Increased unemployment has been the dominant social impact of the crisis in developed economies, but the employment situation in developing countries has been less obvious (UN, 2011). While the informal economy and peasant agricultural sector have absorbed much of the impact of formal sector job losses, large numbers of workers are now subject to more vulnerable employment in developing countries (UN, 2011). The quality of employment deteriorated in both developed and developing countries, as workers were forced to accept reduced working hours and lower wages and benefits (UN, 2011, p. 27). Increased job insecurity has resulted in sustained and devastating impacts on individuals, families, households and their communities. Social workers are concerned with the social impacts of the crisis and the lived human experience. For example, social workers bear witness to the financial and economic hardships that result in people losing their homes to foreclosures and increased poverty, debt and bankruptcy. It is widely acknowledged that work is related to several dimensions of individual well-being, and worsening job and economic insecurity have been associated with increased poor health, psychological hardship and family dissolution (UN, 2011, p. 27). This remains a growing concern given that social protection benefits are often tied to labor market participation in a number of countries.

Loss of access to health care and health insurance. Where access to health care and health insurance is linked to employment, workers who become unemployed not only lose their income, but also lose access to health services, and social services and benefits such as pensions, maternity and family benefits (ILO, 2010). Many governments implemented discretionary health protection measures to help cover the cost of health insurance premiums of low-income workers (such as the United States), and investments on health infrastructure and the extension of health protection coverage (seen in Argentina, Indonesia and the Russian Federation). China extended universal health coverage with the introduction of the New Rural Cooperative Medical Schemes that provides coverage for 91.5% of the rural population by the end of 2008 (ILO, 2010).

Gendered dimensions. Both men and women have experienced adverse impacts due to the crisis, and the effects have also varied across and within regions and countries (UN, 2011). It is important to consider the design and implementation of social protection measures and who can access them, particularly for women. Social insurance programs that are closely tied to formal employment make some assumptions that full-time, formal, life-long employment is the norm, and such programs implicitly discriminate against women (Razavi, Arza, Braunstein, Cook, & Goulding, 2012).

Women tend to be over-represented in vulnerable and informal employment in most countries with access to fewer good-quality jobs within the formal economy than men (UN, 2011). "Women earn less than men, with fewer social security benefits, and are engaged in more precarious work such as domestic service and other care work" (UN, 2011, p. 39). The crisis highlighted a critical gap in social protection, namely, support and protection for informal sector workers who largely comprise poor and vulnerable women (Hossain, Fillaili, Lubaale, Mulumbi, Rashid, & Tadro, 2010). Women workers in developing countries have experienced devastating impacts on their livelihoods, their rights, and their families as a result of the impact of the crisis on their spheres of employment in export manufacturing, garments, electronics and services (Emmett, 2009). There is concern that government responses to the crisis in many countries are inadequate or target overwhelmingly at male employment, as governments provide stimulus packages in the construction and infrastructure sectors, even where women are bearing the disproportionate impact of job losses (Emmett, 2009). Alternatives are possible, and social insurance programs can be made more inclusive of women by making affiliation mandatory and by partially subsidizing their contributions (Razavi et al., 2012).

The impacts of the crisis on income and employment affect household and family dynamics. Gender differences have grown in terms of unpaid work and time use, as women take on even larger shares of unpaid work and caregiving responsibilities in developing countries (UN, 2011). Children face more severe risks than adults during economic crises (Patel, 2009). The effect of the crisis on children has been significant, as parents adjust consumption patterns and reduce health and education expenditures (UN, 2011). During the 1997–1998 Asian financial crisis there was a drop in school enrolment rates while child labor rose among 10–14-year-olds in the Philippines, and there was an increase in the labour exploitation of girls in Indonesia and Thailand (UN, 2011).

Youth unemployment. Youth unemployment has reached alarming levels in developed and developing countries; at the end of 2009, "there were an estimated 79 million unemployed young people 15 to 24 years of age, and the rate of youth unemployment stood at 13.0 per cent globally" (UN, 2011, p. 4). Before the crisis youth already faced higher unemployment rates above those of their older counterparts and a higher risk of low pay. Youth unemployment can have long-term effects on the social trajectory of youth, their families and their communities (IMF & ILO, 2010).

Migrant workers, indigenous groups, older workers, ethnic and religious minorities. As with women and youth, older workers, indigenous peoples, migrant workers and ethnic and religious minorities also face bias in the labor market. Specifically, overseas migrant workers, especially newly arrived migrants, are among the most seriously disadvantaged; in many cases they have invested heavily in being recruited and traveling to work in a foreign country, and are more likely to accept any terms just to retain their jobs (UN, 2011). Migrant workers can be particularly vulnerable because they do not always enjoy the same rights and protection as nationals in the destination country (ILO, 2010). Often they are ineligible for social protection, and when they lose their jobs and work permits, they become illegal or undocumented and forced to turn to income opportunities in the informal economy (UN, 2011). For indigenous groups, unemployment has tended to be higher than the average for the general population, and this situation has worsened since the crisis. Older workers who lose their jobs tend to encounter greater difficulty in finding new work than younger workers, and older persons have seen their incomes shrink as the value of their pension funds has fallen (UN, 2011). Older persons who are not covered by social security or other retirement income schemes are more vulnerable due to the crisis.

Impacts on public health and education

While it is not possible to understand the full social impacts of economic crises on public health and education in the short term, it is possible to draw lessons from past financial and economic crises such as the Great Depression of the 1930s and the 1997/1998 Asian financial crisis. The key lessons from the Asian financial crisis were:

1   to expand established safety net programs rather than create new ones;
2   protect pro-poor spending (health, education and infrastructure);
3   learn from other countries' experiences about how to target social protection; and
4   adopt macroeconomic policies to maintain price stability and employment levels (McCulloch, 2008).

The lack of economic security is often stressful, with the breakdown of social and family structures and the adoption of harmful habits to health (UN, 2011, p. 5). Poverty and unemployment have been linked to crime, gender-based violence, substance abuse and mental illness, including depression and suicide (UN, 2011). Developing policy responses must take into consideration that within national economies some people will have more exposure than others (Institute for Development Studies, 2008).

Impacts compounded by rising food prices

The effects of the crisis were compounded by an increase in food prices in 2007 and 2008 that adversely affected efforts to reduce poverty and hunger. It is estimated that the number of people living in hunger in the world rose to over a billion in 2009, the highest on record (UN, 2011). Food riots and protests threatened governments and social stability in Africa, Asia, the Middle East and Latin American and the Caribbean, and massive public protests erupted in response to higher food prices in diverse countries (Baker, 2008). Increased food prices significantly raised the number of people suffering from hunger and living in poverty in urban and rural areas in both developed and developing countries (UN, 2011). "The most vulnerable bear the brunt of the adverse impacts of high food prices, through malnutrition. Poor households tend to spend a larger share of their income on food and are especially vulnerable to price increases" (World Bank, 2012, p. 63). In developed countries, people who are out of work, have exhausted their savings, or are nearing the end of their unemployment benefits increasingly find themselves having to rely on local food banks and other not-for-profit charitable organizations (UN, 2011). At least 80 countries tried to curb rising food prices and minimize the impact of the food price crisis on the poor by implementing food subsidies, price controls, export restrictions and outright bans on foreign exports in the short term (Lustig, 2009). Additional measures include strengthening food safety nets such as cash transfer programs, food-for-work schemes, school feeding programs and food rationing. A person's capacity to cope varies widely depending on food prices, the state of the local economy, and access to formal and informal sources of support (Hossain et al., 2010).

Development costs

The global crisis and interventions adopted lead to long-term development implications including the regression of the progress made in the Millennium Development Goals (MDGs; which also compromises the success of the newly proposed Sustainable Development Goals) and sustaining (and further solidifying) poverty traps (Otker-Robe & Podpiera, 2013). The first target of the MDGs is halving poverty by 2015, yet sub-Saharan Africa, West Asia and part of Eastern Europe and Central Asia are not expected to attain the poverty target of the Goals, as many countries in these regions have experienced increases in poverty (UN, 2011).

Goal 4 (reduce child mortality), Goal 5 (improve maternal health) and Goal 6 (combat HIV/AIDS, malaria and other diseases) are health-related MDG targets linked to key dimensions of poverty, as people living in poverty are less likely to have access to adequate health care. "While some countries have made impressive gains in achieving health-related targets, others are falling behind. Often the countries making the least progress are those affected by a high level of HIV/AIDS, economic hardship or conflict" (World Health Organization, 2015, para. 3). Several of the MDGs are unlikely to be met, either globally, or by many countries at the national level.

The crisis is slowing progress in human and social development due to the combination of falling incomes owing to job losses and increased vulnerable employment, higher proportions of household expenditure spent on basic needs, worsening nutritional outcomes and more limited coping mechanisms (UN, 2011, p. 46). Economic recovery will not be achieved until the employment situation improves in a sustainable manner in both the formal and informal economies (UN, 2011). Kabeer (2008) argues that:

> there is no clear-but boundaries between formal and informal work, that different activities are located somewhere on a continuum that stretches from highly formalized conditions and relations of work to activities that are not covered by any labour legislation, workers benefits or social protection; and

that such activities may be located within enterprises that are classified as formal.

(p. 52)

The economic crisis will deal significant blows to the progress towards several MDGs in many African countries; these impacts can be long term in many countries even though the economic shock itself may reverse over a short duration, the impact on human development continues to be felt longer.

(Conceição, Mukherjee, & Nayyar, 2011, p. 456)

Individuals, families, communities and societies often adopt coping strategies, such as making changes in expenditure patterns, which negatively influence education, health and nutrition outcomes leading to life-long deficits for children and perpetuating the inter-generational transmission of poverty (UN, 2011). The impact of the crisis was further influenced by "the capacity of Governments to cope with and counteract its consequences, which depended in part on the efficiency and strength of their counter-cyclical macroeconomic policy mechanisms, social protections systems, regulatory frameworks governance structures and political stability" (UN, 2011, p. 2).

Stimulus measures

By mid-2009, many developed countries and some developing countries announced a range of stimulus measures involving monetary, financial, fiscal, and labour market policies of about $2.6 trillion in total (UN, 2009). "On average, in 2008, 48 countries spent about 4.3 percent of their GDP on fiscal stimulus measures" (UN, 2011, p. 85). It is estimated that 25% of the stimulus spending was disbursed on social protection measures in 35 countries of about $654 billion or almost 1% of global GDP in 2008 (Zhang, Thelen, & Rao, 2010). The economies that devoted the largest proportion of their fiscal stimulus package to social protection were South Africa (56%), Singapore (52%), Taiwan Province of China (47%), Finland (43%), United States (39%), France (16%) and Germany (25%) (Zhang et al., 2010). "In absolute terms the two top spenders on social protection were the United States ($310 billion) and China ($135 billion)" (UN, 2011, p. 86). Jia and Liu (2010) found that China's public expenditure package (worth four trillion yuan) provided for major infrastructure spending and that 25% of the package was allocated to post-earthquake reconstruction (cited in UN, 2011). Major stimulus packages were adopted by many governments to halt the downslide and prevent a prolonged recession, with spending on infrastructure, social protection and other specific support measures in direct or indirect health funding, public housing and education. In the Middle East and North Africa, the most popular responses were to subsidize basic food prices, protect wages in some sectors, and improve access to education and health services (UN, 2011). With some early signs of recovery the solidarity of G20 country leaders and their commitment to sustaining stimulus measures began to weaken from mid-2010, with disagreements emerging over mounting public indebtedness at their Summit in Toronto in June 2010. The weakened G20 commitment to international cooperation affects social development in developed and developing countries.

Impacts of austerity measures

Austerity measures in response to high government debt in some advanced economies are also making the recovery more uncertain and fragile (UN, 2011). This is evident in Greece and Spain where austerity threatens public sector employment and social expenditure. The public has reacted strongly with massive, and sometimes violent, protests since February 2010 (UN, 2011). "Protests, rallies and demonstrations have broken out across a number of regions in response to the adverse impacts of the crisis, with documented incidents of civil unrest in at least 44 countries" (UN, 2011, p. 57). Increased pressure for fiscal consolidation and new pressures in response to such debt have severely limited fiscal and policy space in developed economies, and many developing countries are under pressure to cut public expenditure, undertake austerity measures, reduce the scope of government action and further liberalize labor markets (UN, 2011). Policy-makers in Europe and the United States are mainly fixated on reducing fiscal deficits and public debt, and unfortunately, policy responses are highly inadequate with the shift to fiscal austerity (Paddison & Vos, 2012).

The austerity programs of donor countries are likely to result in cuts in their aid budgets at a time when low-income countries have the greatest need for such aid support (UN, 2011). Additional overseas development aid is needed to finance the expansion of social services and programs to meet the MDG targets, and now Sustainable Development Goals (SDGs). International financial institutions are rethinking their approach and acknowledge the importance of stimulus spending, including maintaining and increasing social spending to address the crisis.

It is imperative that governments take into account the social implications of their economic policies. It has been shown that economic policies considered in isolation from their social outcomes can have negative consequences for poverty, employment, nutrition, health and education, which adversely affect long-term sustainable development (UN, 2011). Governments in developed countries should seriously evaluate the social impacts of their austerity measures that reduce social spending and contribute to joblessness (UN, 2011). The crisis offers an opportunity for achieving social progress by making universal social protection a reality, revisiting the social aspects of globalization and ensure a more inclusive and sustained growth in keeping with sustainable development's commitment to achieving economic development, social progress and environmental sustainability (UN, 2011).

Alternative policies that support a recovery for all: the role of social protection

There is growing recognition of the importance of social safety nets in developing countries, and they are becoming more common in the response of governments to recent crises. Several countries expanded existing programs or implemented new ones: The Republic of Yemen extended its cash-for-work and cash transfer programs; the Philippines launched a conditional cash transfer program that was scaled up in response to the crisis; Brazil expanded the Bolsa Família program to include an additional 12 million families and increased the benefit by 10% to compensate for increased food prices (World Bank and IMF, 2010, cited in UN, 2011, p. 54). Conditional cash transfers in Mexico through the Oportunidades [opportunities] program largely prevented a greater increase in poverty, which might have occurred if the full impact of the crisis had been felt in that country (World Bank, 2010). China launched a major reform in December 2009 to introduce a basic pension scheme for 700 million rural residents (ILO, 2010). Social transfers in the form of pensions, family benefits and other cash transfers can contribute to protection household consumption against shocks or crises, thus preventing asset depletion or the adoption of short-term strategies with long-term adverse consequences, such as taking children out of school (ILO, 2010).

The devastating impact of the crisis on so many people underscores the dynamic and multidimensional nature of poverty and the critical importance of social protection for reducing vulnerability (UN, 2011, p. 9). There is an urgent need to halt, if not reverse, the ongoing crisis. Universal social protection systems and active employment generation programs must become permanent measures, not temporary components of national crisis response measures (UN, 2011). Increasing expenditures to expand social protection and improve access to education and health services will help ensure more inclusive development with stronger domestic demand and a more solid foundation for future growth (UN, 2011). The severe shortcomings of the macroeconomic policy agenda to generate employment and eradicate poverty led to renewed interest in social policies and social protection programs (Razavi et al., 2012). Countries that have social protection systems can better mitigate the negative impacts of shocks and prevent people from falling deeper into poverty, and can also help regenerate economic activities and livelihoods (UN, 2011). This means investing in well-functioning and accessible public health, education and care services; public provision of a range of complementary goods and services such as clean water, subsidized food items, sanitation, electricity, transport and housing; and broad-based and redistributive social insurance programs for unemployment, old age and maternity (Razavi et al., 2012).

The *World Social Protection Report 2014/2015* states that:

> still grappling with the economic repercussions of the global financial crisis, the world is faced with a deep social crisis which is also a crisis of social

justice. Social protection measures are essential elements of a policy response that can address those challenges by supporting the realization of the universal human right to social security, but are both a social and an economic necessity.

(ILO, 2015, p. vi)

Universal access to social protection and social services is necessary to break the cycle of poverty and reduce inequality and social exclusion. "The crisis offers an opportunity to rethink the role of social policy and social investment in transforming policy responses to the crisis into opportunities to strengthen social development and to achieve more sustained, inclusive and equitable development" (UN, 2011, p. 10). The crisis serves as a reminder that it is essential for people to be healthy, educated, adequately housed and well fed to contribute to society. Approaches to poverty reduction should be "developmental and holistic, integrating economic and social policies to achieve people-centred development outcomes" (UN, 2011, p. 11).

Social protection includes a range of policy interventions that protect the vulnerable against livelihood risks such as social assistance, social insurance and labor market regulation, typically by the state given the scale of the crisis (Davies & McGregor, 2009). Historically, times of economic crisis also result in social and political unrest, which can drive the development of social protection schemes like the New Deal in the post-Depression United States, or the shrinkage of state protection and a spiral of long-term decline (see the 1984 Ethiopian famine and political failure to address chronic food insecurity) (Davies & McGregor, 2009). Social protection presents an effective and progressive way of responding to crises by addressing short- and long-term development. The chapters in this book highlight international efforts in extending social protection in many developing countries by reducing poverty and vulnerability, redressing inequality and boosting inclusive growth. The international community has identified the critical role of social protection as a priority in the post-2015 development agenda. Finally, social workers are engaged in actions to ensure that people will not face the risk of poverty and insecurity.

References

Addison, T. (2009). Chronic poverty in the global economy. *European Journal of Development Research, 21*, 174–178.

Allan, J. (2003). Practising critical social work. In J. Allan, B. Pease, & L. Briskman (Eds.), *Critical social work: An introduction to theories and practices* (pp. 52–72). Crows Nest: Allen & Unwin.

Atkinson, T. (2014). *Public economics in an age of austerity.* New York: Routledge.

Baker, J. (2008). Impacts of financial, food, and fuel crisis on the urban poor. *Directions in urban development.* Washington, DC: Urban Development Unit, World Bank.

Chronic Poverty Research Centre. (2008). *The chronic poverty report 2008–09: Escaping poverty traps.* Retrieved from www.chronicpoverty.org/publications/details/the-chronic-poverty-report-2008-09.

Chronic Poverty Research Centre. (2014). *The chronic poverty report 2014–15: The road to zero extreme poverty.* Retrieved from http://static1.squarespace.com/static/539712a6e 4b06a6c9b892bc1/t/539b1fe3e4b0d7588ce6ead8/1402675171712/Chronic+Poverty+ report+-+full+report.pdf.

Conceição, P., Mukherjee, S., & Nayyar, S. (2011). Impacts of the economic crisis on human development and the MDGs in Africa. *Africa Development Review, Special Issue: Rethinking African Economic Policy in Light of the Global Economic and Financial Crisis, 23,* 439–460.

Dannefer, D. (2011). Age, the life course, and the sociological imagination: Prospects for theory. In R.H. Binstock, L.K. George, J. Hendricks, & J.H. Schulz (Eds.), *Handbook of aging and the social sciences* (7th ed.) (pp. 3–16). London: Academic Press.

Davies, M., & McGregor, J.A. (2009). *Social protection: Responding to a global crisis.* Institute of Development Studies. Retrieved from www.ids.ac.uk/files/dmfile/Social-ProtectionDaviesandMcGregor.pdf.

Dominelli, L. (2010). *Social work in a globalizing world.* Cambridge: Policy Press.

Dymski, G. (2013). The logic and impossibility of austerity. *Social Research: An International Quarterly, 80*(3), 665–696.

Emmett, B. (2009). *Paying the price for the economic crisis.* Oxfam International Discussion Paper. Retrieved from www.oxfam.org/sites/www.oxfam.org/files/paying-the-price-for-global-economic-crisis.pdf.

Fook, J. (2002). *Social work: Critical theory and practice.* London: Sage Publications.

Hossain, N., Fillaili, R., Lubaale, G., Mulumbi, M., Rashid, M., & Tadros, M. (2010, May). *The social impacts of crisis: Findings from community-level research in five developing countries.* Retrieved from www.ids.ac.uk/files/dmfile/SocialImpactofCrisisreport5.pdf.

Institute for Development Studies. (2008, November 12). *Voices from the South: The impact of the financial crisis on developing countries.* Retrieved from www.ids.ac.uk/ files/Voices_from_the_South_Report.pdf.

International Labour Organization (ILO). (1998). *Labor and social issues relating to export processing zones.* Retrieved from www.ilo.org/wcmsp5/groups/public/--ed_ dialogue/--actrav/documents/publication/wcms_114918.pdf.

International Labour Organization (ILO). (2005). *Globalization and perceptions of social inequality.* Retrieved from www.oit.org/wcmsp5/groups/public/--dgreports/--integration/ documents/publication/wcms_079144.pdf.

International Labour Organization (ILO). (2010). *Employment and social protection policies from crisis to recovery and beyond: Review of experience.* Retrieved from www. ilo.org/public/libdoc/jobcrisis/download/g20_report_employment_and_social_protection_ policies.pdf.

International Labour Organization (ILO). (2012). *Freedom of association for women workers in EPZs.* Retrieved from www.ilo.org/wcmsp5/groups/public/--dgreports/-- gender/documents/publication/wcms_186807.pdf.

International Labour Organization (ILO). (2015). *World social protection report.* Retrieved from www.ilo.org/wcmsp5/groups/public/--dgreports/--dcomm/documents/ publication/wcms_245201.pdf.

International Monetary Fund & International Labour Organization. (2010). *The challenges of growth, employment and social cohesion.* Paper prepared for the Joint IMF-ILO Conference on The Challenges of Growth, Employment and Social Coehsion, Oslo, September 13.

Kabeer, N. (2008). *Mainstreaming gender in social protection for the informal economy.* London: Commonwealth Secretariat.

Kabeer, N. (2010). *Gender and social protection strategies in the informal economy*. New Delhi: Routledge.

Lustig, N. (2009, March 19). *Coping with rising food prices: Policy dilemmas in the developing world*. CGD Working Paper No. 164. Washington, DC: Center for Global Development.

McBride, S., & Merolli, J. (2013). Alternatives to austerity? Post-crisis policy advice from global institutions. *Global Social Policy, 13*, 299–320.

McCulloch, N. (2008). Analysis one: Policy options. In Institute for Development Studies. *Voices from the South: The impact of the financial crisis on developing countries* (pp. 4–8). Retrieved from www.afdb.org/fileadmin/uploads/afdb/Documents/ MCFC_19_EN_Voices%20from%20the%20South%20-%20The%20Impact%20 of%20the%20Financial%20Crisis%20on%20Develoing%20Countries.pdf.

Marshall, V.W. (2009). Theory informing public policy: The Life Course Perspective as a policy tool. In V.L. Bengtson, D. Gans, N.M. Putney, & M. Silverstein (Eds.), *Handbook of theories of aging* (pp. 573–593). New York: Springer Publishing Company, LLC.

Naude, W. (2010). The global economic crisis and developing countries: Effects, responses, and options for sustainable recovery. *Poverty & Public Policy, 2*(2), 211–235.

Otker-Robe, I., & Podpiera, A. (2013). The social impact of financial crises: Evidence from the Global Financial Crisis. Retrieved from www-wds.worldbank.org/external/ default/WDSContentServer/IW3P/IB/2013/11/14/000158349_20131114113429/ Rendered/PDF/WPS6703.pdf.

Paddison, O., & Vos, R. (2012). *Can a protracted slowdown be avoided?* (Policy Brief No. 36). United Nations Department of Economic and Social Affairs. Retrieved from www.un.org/en/development/desa/policy/publications/policy_briefs/policybrief36.pdf.

Patel, M. (2009). Economic crisis and children: An overview for East Asia and the pacific. *Global Social Policy, 9*, 33–54.

Razavi, S., Arza, C., Braunstein, E., Cook, S., & Goulding, K. (2012). *Gendered impacts of globalization employment and social protection* (No. 16). Gender and Development Programme, United Nations Research Institute for Social Development. United Nations Research Institute for Social Development. Retrieved from www.unrisd. org/80256B3C005BCCF9/httpNetITFra.mePDF?ReadForm&parentunid=6E16D1DC3 3F5D82BC12579D000478859&parentdoctype=paper&netitpath=80256B3C005BCC F9/(httpAuxPages)/6E16D1DC33F5D82BC12579D000478859/$file/Dfid paper.pdf.

Schuerkens, U. (2010). Introduction. In U. Schuerkens (Ed.), *Globalization and transformations of social inequality* (pp. 3–30). New York: Routledge.

Shari, I. (2003). Globalization and economic insecurity: A need for a new social policy in Malaysia. *Asian Journal of Social Science, 31*(2), 251–270.

Shelby, T. (2003). Ideology, racism and critical social theory. *The Philosophical Forum, 34*(2), 153–188.

Shrivastava, P., & Statler, M. (2012). Introduction. In P. Shrivastava & M. Statler (Eds.), *Learning from the global financial crisis: Creatively, reliably, and sustainably* (pp. 1–16). Chicago: Stanford University Press.

United Nations. (2009, December). *World economic situation and prospects 2009: update as of mid-2009*. New York: Department of Economic and Social Affairs of the United Nations Secretariat.

United Nations. (2011, June). *The global social crisis: Report on the World Social Situation 2011*. New York: United Nations. Retrieved from www.un.org/esa/socdev/rwss/ docs/2011/rwss2011.pdf.

United Nations Development Programme (UNDP). (1999). *Human development report 1999*. Retrieved from http://hdr.undp.org/sites/default/files/reports/260/hdr_1999_en_nostats.pdf.

World Bank. (2010). *Did Latin America learn to shield its poor from economic shocks? Poverty reduction and economic management team, Latin America and Caribbean region*. Retrieved from www-wds.worldbank.org/external/default/WDSContentServer/WDSP/IB/2011/04/21/000333037_20110421003023/Rendered/PDF/612730WPOWPOBOX351vertyReport01Report01PUBLIC1.pdf.

World Bank. (2012). *Global monitoring report 2012: Food prices, nutrition, and the Millennium Development Goals*. Retrieved from http://siteresources.worldbank.org/INTPROSPECTS/Resources/334934-1327948020811/8401693-1327957211156/8402494-1334239337250/Full_Report.pdf.

World Health Organization. (2015). *Millennium development goals: progress towards the health-related millennium development goals* (Fact sheet No 290). Retrieved from www.who.int/mediacentre/factsheets/fs290/en/.

Zhang, Y., Thelen, N., & Rao, A. (2010, March). *Social protection in fiscal stimulus packages: Some evidence*. UNDP/ODS Working Paper. New York: United Nations Development Programme Office of Development Studies.

4 Social protection

A human right to promote social justice and equity

Sekar Srinivasan, Malakkaran Johny Jino and Edakkat Subhakaran Sriji

Introduction

All countries have a duty to guarantee the right to social security and social protection as enshrined in international treaties, national legislations and respective constitutional provisions. Social protection is a central tenet of social contracts that aim to protect the vulnerable in society. In Article 9 of the International Covenant on Economic, Social and Cultural Rights, the Committee on Economic, Social and Cultural Rights (CESCR) defined the right to social security in its General Comment No. 19 as:

> encompassing the right to access and maintain benefits, whether in cash or in kind, without discrimination in order to secure protection, inter alia, from (a) lack of work-related income caused by sickness, disability, maternity, employment injury, unemployment, old age, or death of a family member; (b) unaffordable access to health care; (c) insufficient family support, particularly for children and adult dependents.
>
> (p. 2)

Further, the right to social security includes the right not to be subject to arbitrary and unreasonable restrictions of existing social security coverage, whether obtained publicly or privately, as well as the right to equal enjoyment of adequate protection from social risks and contingencies. The term social security is often used in the same way as social protection in the literature and international treaties, and although the two terms are used interchangeably, social security is primarily used in the field of social policy, while social protection is favored in social development circles. While social security is associated with government social insurance and social assistance schemes, social protection has a broader scope and includes a variety of programs operated by NGOs and grassroots organizations (Midgley, 2014).

While there are diverse perspectives on social protection, it is a term used to understand various forms of public assistance, social insurance, developmental strategies and public policies. The importance of social protection initiatives is evident in developed and developing countries (Gentilini & Omamo, 2011).

Issues of economic inequality and social justice have come to dominate global debates, together with rising levels of social unrest and worldwide discontent. Further, unstable economic conditions and increased globalization have intensified the necessity of social protection. Social protection has attracted global attention and global relevance given the importance of addressing complexities associated with preventing, reducing and eliminating economic and social vulnerabilities related to poverty and deprivation (Srivastava, 2013). Despite recent developments and avenues for growth, there continues to be many people in the world still vulnerable to poverty and deprivations. Social protection contributes to the assurance of basic needs for human survival and contributes to one's quality of life through structural change, upward stability, and advancing social justice and economic redistribution (Garcia & Gruat, 2003). Our world continues to experience increasing and recurrent natural disasters, armed conflicts, financial crises, and political and economic transitions that destabilize many countries and their systems of social protection where they exist. With the continued threat to human life and human development there is an urgent need to consider social protection and welfare measures to mitigate and reduce people's vulnerability to poverty and deprivations. A human rights perspective on social protection establishes the hope that human rights enshrined in the Universal Declaration of Human Rights, international conventions and national constitutions can uphold rights to social protection. The United Nations (UN) Social Protection Floor initiative aims to ensure that social security will contribute to the broader goal of human development (Srivastava, 2013). The increasing interest in social protection programs across the globe demonstrates the importance of considering the social dimensions of major economic crises or risks from a human rights perspective. This universal acceptance of social protection has created avenues to draw insights from different perspectives and to understand how these have been incorporated in countries' growth and sustainable development plans. This chapter will consider social protection initiatives through a right-based approach. A rights-based approach entrusts people to claim and demand their rights to be enacted rather than bestowed by others. This chapter considers the role of human rights, social justice and equity approaches in social protection.

Characteristics of social protection

Social protection initiatives are, in general, directed or designed broadly based on three perspectives: promotional, preventive and protective measures (World Bank, 2011). Promotional measures are aimed to improve incomes, both in terms of short- to medium-term through livelihood intervention programs, and in the long-term through human capital approaches such as subsidy assistance, nutritional or food security, or other specific programs to address the needs of the poor (World Bank, 2011). Preventive measures are aimed to prevent or avoid vulnerability and deprivations through social security or social insurance programs (World Bank, 2011). Preventative measures work to prevent people from unexpected risks and shocks in their lives and can act as a protective layer to ensure minimum basic needs during times of crisis and discontent. Protective measures are aimed at providing relief to the deprived in order to improve their conditions in the aftermath of crisis (World Bank, 2011). This can be achieved through targeted relief programs, economic activities for the rural poor, nutritional supplement programs for the malnourished children, and so on (World Bank, 2011).

Social protection systems

There is evidence of social protection in all countries. Interestingly, middle-income and low-income countries are proactive in social protection implementation and institutionalization in their respective countries (Gentilini & Omamo, 2011). The existing literature classifies social protection systems as "consolidated," "emerging" and "limited" (Gentilini, 2009; Gentilini & Omamo, 2009), and these are widely considered and discussed. This provides a wide spectrum to understand the positions of different nations and their path toward achieving social protection.

Countries with "consolidated" systems are comprised of Organization for Economic Cooperation and Development (OECD) countries and developed economies. In this system, social protection is institutionalized in their national budgets, structures, socio-cultural and political processes. In these countries, social protection is financed domestically. They operate largely through formal labor markets and entrusted with insurance. Further, there are non-contributory safety net programs as well (Gentilini & Omamo, 2011). Upgrading and upholding the quality of life through social security, welfare provisions and maintaining economic equity are high priorities of these countries despite recent austerity measures.

Countries with "emerging" systems are those countries who are proactive for social protection and beginning to institutionalize social protection in their processes and policies. Examples include South-East Asian, Middle-Eastern and Latin American countries. In these countries, international assistance is limited and social protection initiatives are largely domestically funded. In many countries, national constitutions have enshrined provisions for comprehensive social protection systems. For example, in India, social protection is mandated by law; the constitution has enshrined provisions for social protection through fundamental rights and through its directive principles of state policies. India has shown its commitment for social protection through its recent enactment of legislations and its active implementation ensures citizens a minimum and desired social security. Legislations include the Mahatma Gandhi National Rural Employment Guarantee Act, 2005, and the Right of Children to Free and Compulsory Education Act, 2009. More recently, through the National Food Security Act, 2013, the government has recognized the right to food for all people. Further, the National Rural Health Mission, 2005, has entrusted that people have better access to health care with the intention to provide enhanced and institutionalized maternal care in order to reduce maternal mortality and infant mortality rates (Srivastava, 2013).

Countries with "limited" social protection systems are those with more attention on poverty reduction, food insecurity and high malnutrition rates. These countries have very limited domestic funding for social protection than external funding to enact and implement social protection schemes. These constraints highlight the importance of external interventions and governmental bodies to join hands to extend social security and insurance assistance to safeguard the basic needs of the people. The limited capacity of these countries is challenged by recurring economic crises, internal political crises, militant threats, unsafe social conditions, and so forth. International bodies such as United Nations and many non-governmental bodies are committed to ensuring minimum basic needs to everyone without any disparity or inequality (Gentilini & Omamo, 2011).

There is no common social protection system across all countries. There is a distinct difference in the approaches and arrangements of each country's social protection system. The complex economic growth and rapid globalization have intensified the need for better understanding on how social protection can be achieved and how people access the benefits. In this process, multiple domains including the profession of social work play a role in the attainment of this goal. This chapter reviews how human rights, social justice and equity approaches contribute to social protection. The following sections consider how each of these dimensions contribute to understanding the right to social protection and how that has been reflected in the implementation of social protection programs.

Human rights

In 1948, the United Nations' Human Rights Commission set out to draft the Universal Declaration of Human Rights; it was adopted by the United Nations on December 10, 1948. In its preamble and in Article 1, the Declaration unequivocally proclaims the inherent rights of all human beings: "human beings shall enjoy freedom of speech and belief and freedom from fear and want has been proclaimed as the highest aspiration of the common people." The Declaration places emphasis on equality as an approach toward human rights. "All human beings are born free and equal in dignity and rights" (Article 1). The Member States of the United Nations pledged to work together to promote the 30 articles of human rights, and in consequence, many of these rights, in various forms, are today part of the constitutional law of democratic nations ("Universal Declaration of Human Rights," n.d.).

How are human rights guaranteed and expressed?

Universal human rights are legally guaranteed by international human rights law (United Nations, n.d.). They are expressed in treaties, customary international law, bodies of principles and other sources of law. International human rights law lays down obligations on countries to act in certain way or to refrain from certain act, in order to promote and protect human rights and fundamental freedoms of individuals or groups. Further, any country should comply with human rights in the course of the design, implementation and evaluation of any public policies. However, the role of treaties and other sources of law limits to protection of human rights formally, not in its establishment.

Since 1945, a series of treaties and instruments have emerged, conferring a legal form of inherent human rights. The creation of the United Nations provided an ideal forum for the development and adoption of human rights instruments. Most countries have also adopted constitutions and other laws which formally protect basic human rights. For instance, the constitution of India enshrined the right to equality, right to freedom, right against exploitation, right to freedom of religion, cultural and educational rights in fundamental rights; and rights related to social justice and economic welfare are protected through directive principles of state policy.

Human rights and social protection

Social security is recognized as a fundamental human right by the international community. The CESCR, which monitors the implementation of the International Covenant on Economic, Social and Cultural Rights (ICESCR), has progressively developed the content of the right to social security. Specifically, General Comment 19 (Article 9 of the covenant) of the committee emphasized the right to social security. In the introduction, it states that:

> Article 9 of the International Covenant on Economic, Social and Cultural Rights (the Covenant) provides that, "The States Parties to the present Covenant recognize the right of everyone to social security, including social insurance." The right to social security is of central importance in guaranteeing human dignity for all persons when they are faced with circumstances that deprive them of their capacity to fully realize their Covenant rights.
>
> (International Covenant on Economic, Social and Cultural Rights, 1976, p. 2)

Article 9 of the ICESCR identifies social security as an economic, social and cultural right. This qualifies the right to social security as international human rights, and thus is a legal obligation on countries rather than a policy option. The CESCR often uses the conventions and recommendations adopted by the International Labour Organization (ILO) to interpret the right to social security, specifically the Social Security (Minimum Standards) Convention, 1952 (No. 102).

On May 30, 2012, the General Conference of the ILO reaffirmed that the right to social security is a human right. It also emphasized the importance of social security and adopted the Social Protection Floor Recommendation considering the relevance of earlier established standards such as the Universal Declaration of Human Rights, in particular Articles 22 and 25, the ICESCR, in particular Articles 9, 11 and 12, ILO social security standards, in particular the Social Security (Minimum Standards) Convention, 1952 (No. 102), the Income Security Recommendation, 1944 (No. 67), and the Medical Care Recommendation, 1944

(No. 69). The Social Protection Floor Recommendation was adopted by the ILO to assist governments in providing social protection (Social security standards of the International Labour Organization, n.d.).

Social protection practices and human rights hold reciprocal benefits. Countries that have social protection practices not only comply with social security obligations of human rights, but also comply with other human rights obligations. By providing resources to the deprived or vulnerable beneficiaries, social protection programs help in the realization of a number of economic, social and cultural rights, such as the right to an adequate standard of living – including the right to adequate food, clothing and housing as well as rights to education and health. For example, the Mahatma Gandhi National Rural Employment Guarantee Act (MGNREGA) is one scheme that ensures a right to social security in India. It is a scheme that ensures a legal guarantee for 100 days of employment in every financial year to all rural households with skilled or unskilled workers. It also provides rural employment through public works with a minimum fixed wage per day. Over the years, MGNREGA has become an instrument for equitable growth, gender parity and social security, thus realizing other human rights (Srivastava, 2013).

A human rights-based approach for social protection

A human rights-based approach (HRBA) is a conceptual framework that is normatively based on international human rights standards and operationally directed to promoting and protecting human rights. When plans, policies or programs are anchored in a human rights-based approach, it demands compliance with international law. This is necessary to ensure sustainability and efficiencies of those initiatives.

When social protection systems adopt a human right approach, it helps not only to respond to international obligations and commitments, but also to improve the effectiveness of efforts toward poverty reduction. The beneficiaries who are in need of resources can be effectively identified with a human rights-based social protection program. The next section outlines the essential principles of the human rights approach applicable to social protection programs.

H2-universality of protection

One of the features of human rights is the principle of universality, meaning it applies to all people. All human beings are holders of human rights, independent from what they do, where they come from, where they live and from their national citizenship, or community (Kirchschlaeger, 2011). In a social protection context, the principles of universality suggest that social protection programs must be available to all individuals. Universal social protection systems are the initiatives that benefit all residents without conditions (Social Protection and Human Rights, n.d.).

H2-dignity and autonomy

Personal dignity and autonomy form the basis of human rights. Thus, states need to ensure it through policies and other initiatives. In social protection systems, all actors need to recognize the efforts taken by the beneficiaries to improve their lives. This may get violated when conditionalities or co-responsibilities are imposed in social protection initiatives.

Social protection programs such as conditional cash transfers (CCTs) require beneficiaries to fulfill one or more conditions. Such conditionalities in social protection programs assume that they strengthen human capital, and in the long term, contribute to breaking the inter-generational transmission of poverty. The imposition of conditionalities may suggest that people who are living in poverty would not make conscious allocation of available resources to improve their livelihoods. This violates the right to dignity of the poor. Also, individual autonomy is denied. Conditionalities deprive the poorest the freedom to make a decision for themselves and their family welfare and to regulate the course of their own lives. Under international human rights treaties such as the ICESCR and the Convention on the Rights of the Child (CRC), states parties are obliged to immediately meet minimum essential levels to the rights of food, health, housing, education and social security. These are inherent human rights and not conditional on the performance of certain actions or meeting requirements. When conditionalities are imposed, it demands additional monitoring and administration work, which demands extra costs. Further, beneficiaries need to incur private costs to comply with them. These requirements affect the cost-effectiveness of any program. A HRBA suggests that countries should refrain from imposing conditionalities to meet minimum essential levels to various rights (Social Protection and Human Rights, n.d.).

H2-equality and non-discrimination

Another principle of human rights is non-discrimination. Principles of equality regard all human beings as born free and equal in dignity and rights. Article 2 of the Universal Declaration of Human Rights states "all the rights and freedom are applicable to every single human being without distinction as to race, sex, national or ethnic origin, colour, religion, language, or any other status" ("Universal Declaration of Human Rights," 1948). Similarly, the International Covenant on Civil and Political Rights (ICCPR) and the ICESCR demand requirements on the respective states parties so as to guarantee the enjoyment of all rights without discrimination of any kind. These have specific provisions for the equal right of men and women in the enjoyment of all rights. Other conventions that uphold the prohibition of discrimination in the enjoyment of the rights include the Convention on the Elimination of All Forms of Discrimination against Women (CEDAW, Articles 11e and 14), the International Convention on All Forms of Racial Discrimination (CERD, Article 5) and the Convention on the Rights of Persons with Disabilities (CRPD, Article 28). This prohibition of discrimination is applicable to the right to social security as well. The right to equality and non-discrimination with respect to social protection has been underlined by ILO social security standards.

Integration of equality and non-discrimination principles in social protection systems has additional benefits because it assures human rights protection of the beneficiaries and improvement of effectiveness of social protection systems. However, implementation of these principles requires countries to eliminate any forms of discrimination, and to protect the most vulnerable segments of society as a matter of priority (Equality and Non-Discrimination, n.d.).

Equality and non-discrimination can be achieved by ensuring inclusion of vulnerable and disadvantaged groups. This is in line with the obligations imposed by the CEDAW, CRC, CRPD and International Convention on the Protection of the Rights of All Migrant Workers and their Families. Second, accounting for differences in the experiences of men and women while designing, implementing and monitoring social protection programs can be achieved by comprehensive and disaggregated gender analysis (Recommendation No. 202, para. 21). This ensures incorporation of gender perspectives. Finally, ensuring that social protection programs meet the standards of accessibility, adaptability, acceptability and adequacy for all rights holders is found in General Comments 13, 14 and 19 of CESCR (Sepulveda & Nyst, 2012).

H2-ensure transparency and access to information

Transparency and access to information need to be ensured by all social protection interventions based on human rights. The General Comment 19 of the UN CESCR states that transparency is integral to national social security programmes and action plans (CESCR, 2007). The ILO's Recommendation No. 202 (para. 3j) echoes the need to ground the financial management and general administration of social security systems in the principles of transparency and accountability. Further, Article 19 of the ICCPR notes that the right to freedom of expression includes the freedom to seek, receive and impart information from the state. The compliance with all these obligations demands transparency and access to information. Transparency and access to information ensures access and participation, and reduces corruption, clientelism and inefficiency. It is also necessary to ensure that personal information about rights holders are kept confidential and thus the right to access public information does not breach the right to privacy. This demands the process to follow international standards of privacy and confidentiality (Ensure Transparency and Access to Information, n.d.).

H2-ensuring meaningful and effective participation

Human rights norms such as Article 25 of the ICCPR emphasize the right to participate in public life. The CESCR (General Comment 19), and the ILO's social security conventions and recommendations have also highlighted the necessity to participate in the formulation and administration of social protection programs.

Participation allows beneficiaries to feel respected and promoted. This is necessary for the better involvement of beneficiaries in any program and thereby contributing to its success. A proper representation of the group that has taken into account existing asymmetries of power, patterns of marginalization and gender inequalities that exist within the household and the community, will ensure effective participation. For example, initiatives like "quota based on gender" may ensure a true representation (Ensure Meaningful and Effective Participation, n.d.).

H2-ensuring access to accountability mechanisms and effective remedies

Accountability ensures effectiveness of any initiative. This is equally applicable to a human rights approach as well, where accountability is one of the central pillars. Right-based social protection demands accountability and judicial reviewable decisions. This is to comply with human rights standards that emphasize individual right to effective remedy when his or her rights have been violated. Effective accountability mechanisms enhance protection for beneficiaries, improve efficiency of social programs, minimize wastage and mismanagement, and strengthen the public support of social protection schemes.

Accordingly, right-based social protection programs must incorporate accessible and effective complaints mechanisms which guarantee anonymity, allow for individual and collective complaints, and are sufficiently resourced and culturally appropriate. The need for the provision to effective remedy is outlined in Article 8 of the Universal Declaration of Human Rights (UDHR) and Article 2(3) of the ICCPR.

Finally, Sepulveda and Nyst (2012) suggest a periodic review of social protection programs to monitor its effectiveness and also to control deviations, if any. In their opinion, this periodic review may comprise following features. First, it should ensure the procedures used to register beneficiaries are correct. This will help to address possible wrongful exclusion of beneficiaries. Second, it should see to it that the various levels of implementation are proper. This will monitor possible abuses in the existing system and effective measures that can be taken. Third, it should protect overall payment procedures. This will expose possible misappropriation of financial resources. Periodic reviews should cover the initiation process to implementation in order to identify deviance at the earliest and facilitate corrective measures.

Adequate legal instrument and institutional framework

A legal instrument is a formal or legal written document. It creates an entitlement of benefits, ensures the permanence of the initiatives, and gives rightholders the legal ability to invoke their rights. This is mandatory for any social protection programs based on human rights. For example, the CRPD 2006 in Article 28 calls for countries to ensure an adequate standard of living and social protection for disabled persons.

An institutional framework refers to a system of formal laws, procedures, rules, and informal customs and norms. The institutional framework serves as a guide in the implementation of a program or project. Institutional frameworks along with legal aspects play an integral role to ensure that beneficiaries can demand their entitlements and protest in case of any violation of their rights. This will ensure that social protection programs will outlive political cycles and manipulations of political nature, and the long-term involvement of state authorities. For example, Social Security Act 1991 was established in Australia to regulate the payment of benefit schemes such as pensions, benefits and allowances (Social Security Act 1991, n.d.).

Comprehensive, coherent and coordinated policies

One of the characteristics of human rights is its indivisible, interrelated and interdependent nature. Thus, when social protection systems are implemented, other human rights obligations will also be met. This should not be inferred that social protection programs are a panacea for all economic and social issues, but rather an important element within a broad development strategy aimed at overcoming poverty and realizing other human rights, including economic, social and cultural rights such as the rights to education, adequate food and housing (Sepulveda & Nyst, 2012). For the effective implementation of social protection programmes and initiatives, countries strive for comprehensive and coherent policies. A comprehensive and coherent policy along with a proper coordination of programs and initiatives strengthens its cost-effectiveness and its responsiveness to risks. Coordination indicates the allocation of responsibility or the accountability of a task. Its absence restricts the identification of who is accountable for which aspects of implementation, which weakens any program or initiative. The need for coherent policy is indeed recognized by ILO Recommendation No. 202 (para. 3(l)) (R202 – Social Protection Floors Recommendation (No. 202), 2012).

Social justice

Social protection is oriented toward the social development of members in a society (Midgley, 2012). Proactively, social protection targets the empowerment of social actors to insulate themselves from possible exploitations and economic contingencies. Justice, a principle based theory, gives way to a number of theoretical perplexities and practical confusions. Theoretical complexity in the concept has given room for proposing many definitions and interpretations. For instance, Mathew (2005) reviews justice as proportion in distribution and retribution (Aristotelian view) and the disposition of the will to give each one his [her] due (Ulpian, a Roman jurist's view) and states the difficulty for coming up with a single definition for justice. The absence of a homogeneous idea of justice as well as the presence of many theories, definitions and interpretations prove the unique richness of the concept along with the possibility of universal applicability of the concept, considering the various contextual and cultural factors relevant to the situation. However, justice needs a more socially integrated approach to deal with situations where individual interest conflicts with social interest.

Social justice is a key principle and is fundamental to the profession of social work ("Statement of Ethical Principles," n.d.). Jost and Kay (2010) define social justice as:

> a state of affairs in which (a) benefits and burdens in society are dispersed in accordance with some allocation principle (or set of principles); (b) procedures, norms, and rules that govern political and other forms of decision making preserve the basic rights, liberties, and entitlements of individuals and groups; and (c) human beings (and perhaps other species) are treated with dignity and respect not only by authorities but also by other relevant social actors, including fellow citizens.
>
> (p. 1122)

Individual right-based approach is the key focus of this definition that contributes to an ideal situation of justice, as it is viewed from theories of justice (e.g., distributive justice and procedural justice). The National Association of Social Workers (NASW) explains social justice as "the view that everyone deserves equal economic, political and social rights and opportunities. Social workers aim to open the doors of access and opportunity for everyone, particularly those in greatest need" (NASW, n.d.). The International Federation of Social Workers (IFSW) asserts that social workers have a responsibility to promote social justice, in relation to society generally, and in relation to the people with whom they work, by challenging negative discrimination, recognizing diversity, distributing resources equally, challenging unjust policies and practice, and working in solidarity (IFSW, 2012). The two critical features that make the definition of social justice unique are that "everyone deserves" (right-based justice) and "open the doors of access" (duty based justice). Morgaine (2014) describes this definition as grounded in social justice with a strong individual focus. Thus, the philosophical underpinnings of social justice mark it as a core value of social work.

Historically, social justice received significant attention among researchers who belonged to the discipline of social psychology. Many events like fascism in Europe, war, terrorism and denial of mutual dignity and respect at individual and group level triggered this search for the meaning of social justice (Jost & Kay, 2010). However, today the situation is dire with religious fanaticism, terrorism, domestic violence, oppression and discrimination based on gender, race and income, in which the meaningful existence of individuals is challenged. This emerging context warrants social workers to refocus "their attention to peace and anti-war movements and a variety of identity-based movements such as women's rights, civil rights, LGBTQQI[1] rights, among others" (Morgaine, 2014, p. 3). It also throws light onto the evolving nature and dynamic interpretation of social justice as the context and times change. For instance, the recent study by Bakshi et al. (2015) attempts to integrate social justice to medical professionalism. The main focus here is to ensure equity, quality and ethics in the access to and provision of health care in current society.

Justice motive

Broadly, many social protection programs are carried out for the alleviation of poverty, for the accessibility to sufficient food, health and income. In recent years, adaptive social protection aims to support social protection in the context of climate change and disasters, as well as the role of infrastructure development in post-disaster recovery, among others. Social protection, as a human right, is a powerful tool to address many social, economic and environmental evils. In this context, fairness of social protection programs becomes crucial. If the bundle of social protection programs happened to untie without the essence of justice, it will counterfeit the purpose of social work. A reason for this forecasted failure would be the nature of the target group (e.g., the social, political and economic vulnerability of the target group). In addition, this aspect of social work involves the vast distribution of public resources and an enormous amount of accountability. In the absence of justice, these progressive activities will remain ineffective and lame. In this context, we discuss different justice theories that inspire the effective execution of social protection programs through the hands of social workers.

There are a number of theories in ethics that support this idea of fairness in relationship. Social workers adopt a holistic approach in their practice to assess and evaluate each case or situation. Insights offered by Robin and Reidenbach (1987) describe the major traditions in moral philosophy as deontology, utilitarianism and virtue ethics (character-based theory). Deontology holds that "there are *prima facie* ideals that can direct our thinking" (p. 46). These ideals or rules are absolute in nature. But at the same time, modern interpreters, in contrast to the early thinkers, do not admit the non-absolute nature of rules. Modern interpretations suggest that these ideals can be "universal" but not necessarily "absolute" (Robin & Reidenbach, 1987; Ross, 1930). For instance, there can be some situations where one or more universal statements of "right" or "wrong" might be inappropriate. For example, in a situation of war, the ideal "do not kill" is challenged or even violated and still justified. Thus the ideal alone would be inadequate to justify "killing the enemy." Situational nuances such as the nature of enemy, the potential harm and security of many nationals would explain better why an ideal like "do not kill" should be universal, but not absolute. In the same situation, the medical aid movements and people involved are protected and not considered as enemies.

Further, utilitarianism anchors around the golden rule of the "greatest good for the greatest number of people" (Robin & Reidenbach, 1987, p. 46). Robin and Reidenbach suggest the performance of social cost–benefit analysis to assess the "greatest good for the greatest number of people" (p. 46). All benefits minus all costs can give either positive or negative results, based on which an action could be morally acceptable or not. Thus, an action can be judged as right or wrong depending on the value it generates. Another quite ancient but still respected tradition of moral philosophy is "virtue ethics." This derives from Aristotelian moral philosophy where "golden mean" is the basis of choice. It is moderation or prudence that defines how one should choose a virtuous stand in behavior. It focuses on the person, who does the action, rather than the individual acts (Mathew, 2005).

Apart from these three, *liberal individualism* (I act in a particular way, since it is my right), *justice-based theory* (broadly depending on the subject and the object of the right or the due at stake) and *ethics of care* (a relationship based theory which associates moral obligation with whom we have significant relationships) are other ethical theories (Mathew, 2005). In general, the *consequentialist teleological theories* and the deontological theories on rights or justice represent the principle-based theories, whereas virtue ethics like *ethics of care* represent more context-oriented approaches (Gu & Neesham, 2014). Though justice-based theory is counted as one among many ethical theories, it would be reasonable to argue that all these theories directly or indirectly add value to the fairness in society. In sum, ethical theories may not be considered as absolute in nature. But it has a universal application. While we evaluate the issue of poverty in developed countries the focus could be the implications of procedural justice whereas the same issue in a lesser developed country may need to be considered from a distributional aspect of justice. In general, different aspects of justice theories bring the synergy of "justice motive" in a given social context.

In addition, there can be different reference points, while evaluating an action. Three such principles are ethical egoism, utilitarianism and altruism. These three approaches agree on the notion of "create the greatest good." But they may not always agree on the notion of "greatest good for whom." Ethical egoism focuses on creating the greatest good for oneself, utilitarianism for the greatest number, and altruism for the greatest interest of others (Peter, 2007). The same approach is seen in proposing three ethical criteria (Victor & Cullen, 1988) for ethical climate perception. They are egoism (maximizing the self-interest), benevolence (maximizing joint interest) and adherence to a principle that follows the deontological (an action is justifiable in itself) understanding of morality. Thus, seeking self-interest in itself need not be in contrast to social justice. In many instances, maximizing self-interest would be justifiable. For example, in a context of gender discrimination and torture, a person is fighting to uphold his/her self-dignity and personal integrity. In short, justice and self-interest need not always be contradictory. Nevertheless, selfless activities or sacrificing self-interests for protecting others from the effects of unfairness could be clear evidence of justice motive (social justice). Social protection, while being a right of an individual, also becomes a duty of each co-habitant to uphold. It is the inherent responsibility of all to protect others from vulnerabilities and also to improve their conditions of life.

Social implications of justice theory

Justice as one of the foundations of social protection provides significant implications in our lives, which is philosophically and practically different from situation to situation. These different contexts of life implicate different theories of social justice as and when we start practicing social work (Morgaine, 2014). The major theories of justice are discussed in the next section, and vary their implications according to the specific characteristics of each situation.

First, distributive justice refers to fair or proportionate distribution of resources. Aristotle put forth just distribution of scarce resources for a just society. This view brings the traditional definition of justice to discussion. Justice refers to providing what is due to others. It regulates the relation of a society as a whole to its members (Mathew, 2005). An impartial distribution by "treating equals as equals" would constitute fairness in society. It is the perceived fairness outcome distribution (Victor, Trevino, & Shapiro, 1993). However, the difficult tasks would be to determine what is due, to identify the criteria for equality and finally to fix the distributor (Mathew, 2005). The determination of "what is due" would be detailed in our discussion about human rights. Similarly, the notion of equity, which is different from equality, will be explained in our discussion on equity theory. The Aristotelian concept of proportionality is reasonably argued as the basis of equity theory. Regarding the role of distributor, the debate is not yet concluded on whether it is the state, a collective body of individuals or an individual. However, in the context of social protection, specifically in the activities to provide assistance to the deprived, distributive justice helps social workers to determine the distributor and beneficiaries. The quantification of "what is due" will be determined by an equity approach that ensures the just distribution of resources.

Second, procedural justice refers to the fairness that is achieved or maintained in the processes of decision-making. Drawing insights from the nuances of natural justice, procedural justice insists on the requirement of being heard or submitting all possible evidence before taking a decision. It also includes the possibility of effective involvement in the process of decision-making. For instance, a livelihood intervention (compensation) system in a company needs to be procedurally robust in which every employee gets a reasonable platform to submit evidence for his/her views on and opportunities to revisit the decision.

Third, Amartya Sen, the Nobel Laureate, stated in his book *The Idea of Justice* that "the success of democracy is not merely a matter of having the most perfect institutional structure that we can think of. It depends inescapably on our actual behaviour patterns and the working of political and social interactions" (Sen, 2011, p. 354). The injustices that are peeping into the fabric of society are not only due to the failures on the part of the state or system. Rather, these injustices are associated with how individual members of the society treat each other. In other words, a character-based justice theory would focus on the person who performs the action rather than the act itself (Mathew, 2005). The fairness depends upon how individuals tend to treat each other in the context of socio-political factors. A virtue-based ethics would be recommended for social workers while working toward the welfare of the society.

Fourth, retributive justice seeks the justification for punishments. Retributive theory of justice would prevent the tendencies to violate the rules and regulations that exist to protect the meaningful exercise of human rights. The execution of punishments is justified from the utilitarianism perspective; it is for the larger good of the society. The people who are involved in the activities of harming others need to be incapacitated to keep the rights of individuals safe and secure. Another major justification would be the effect of deterrence. Once the perpetrator receives punishment for what he or she has done this would deter him/her from becoming involved in such activities in future. Thus it is meant to reduce the risk of damaging the welfare of individuals, which is the purpose of social protection programs.

Finally, John Rawls's *Theory of Justice* has attracted wide attention and discussion among academic scholars for the past years. He has envisioned an egalitarian society, where each citizen is aware of their rights and able to take decisions using free will; emphasizing their mutual cooperation in their economic system (Wenar, 2013). Apart from sophisticated arguments, the Rawlsian idea of justice as fairness places justice as the maximal moral standard of a society. He holds the idea that citizens are free and equal to cooperate with each other for the welfare of each member, and in turn the common good of the society. Justice as fairness proposes a fair rearrangement or restructuring of various institutions of a liberal society such as political, social and legal associations and so on. The benefits and burdens of cooperation need to be distributed among the members. Rawls put forth "equality based reciprocity" to divide social goods equally among its members (Wenar, 2013). However, Rawls's view on justice seeks high moral uprightness and individual virtuosity to accomplish this idea of fairness in today's social life, irrespective of political, economic and social boundaries.

In summary, justice theories contribute in the design and fulfillment of social protection. Social protection aims to improve quality of life by an effective application of social welfare measures in order to reduce people's vulnerability to poverty and deprivation. The three steps characteristics (World Bank, 2011) are built on the aforementioned theories. For example, the promotional characteristic of social protection focuses on the improvement of income. Distributive justice guides the various livelihood interventions to be fair in the process of distributing resources and promoting the availability of resources required. However, the purpose may stand unachieved if the procedures applied to select the needy or the right beneficiaries in providing relief are corrupt. All the more, we need virtue-based individuals to implement quality social protection programs. Thus, a holistic approach of justice theories assists social workers to realize the goals of social protection and social development in contemporary society.

Equity

Equity is linked and understood with concepts of "fairness, justice and equitable distribution" (Svara & Brunet, 2005, p. 2). Equity is dealt with distributive justice and procedural fairness. Falk and colleagues describe equity in this broader perspective:

> Equity derives from a concept of social justice. It represents a belief that there are some things which people should have, that there are basic needs that should be fulfilled, that burdens and rewards should not be spread too divergently across the community, and that policy should be directed with impartiality, fairness and justice towards these ends.
> (Falk, Hampton, Hodgkinson, Parker, & Rorris, 1993, p. 2)

In summary, everyone should be ensured with a minimum level of income below which nobody falls. The agenda has been institutionalized in many countries through national legislations, which mandate payment of minimum wages that are compulsory and proportionately fixed on factors such as geographical regions and economic fluctuations. For instance, India's Minimum Wages Act, 1948, is widespread in its implementation and minimum wages are fixed at regular revisions.

In addition, equity further iterates that no particular communities or groups should be asked to undergo more burdens than others through governmental actions. Equity implies a need for fairness, not necessarily equality, in the distribution of gains and losses, and entitles everyone to a better quality of life and standard of living. Equity has found its significance in international law and conventions, and according to Weiss (1990) "recognition of the inherent dignity and of the equal and inalienable rights of all members of the human family is the foundation of freedom, justice and peace in the world" (p. 20).

An equity approach aims to reach the most marginalized and deprived people first, rather than benefit a larger number of people (Equity for Children, 2013). In contrast, social equity concerns how particular groups or communities are protected from vulnerability and deprivations. Distributive justice provides a foundation for equity based on how provisions or resources are distributed to individuals, groups or communities by considering their proportionality of needs rather than the equality principle of distribution of resources equally across the different groups and communities.

The concept of equity has been highly appreciated and its inclusion found in many initiatives of international bodies such as World Bank, International Labour Organization (ILO), Asian Development Bank, and national level programs in many countries (Smyth, 2014, p. 2). The World Bank and ILO recently issued a statement about their joint mission to ensure social protection to everyone through their new initiative called Universal Social Protection (World Bank, 2015). It is designed to integrate a set of policies to ensure minimum income security and provide support to all people, in particular those who are poor and vulnerable.

Universal social protection aims to protect the best interests of children, women, people with disability, people without jobs, and pensions for all older persons. This protection can be provided through social insurance, tax-funded social benefits, social assistance services, public works programs and other schemes guaranteeing basic income security (World Bank, 2015).

Equity is an ethical concept grounded in distributive justice (Bravemen & Gruskin, 2003). It aims to reduce unequal opportunities, especially to reduce the disparities among the most disadvantaged and underprivileged. Many view an equity approach as a tool to address the growing inequalities and serve as a guiding principle for the redistribution of wealth and access. Equity and human rights go hand-in-hand since both of them strive to make people attain their desired standards by reducing discrimination and inequalities (Bravemen & Gruskin, 2003). International human rights instruments set the platform for legal obligations to protect the rights of people to reduce poverty and inequity (Bravemen & Gruskin, 2003). Some of the important international human rights instruments which promote social protection are (UN Human Rights Instruments, n.d., section 1–10):

1   Universal Declaration of Human Rights, 1948
2   International Covenant on Economic, Social and Cultural Rights (ICESCR), 1966
3   Convention on the Elimination of All Forms of Discrimination against Women, 1979
4   Convention on the Rights of the Child, 1989
5   Convention on the Elimination of All Forms of Racial Discrimination, 1965
6   International Convention on the Protection of the Rights of All Migrant Workers and their Families, 1990
7   Convention on Rights of Persons with Disabilities, 2006
8   Convention relating to the Status of Refugees, 1951 and Convention relating to the Status of Stateless Persons, 1954.

Equity approach and human rights are directed toward reducing disparities and protecting the rights of the underprivileged and most marginalized groups in society (Bravemen & Gruskin, 2003). Equity and human rights frameworks strive to uplift the disadvantaged and maintain parity in society. Social protection and social security become an integral part of the state's legal obligations to meet its agenda to ensure equal opportunity and access to better resources. International agreements, covenants, conventions and treaties impose the signatory countries to orient their local policies and legislations to uphold the social protection (Smyth, 2014).

The concepts of equity and equality traced their presence in social justice and fairness, from a time when the redistribution of wealth and service was practiced (Equity for Children, 2013). The theoretical foundation for equity arose from social justice theory; the most prominent theory which laid the theoretical framework for equity was John Rawls's concept of justice as fairness, which changed the direction of distribution to the greater society rather than for individuals (Rawls, 1971). John Rawls established a principle approach to combat inequity by addressing the most disadvantaged. He insisted on two central principles to encompass this philosophy. First, the "equal liberty principle" holds the view that individuals are entitled to the maximum amount of liberties as long as it assures greater good for the society and it can be applied to all individuals. The equal liberty principle has been largely found in most of the constitutional provisions, which provides liberties and fundamental rights to individuals that protect them from deprivations and exploitations. It is individually focused and is not applied for any large group or communities. Next, the "difference principle" insists that inequalities are acceptable only if they are addressing the inequalities of the marginalized and to the greatest benefit of the most disadvantaged. The difference principle found its place in most social protection programs and human capital provisions such as subsidy to the marginalized, midday meals scheme for people living below the poverty line, and housing schemes for the homeless and landless.

Rawls's principles to deal with inequalities are in alignment with the principle of equity because he aims to redress the inequalities and disadvantages among the most vulnerable and marginalized. The equity paradigm derives from the concept of a fair equality of opportunity from Rawls's second principle (Equity for Children, 2013). The "difference principle" then permits the inequalities in outcomes as long as equality of opportunity exists. Rawls claims that "undeserved inequalities call for redress; and since inequalities of birth and natural endowment are undeserved, these inequalities are somehow to be compensated for" (Rawls, 1971, p. 86). In Rawls's view, individuals in the society should be treated as equal and no disparity should be shown among people based on any identities. Under the social equity paradigm in the development context, priority can be placed on the most disadvantaged and marginalized over other groups in society. The inequalities in this approach maintain an ability to redress the large gap existing between the privileged and underprivileged groups in society. The equity approach is not in violation of the equality principle as long as it meets the basic needs of the marginalized. As discussed earlier in this chapter, equity and human rights share a very close agenda to ensure minimum basic standards of living to all human beings. An equity approach strives to reduce poverty through differential treatment to underprivileged and privileged groups; while a human rights approach strives to ensure protection through legal obligations. However, both equity and human rights approaches direct respective bodies to establish social protection programs and social security schemes to implement their agenda.

A human rights framework asserts that equality, non-discrimination, participation, transparency and accountability are maintained at different phases of social protection programs from planning to evaluation (Piron, 2004). Further, international human rights establish the right to an adequate standard of living (including the right to adequate food and housing), the right to social security, the right to education and the right to the highest attainable standard of health

(Sepulveda & Nyst, 2012). "Social protection as the set of public and private policies and programmes aim[s] at preventing, reducing and eliminating economic and social vulnerabilities to poverty and deprivation" (Integrated social protection systems: enhancing equity for children, 2012, p. 4). An analysis of social protection and human rights obligations provide a clear perspective that human rights obligations can be realized through implementation of social protection programs. Along with the programs, the process of its implementation can contribute to an inclusive development agenda in the course of its planning and actions (Sepulveda & Nyst, 2012).

Human rights, social protection and equity

A human rights perspective of social protection aims at the realization of human rights; it empowers people to claim their rights rather than being just a receiver (Piron, 2004). It is identified that social protection is recognized as one of the most important human rights in international human rights instruments by way of incorporating a right to social security. The Universal Declaration of Human Rights has enshrined specific provisions related to social protection; the following articles have conferred the right to social security:

> Article 22: Everyone, as a member of society, has the right to social security and is entitled to realization through national effort and international cooperation and in accordance with the organization and resources of each state, of the economic, social and cultural rights indispensable for his dignity and the free development of his personality.
>
> (United for Human Rights, n.d., section 2)

> Article 23.3: Everyone who works has the right to just and favourable remuneration ensuring for himself and his family an existence worthy of human dignity, and supplemented, if necessary, by other means of social protection.
>
> (United for Human Rights, n.d., section 3)

> Article 25: Everyone has the right to a standard of living adequate for the health and well-being of himself and of his family, including food, clothing, housing, and medical care, and necessary social services, and the right to security in the event of unemployment, sickness, disability, widowhood, old age or other lack of livelihood in circumstances beyond his control. Motherhood and childhood are entitled to special care and assistance. All children, whether born in or out of wedlock, shall enjoy the same social protection.
>
> (United for Human Rights, n.d., section 5)

Social protection is one of the international human rights, and it is obliged to uphold the important principles of human rights: inclusion, equality and non-discrimination in its approach and manifestation of social protection programs.

When social protection targets services and programs for the betterment of the poor and vulnerable, it may contradict the principle of equality (Piron, 2004). However, it is advised that when promoted as a right rather than a charity, it would amplify its significance more vividly. Social protection cannot be treated in isolation from human rights, since human rights guide social protections policies from planning to implementation and evaluation. Human rights promote social protection to fulfill and meet the minimum standards of living such as access to resources, education, health care and affordability of people. Thus, human rights forms an integral part of social protection programs that assure that the poor and vulnerable are prevented, mitigated and relieved from economic inequalities and deprivations.

Conclusion

Social protection has attracted great interest in the field of social development in recent years. While scholars find it difficult to define the term, there is agreement that social protection contributes to social development. It is larger in scope than existing social security schemes. Social protection follows an empowerment approach rather than an "occupationalist" approach (Midgley, 2012). In other words, it is not a reactionary measure to insulate or protect a member of society from the contingencies that affect him/her negatively. Rather, it is proactively strengthening the member to protect himself/herself from the vulnerabilities of existence. In short, the meaning of social protection is gradually moving beyond the limitations of income maintenance toward a more holistic and integrated approach.

In the profession of social work today, social protection initiatives are supported. While the Universal Declaration of Human Rights (1948) states social security as a human right (Article 22) from a developmental perspective of society, the term social protection is more frequently used today. This chapter interweaves concepts such as human rights, justice and equity with social protection from a rights-based approach. Accordingly, human rights guide social protection from its design to implementation; justice takes a major role in the delivery of social protection programs and principles of equity ensure a proportionality approach in the realization of social protection measures.

Social protection thus aims to achieve its objectives in and through human rights, justice and equity based approaches. Human rights-based social protection interventions reduce the risk of poverty, unreasonably low income, medical inaccessibility and similar socio-economic phenomena. This chapter has discussed important rights which exclusively focus on social protection and various initiatives of governmental bodies to protect members of society from unexpected risks, natural calamities and economic crises. When social protection programs are based on human rights, it demands compliance with international human rights and respective national legislations. Human rights-based social protection programs also ensure universality, equality, non-discrimination, transparency, accountability and accessibility to resources. Thus, social protection programs with a right-based approach establish a comprehensive framework that not only protects the rights of the people, but also redress the inequalities.

Justice as fairness in transactions and interactions pose the greatest challenge in the process of achieving social protection. Any transaction of goods and services is initiated on some presumed values. However, the demands of justice are unclear when many claimants are involved, such as employer, employee and the wider society, including the unemployed (Mathew, 2005). The boundaries of "fairness or what is due" are not clearly determined by the law or theories, though it is always guided by them. In ambiguous situations, judicial bodies are entrusted with the responsibility to interpret and define the boundaries of fairness or what is due, which will set the standard. Thus, it would be the responsibility of the state as well as the concerned authorities who are involved in the process of distribution or redistribution of resources. The distributive, procedural and interactional theories of justice provide an integrative guidance to society to protect its members from the deprivation of wealth, safety and freedom. Justice as a principle-based theory guides political and legal institutions to formulate various policies and programs for the alleviation of poverty, discrimination based on caste, colour, creed, sex and so on. Common policies and treaties that are formulated within a nation or between nations or in any such international decision-making bodies are required to reflect this fairness for a decent society. Thus, it is necessary for any social protection programs to integrate the principles of justice, for a fair distribution and redistribution of resources to maintain parity and to reduce the inequalities.

The significance of equity in right-based social protection has been found in its principles and approach. An equity principle brings a broader perspective to social protection through its element of justice and fairness in distribution. Since the equity theory incorporates the differences principle that appreciates inequalities in services and among the members of the society, it has received a larger meaning than equality (Piron, 2004). Beyond uniformity, equity tries to find a fair balance between differences among individuals and distribution of scarce resources and services. The different patterns and dimensions of distribution under equity principles ensure that required proportionality is maintained over equality so as to keep the access of resources to the marginalized sections of the society.

The fundamental goal of social protection is to reduce vulnerability and deprivation. To ensure the realization of social protection, equity plays a pivotal role in establishing a system of fairness, and procedural and distributive justice. Equity is not an independent concept in itself, as it integrates social justice, human rights and fairness to attain its goals. In this context, it is important to consider the differences among the groups/society/community; the differences in the socio-economic conditions of people and their level of access to resources. This difference delineates and classifies people as disadvantaged and privileged. Thus, the equity approach strives to reduce the gap between advantaged and most disadvantaged through its proportionate distribution of wealth and services.

This chapter reviewed social protection with respect to human rights, social justice and equity. Social protection reflects a right-based approach in the social life of a person. All these concepts are interlinked and interdependent, and thus the combination of these concepts to establish social protection programs would be most effective in contributing to the quality of social life. Effectively implemented interventions promote economic welfare, prevent social vulnerabilities, ensure minimum basic needs, and improve living conditions. In summary, right-based social protection programs contribute to the realization of human rights, upliftment of marginalized groups and reduction of economic inequalities. As human rights advocates, social workers play a critical role in the delivery, implementation and evaluation of social protection initiatives.

Note

1 The acronym LGBTQQI stands for Lesbian, Gay, Bisexual, Transgender, Queer, Questioning, and Intersex (LGBTQQI, n.d.).

References

Bakshi, S., James, A., Hennelly, M.O., Karani, R., Palermo, A.-G., Jakubowski, A.,…., & Atkinson, H. (2015). The human rights and social justice scholars program: A collaborative model for preclinical training in social medicine. *Annals of Global Health, 81,* 290–297.

Bravemen, P., & Gruskin, D. (2003). Poverty, equity, human rights and health. *Bulletin of the World Health Organization, 81,* 539–545.

CESCR. (2007). General comment NO. 19: The right to social security (art. 9). Retrieved on September 16, 2015, from http://socialprotection-humanrights.org/wp-content/uploads/2015/06/CESCR-General-Comment-19.pdf.

Ensure Meaningful and Effective Participation. (n.d.). *Ensure meaningful and effective participation @ Social protection and human rights.* Retrieved September 16, 2015, from http://socialprotection-humanrights.org/framework/principles/ensure-meaningful-and-effective-participation/.

Ensure Transparency and Access to Information. (n.d.). *Ensure transparency and access to information @ Social protection and human rights.* Retrieved on September 14, 2015, from http://socialprotection-humanrights.org/framework/principles/ensure-transparency-and-access-to-information/.

Equality and Non-Discrimination. (n.d.). *Equality and non-discrimination @ Social protection and human rights.* Retrieved on September 14, 2015, from http://socialprotection-humanrights.org/framework/principles/equality-and-non-discrimination/.

Equity for Children. (2013). *Equity and social justice: A short introduction.* Retrieved from www.equityforchildren.org/wp-content/uploads/2013/07/FinalPaper-EquityandSocialJustice-AnIntroduction-1.pdf.

Falk, J., Hampton, G., Hodgkinson, A., Parker, K., & Rorris, A. (1993). *Social equity and the urban environment.* Canberra: A.G.P.S.

Garcia, A.B., & Gruat, J.V. (2003). Social protection: A life cycle continuum investment for social justice. *Poverty Reduction and Sustainable Development. Paper for International Labour Organization.*

Gentilini, U. (2009). Social protection in the "real world": Issues, models and challenges. *Development Policy Review, 27,* 147–166.

Gentilini, U., & Omamo, S.W. (2009). *Unveiling social safety nets.* Rome: World Food Programme.

Gentilini, U., & Omamo, S.W. (2011). Social protection 2.0: Exploring issues, evidence and debates in a globalizing world. *Food Policy*, *36*, 329–340.

Gu, J., & Neesham, C. (2014). Moral identity as leverage point in teaching business ethics. *Journal of Business Ethics*, *124*, 527–536.

Integrated social protection systems: Enhancing equity for children. (2012). Retrieved on September 14, 2015, from www.unicef.org/socialprotection/framework/files/Full_Social_Protection_Strategic_Framework_low_res%281%29.pdf.

International Covenant on Economic, Social and Cultural Rights. (1976). Retrieved on September 14, 2015, from www.ohchr.org/EN/ProfessionalInterest/Pages/CESCR.aspx.

Jost, J.T., & Kay, A.C. (2010). Social justice: History, theory, and research. In S.T. Fiske, D.T. Gilbert, & G. Lindzey (Eds.), *Handbook of social psychology* (pp. 1121–1165). Hoboken: John Wiley & Sons, Inc.

Kirchschlaeger, P. (2011). *Universality of human rights*. Retrieved on September 14, 2015, from http://theewc.org/uploads/files/Statement%20Series%20First%20Issue-Final%20WEB.pdf#page=22.

LGBTQQI. (n.d.). *LGBTQQI @ Urban dictionary*. Retrieved on September 21, 2015, from www.urbandictionary.com/define.php?term=LGBTQQI.

Mathew, I. (2005). *Business ethics*. Kottayam: Macfest.

Midgley, J. (2012). Social protection and social policy: Key issues and debates. *Journal of Policy Practice*, *11*, 8–24.

Midgley, J. (2014). *Social development: Theory and practice*. London: Sage.

Morgaine, K. (2014). Conceptualizing social justice in social work: Are social workers "too bogged down in the trees?" *Journal of Social Justice*, *4*, 1–17.

NASW. (n.d.). *Social justice*. Retrieved on September 1, 2015, from www.socialworkers.org/pressroom/features/issue/peace.asp.

Peter, N.G. (2007). *Leadership: theory and practice* (4th ed.). India: Sage Publications.

Piron, L.H. (2004). *Rights-based approaches to social protection*. London: Overseas Development Institute. Retrieved on September 14, 2015, from www.odi.org/sites/odi.org.uk/files/odi-assets/publications-opinion-files/1700.pdf.

R202 – Social Protection Floors Recommendation (No. 202). (2012). *Social protection floors recommendation @ International labour organization*. Retrieved September 14, 2015, from www.ilo.org/dyn/normlex/en/f?p=NORMLEXPUB:12100:0::NO::P12100_INSTRUMENT_ID:3065524.

Rawls, J. (1971). *A theory of justice*. Cambridge, MA: Harvard University Press.

Robin, D.P., & Reidenbach, R.E. (1987). Social responsibility, ethics, and marketing strategy: Closing the gap between concept and application. *Journal of Marketing*, *51*, 44–58.

Ross, W.D. (1930). *The right and the good*. Oxford: Oxford University Press.

Sen, A. (2011). *The idea of justice*. Cambridge, MA: Harvard University Press.

Sepulveda, M., & Nyst, C. (2012). *The human rights approach to social protection*. Merikasarmi: Ministry of Foreign Affairs of Finland.

Smyth, I. (2014). Anticipatory social protection claiming dignity and rights. *Gender & Development*, *22*, 401–402.

Social Protection and Human Rights. (n.d.). *Dignity and autonomy*. Retrieved on September 14, 2015, from http://socialprotection-humanrights.org/framework/principles/dignity-and-autonomy/.

Social Security Act 1991. (n.d.). *Social security act 1991 @ Social protection and human rights*. Retrieved on September 14, 2015, from http://socialprotection-humanrights.org/instru/social-security-act-1991/.

Social security standards of the International Labour Organization. (n.d.). *Social security standards of the International Labour Organization @ Social protection and human rights*. Retrieved on September 8, 2015, from http://socialprotection-humanrights.org/social-security-standards-of-the-international-labour-organization/.

Srivastava, R.S. (2013). *A social protection floor for India*. Geneva: International Labour Office.

Statement of Ethical Principles. (n.d.). Retrieved September 12, 2015, from http://ifsw.org/policies/statement-of-ethical-principles.

Svara, J.H., & Brunet, J.R. (2005). Social equity is a pillar of public administration. *Journal of Public Affairs Education, 3*, 253–258.

Weiss, E.B. (1990). In fairness to future generations. *Environment: Science and Policy for Sustainable Development, 32*(3), 6–31.

World Bank. (2011). *Social protection for changing India*. Washington, DC: World Bank.

World Bank. (2015). *Joint statement by World Bank group president Jim Yong Kim and ILO director general Guy Ryder*. Retrieved on September 7, 2015, from www.world-bank.org/en/news/press-release/2015/06/30/joint-statement-world-bank-group-president-ilo-director-general-guy-ryder.

UN Human Rights Instruments. (n.d.). *UN human rights instruments@Social protection and human rights*. Retrieved on September 14, 2015, from http://socialprotection-humanrights.org/legal-depository/legal-instruments/un-human-rights-instruments/.

United for Human Rights. (n.d.). *Universal declaration of human rights*. Retrieved on September 8, 2015, from www.humanrights.com/what-are-human-rights/universal-declaration-of-human-rights/articles-21-30.html.

United Nations. (n.d.). *Human rights: A basic handbook for UN staff*. Retrieved on August 9, 2015, from www.ohchr.org/Documents/Publications/HRhandbooken.pd.

Victor, B., & Cullen, J.B. (1988). The organizational bases of ethical work climates. *Administrative Science Quarterly, 33*, 101–125.

Victor, B., Trevino, L.K., & Shapiro, D.L. (1993). Peer reporting of unethical behavior: The influence of justice evaluations and social context factors. *Journal of Business Ethics, 12*, 253–263.

Wenar, L. (2013). John Rawls. In E.N. Zalta (Ed.), *The Stanford encyclopedia of philosophy*. Retrieved from http://plato.stanford.edu/archives/win2013/entries/rawls/.

5 Key concepts and definitions of social protection, social development, and related terms

Tiffany Sampson and Julie Drolet

Introduction

Living in a precarious world as we do, people encounter any number of shocks, stresses, and hardships throughout their lifetime such as illnesses, loss of livelihoods, loss of assets (e.g., housing, savings, investments), and so forth that can be due to one or more causes, including: personal, social, economic, political, and environmental. The concept of social protection is concerned with providing public and private supports for individuals and households to not only cope with adversities but to overcome them. While there is no generally agreed upon definition for the term "social protection" it is necessary to explore meanings and understandings using the relevant literature. It has been said that a "remarkable feature of writing on social policy is its lack of theoretical and conceptual underpinnings beyond the general suggestions that social policy must be somehow holistic and integrated with economic policy" (Mkandawire, 2004, p. 4). The chapter begins by defining the term "social protection" and its main components. A social development perspective and approaches is traced through policies, programs, and initiatives. The origins of the term "sustainable development" that linked economic, social, and environmental dimensions in international policy and initiatives are presented, and the newly adopted Sustainable Development Goals in the post-2015 development framework. The concept of livelihoods, and related approaches and strategies, is highlighted, as well as the term "sustainable livelihoods" given the need for people to earn a living. A gender perspective that considers gender equality, gender equity, and gender inequality is necessary for transformative social protection. Finally, the chapter considers varied definitions of poverty relevant to social protection initiatives. A multidimensional approach to eradicating poverty is required with social protection systems and floors.

Defining social protection

The term "social protection" is understood in many ways. With that said, several authors describe social protection as involving public and/or private actions, initiatives, or interventions to address economic risks and vulnerabilities, particularly of the poor in order to reduce or protect against economic and social deprivation (Conway, de Haan, & Norton, 2000; Devereux & Sabates-Wheeler, 2004; Roelen & Devereux, 2013; Sabates-Wheeler & Devereux, 2007). Others suggest that social protection comprises of policies and/or programs (Ortiz, 2001; Social protection, poverty reduction and pro-poor growth, 2008; United Nations Children's Fund, 2012; United Nations Economic and Social Council, 2001a) designed to protect individuals and households from deprivation or slipping further into poverty. Social protection is also referred to as a broad concept covering social security and non-statutory schemes (International Labour Organization, 2001). Midgley (2012) points out that social security tends to be used synonymously with social protection. Standing (2007) argues that these two terms are in fact different since social protection "[signifies] the full range of protective transfers, services, and institutional safeguards supposed to protect the population 'at risk' of being 'in need'" whereas social security covers a statutory scheme system that guards against unforeseen risks (p. 512). As for the goal of social protection, Devereux and Sabates-Wheeler (2004) suggest that it is to decrease vulnerabilities of those living in poverty. Midgley (2012) proposes that the purpose of social protection is to safeguard people's incomes with the overall objective to prevent poverty. Finally, the International Labour Organization (2001) maintains that humanitarian principles of social inclusion and human dignity are the goal of social protection. According to Devereux and Sabates-Wheeler (2004) three categories of people can benefit from social protection, including: the chronically poor; the economically vulnerable; and the socially marginalized. Furthermore, developing and developed countries both benefit from a social protection floor approach that comprises of "essential services and social transfers" (International Labour Organization & World Health Organization, 2009). The International Labour Organization (2011) suggests that for countries in the Global South, a social protection floor approach is the first step in protecting the most vulnerable citizens; whereas for countries in the Global North with established social welfare systems a social protection floor approach is necessary in order to address the coverage gap by reaching vulnerable populations.

Although social protection has a number of components, there are two main components. The first is social assistance, which covers public actions, both governmental and non-governmental, that are intended to transfer resources to groups of people considered eligible due to their deprivation status (Conway et al., 2000). Social insurance is the second main component that is in effect social security, whereby individuals or households use the insurance principle to safeguard themselves against risks by pooling their resources with those facing similar vulnerabilities (United Nations Economic and Social Council, 2001a). Social insurance is financed from the regular contributions of those who participate in these schemes such as pensions, severance payments, health insurance, and unemployment compensation. These programs are often limited to a relatively small number of formal sector workers. In addition to social assistance and social insurance, Gentilini and Were Omamo (2011) suggest that social services and legislation are integral elements in social protection, particularly the latter since it empowers marginalized populations through legislative standards such as labor laws. The International Labour Organization (2001) proposes that microinsurance is also a mechanism of social protection. The state is primarily responsible for developing and implementing the components mentioned above; nonetheless there are other actors involved in activities related to social protection such as international agencies, civil society groups, non-profit organizations (NGOs), employers' and workers' organizations, and private enterprises.

Policies and programs are considered a central part of social protection in terms of delivering supports and services to minimize vulnerabilities and eliminate risks that if not addressed could lead to poverty or further entrench those already poor. Ortiz (2001) proposes five key activities linked to social protection, including:

1   labor market policies and programs facilitating labor market stabilization and adjustments;
2   social insurance programs buffering against livelihood risks connected to unemployment, illness, and work-related injuries;
3   social assistance and services providing a floor of basic needs for vulnerable populations lacking any means of support;
4   agricultural insurance buffering against risks such as crop failure or disruptions; and
5   social funds and employment programs at the community level offering short-term opportunities for individuals to earn an income.

Devereux and Sabates-Wheeler (2004) identify four sets of social protection interventions with respect to policies and programs, which include the following: protective measures that buffer against deprivation; preventive measures that avert deprivation; promotive measures that enhance human development; and transformative measures that address human rights issues of social equity and exclusion. Ortiz (2001) states that "social protection should therefore be seen as one of several measures that work together to promote socially inclusive human development" (p. 58). Overall, social protection is concerned with risks and vulnerabilities that impact human development and therefore encompasses a multidimensional approach to protect individuals and households from shocks, stresses, and deprivation through an array of interventions to enhance livelihood security, social inclusion, and above all human dignity.

Defining social development

Social development is first and foremost a developmental perspective that is concerned with both people's well-being and progressive social change. As a theory and an approach that is widely applied today by international agencies such as the United Nations, World Bank, and the International Monetary Fund as well as countries in the Global South and Global North, social development has its roots in social welfare programs and policies that were used by British bureaucrats in

Africa during the early to mid 20th century to improve education levels, health, and livelihoods through community and economic development (Midgley, 1995). Although social development has evolved over the decades, interconnecting social and economic systems to improve people's well-being continues to be a prominent feature of this perspective (Elliott, 1993; Gray, 2006; Lunt, 2009; Midgley, 2014). Midgley (1995) states that "Social development cannot take place without economic development and economic development is meaningless unless it is accompanied by improvements in the social welfare for the population as whole" (p. 23). Thus, social development and economic development are both essential in order to elevate people's welfare and foster structural change in society.

Presently, there is no universal definition of social development. Nonetheless, there are several notable components of social development that are identified in the academic literature. One important aspect of social development is that it is a process (Cetingok & Rogge, 2006; Midgley, 1995; 2014; Mosher, 1979; Paiva, 1977; Remion, 1995). According to Cetingok and Rogge (2006), social development is a "multifaceted process" that involves distributing resources, including economic, social, and environmental, in equitable and sustainable ways (p. 10). Midgley views planned actions and activities as part of the process of social development (Midgley, 1995), which involves the implementation of policies and practices at micro and macro levels (Midgley, 2010). The developmental process of integrating social and economic systems aims to improve the living standards of individuals, households, and communities. Another critical component of social development is that it is concerned with outcomes. Improving the well-being of people and society is an outcome of social development (Cox & Pawar, 2006; Gray, 2006; Midgley, 1995, 2014; Mosher, 1979; Omer, 1979; Paiva, 1977). Cetingok and Rogge (2006) explain that the outcome of social development is "defined as the existence of a developed state of human well-being in the political, civil, social, economic, and environmental dimensions of life in a nation" (p. 10). The social development perspective recognizes that not only people's basic needs must be met but also their full potential realized. At the United Nation's World Summit for Social Development in Copenhagen in 1995, governments from around the world acknowledged the necessity of social development to address people's needs and aspirations as well as to take action against extreme poverty, social injustices, and social inequalities (United Nations, 1995). The Copenhagen Declaration of Social Development recognizes that social development is people-centered development. With a broad framework for action, the Declaration has a number of commitments, which include: ensuring an enabling environment in all dimensions (e.g., economic, political, social, cultural, and legal); eradicating poverty; promoting full employment and sustainable livelihoods for men and women; promoting social integration and human rights; achieving gender equality and equity; and attaining universal education and health care (United Nations, 1995). As a people-centered approach, social development requires a multifaceted approach in terms of utilizing a variety of strategies alongside designing and implementing policies and programs to meet people's needs, to promote people's aspirations, and uphold people's dignity.

A myriad of approaches are employed under the umbrella of social development through policies, programs, and initiatives. One approach is social investment that provides support and inputs for individuals and households to build their capacities and skills in order to participate in the labor market. Gray (2010) states that social investment is strengthened by financial resources such as microcredit and microfinance, defining the former as "small loans to help the poor engage in productive activities or businesses" and the latter as "microcredit plus other financial products, including savings, remittances and insurance designed for use by the poor" (p. 466). Small businesses owned and operated by individuals or groups of people who are poor are known as microenterprises (Midgley, 2008). These businesses are generally sponsored by nonprofit organizations that provide microcredit, expertise, and support to business owners. The Grameen Bank in Bangladesh, the Bangladesh Rural Advancement Committee (BRAC) also in Bangladesh, and the Self-Employed Women's Association (SEWA) Bank in India are just a few examples of innovative organizations that provide microcredit and microfinance to people in poverty, particularly women, to help them become self-employed, to provide livelihood security, and to help build their assets. Furthermore, asset development is another function of social development. Through asset-building programs, people living in poverty have the opportunity and support to accumulate resources at market value. Midgley (2014) explains that asset building for the poor allows them to "store or stock … resources which can be utilized in the future" (p. 156). Asset development contributes to a level of financial security by providing protection against risks, shocks, or stress from natural disasters, loss of livelihoods, or illnesses. For social development there is no one approach but rather a number of different approaches to consider for designing and implementing policies and programs that are contextually appropriate (e.g., economic, social, political, cultural, and environmental). Social development needs to be practiced locally, regionally, nationally, and internationally as it involves structural changes at the micro, mezzo, and macro level. Cox and Pawar (2006) suggest that social development also involves different sectors of society, including: individual/family/community sector; the civil society sector; the corporate sector; and the state sector. Too often development initiatives by governments, international agencies, and NGOs are viewed as a way to "'develop' other people" rather than a way to engage in a participatory practice working collaboratively with individuals, groups, and communities with space for them to voice their needs, develop a shared vision, discover solutions together, and become empowered as a result (Global Agenda for Social Work and Social Development, 2014, p. 7). Social development cannot be narrowly defined but as Remion (1995) states, "in its broadest and richest sense," social development "[reconciles] the social and economic aspects, and [re-invents] the relationship between humans and their own selves, between humans and others and between humans and their environment" (p. 296).

Defining sustainable development

In the 1960s, the concept of "sustainable development" was first suggested in Rachel Carson's published study *Silent Spring* that interlinked the environment, economy, and social well-being (International Institute for Sustainable Development, 2012). Nonetheless, it is the 1987 report of the World Commission on Environment and Development, commonly known as the Brundtland Commission, in which the definition of "sustainable development" became internationally recognized and often referenced. The World Commission on Environment and Development (1987) defines sustainable development as "[meeting] the needs of the present without compromising the ability of future generations to meet their own needs" (p. 43). The World Commission on Environment and Development (1987) also postulates that sustainability ought to be part of both developed and developing countries' economic and social development objectives. Kates, Parris, and Leiserowitz (2005) describe sustainable development as a way to "preserve the basic life support systems of the planet" within the demand of development goals (p. 20). Similarly, Barker (2003) asserts that sustainable development occurs when economic well-being is achieved while maintaining the environment. Grist (2008) explains that issues around intergenerational equity along with concerns regarding environmental degradation have been a focus of mainstream sustainable development, while at the same time incorporating solutions for environmental change based on technology and the market economy. Over the last two decades, the idea of sustainable development has been redefined, adapted, and expanded upon; yet, there is no universally accepted definition (United Nations Conference on Sustainable Development, 2012a). With that said, the concept of sustainable development is widely accepted around the globe by governments, scientists, academics, international agencies, and civil society groups.

At the core of sustainable development is the concern with social well-being, particularly basic needs, equity for all (Holden, Linnerud, & Banister, 2014) and economic growth (Kates et al., 2005), in relation to the physical environment in order to preserve and sustain it for the long term. Thus, the social, economic, and environmental dimensions are central to the framework for sustainable development (Peeters, 2012; Rogers, Jalal, & Boyd, 2006; Zaccai, 2012). Although these three pillars are important for framing the sustainable development approach, it is important to also consider sustainable development as an ongoing process encompassing change, growth, and renewal (Estes, 1993; Newman, 2006; Rogers et al., 2006). Estes (1993) explains that the process that occurs within sustainable development is the "means of practice" (p. 12). According to Estes (1993) the practice within sustainable development involves development interventions at institutional levels, including micro, mezzo, and macro, which support and improve human well-being while sustaining the physical environment. For Kates et al. (2005) sustainable development practice entails more than interventions. These authors state (2005):

> The practice includes the many efforts at defining the concept, establishing goals, creating indicators, and asserting values. But additionally, it includes

developing social movements, organizing institutions, crafting sustainability science and technology, and negotiating the grand compromise among those who are principally concerned with nature and environment, those who value economic development, and those who are dedicated to improving the human condition.

(pp. 17–18)

Sustainable development requires the collective action of all.

The concept of the Sustainable Development Goals (SDGs) is part of sustainable practice in international and local development. In 2012, the United Nations Conference on Sustainable Development, commonly referred to as Rio+20, was held in Rio Janeiro, Brazil. What emerged from Rio+20 was a sustainable development policy framework called "The Future We Want," which included the recognition and commitment to developing and implementing SDGs in order to build upon the Millennium Development Goals (MDGs), which have a target date of 2015 (United Nations Conference on Sustainable Development, 2012b). In January 2013, a working group, appointed by the United Nations General Assembly, was established to propose a set of specific sustainable development goals (United Nations Department of Economic and Social Affairs, 2014). The 30-member Open Working Group, in July 2014, submitted to the General Assembly 17 proposed goals with 169 targets addressing social, economic, political, and environmental issues for all people, including: ending poverty; ending hunger, achieving food security, and promoting sustainable agriculture; ensuring water and sanitation; ensuring health and well-being; achieving gender equity and empowering women and girls; ensuring quality education and learning opportunities; ensuring affordable and sustainable energy; promoting sustainable economic growth and decent work; building sustainable and innovative industry sectors; reducing inequality in and between countries; ensuring sustainable consumption and production; combating climate change and its impacts; conserving oceans and sustainable use of marine biodiversity; protecting and restoring terrestrial ecosystems; promoting peace, providing access to justice, and accountable institutions; and strengthening global partnership for implementing and achieving sustainable development (United Nations Department of Economic and Social Affairs, 2014). Ultimately, the SDGs are a framework for purposeful planning and implementation of policies, programs, and projects at regional, national, and international levels to enhance social well-being and economic development while at the same time not only protecting the physical environment for future generations but addressing present environmental issues and challenges.

Defining livelihoods

For millions of people around the world, a livelihood is a vital part of their life that allows them to earn an income, meet basic needs, build assets and investments, and engage in work that is both professionally and personally fulfilling. A livelihood in simple terms is a way for people to make a living (Chambers & Conway,

1991). It is a way to secure the means to provide for life's basic necessities such as food, clothing, and shelter for one's self and household. Midgley (2014) suggests that livelihoods do not only entail economic activities but also non-productive activities such as caring for children, older people, and relatives as well as creating social bonds. Livelihoods approaches are commonly practiced in the development sector by international agencies, governments, particularly in the Global South, and local NGOs to address issues such as poverty, sustainability, and well-being. Assets are a component of livelihoods. They can be material or non-material, including: financial, social, institutional, or physical resources (Ting, 2013; United Nations Development Programme & International Recovery Platform, 2010). Ting (2013) states that "assets can enhance efforts to maintain resources and can be used to develop other forms of assets" (p. 191). Assets assist individuals and households in establishing, maintaining, diversifying, and protecting their livelihoods. Another important component is livelihoods strategies that look at how individuals and households organize and use their assets as well as what types of activities they engage in to make a living. In Scoones's (1998) analysis of rural livelihoods, the author identified three common strategies of households, including: agricultural intensification/extensification, livelihood diversification, and migration. Heltberg, Siegel, and Jorgensen (2009) note that livelihood strategies such as "employment generation, asset transfers and asset building, livestock restocking, seed transfers, training and skills development, micro finance initiatives, and more orderly migration and access to safe and easy remittances" require a social protection approach and multi-sector support (p. 97). Finally, livelihoods are situated in economic, social, political, cultural, and environmental contexts. These dynamic contexts either contribute to opportunities to boost individuals and households' livelihoods or constraints that inhibit their growth (Sabates-Wheeler & Devereux, 2011; United Nations Development Programme & International Recovery Platform, 2010).

Since the 1980s, the sustainable livelihoods approach has informed development discourse, which has recognized that livelihoods are a major component in poverty reduction. The sustainable livelihoods approach is concerned with factors and processes, including economic, social, and environmental, that affect people's livelihoods and ultimately their quality of life. Lawrence (2012) states that even though economic development is an important component in the sustainable livelihoods approach, structural barriers also need to be addressed in order to improve the quality of people's lives. Chambers and Conway (1991) define a livelihood as sustainable when it can "cope with and recover from stress and shocks, maintain or enhance its capabilities and assets, and provide sustainable livelihood opportunities for the next generation" (p. 6). For people living in poverty, their ability (in terms of what they have for assets and means) to manage risk and/or recovery from any stress, shock, or crisis, is minimal. Heltberg et al. (2009) explain that climate change can have a significant impact on people living in poverty, particularly those whose livelihoods rely on agriculture, livestock, and fisheries, since their capacity to manage risk is severely inhibited by impoverishment, leaving them vulnerable to the effects of climate change. As a development approach, sustainable livelihoods incorporate a number of components such as adaptive strategies and technologies, community resources, cross-sector policies, and institutional investments to not only improve people's livelihoods but also to achieve sustainable development (International Institute for Sustainable Development, n.d.). The sustainable livelihoods approach interconnects livelihoods, poverty, and ecology emphasizing the need to consider different solutions for livelihoods that depend on natural resources in order to sustain the environment in the short term as well as for the long term (Scoones, 1998; World Commission on Environment and Development, 1987). Interventions are an integral aspect of the sustainable livelihoods approach consisting of protective (providing basic needs), preventive (guarding against asset loss), and promotion measures (developing abilities, capabilities, and assets) (Davies, Béné, Arnall, Tanner, Newsham, & Coirolo, 2013; Sabates-Wheeler & Devereux, 2011; United Nations Development Programme & International Recovery Platform, 2010). Scoones (1998) provides five indicators of the sustainable livelihoods framework, including:

1   creation of working days;
2   poverty reduction;
3   well-being and capabilities;
4   livelihood adaptation, vulnerability, and resilience; and
5   natural resource base sustainability.

These five indicators summarize the broad objectives of the sustainable livelihoods approach that aim to reduce poverty through creating work opportunities to increase people's resiliency and capacities as well as improve well-being, while sustaining the environment.

Although sustainable livelihoods continue to be an important approach, the issue of decent work has become an increasingly prominent topic, specifically in the global conversation of the post-2015 development agenda. According to the International Labour Organization (2013) the annual increase for the world's labor force in 2030 will likely average to 31 million per year. The International Labour Organization (2013) states that in order "to keep pace with the growth of the world's labour force, some 470 million new jobs will be needed over the fifteen-year period from 2016 to 2030" (p. 2). It is not enough for an individual to just have a "job," his or her economic participation needs to be "meaningful, remunerative, and satisfying" (Midgley & Conley, 2010, p. 200). The United Nations Development Group (2013) points out that the issue of jobs was raised consistently throughout its consultations with different nations around the world. Building on the MDGs, the International Labour Organization (2013) proposes several potential targets for the post-development 2015 development goals, including: improved livelihoods for those individuals and households most vulnerable; increased portion of "good jobs"; increased economic participation of women and youth; and coverage of social protection floor. As mentioned previously, the Open Working Group's 17 proposed SDGs include a target (goal 8) that is to "promote sustained, inclusive and sustainable economic growth, full and productive employment and decent work for all" (United Nations Department of Economic and Social Affairs, 2014, p. 10). Having a goal that directly commits to sustainable and decent employment for all requires social and economic policies that support livelihood capabilities through infrastructure and services, prioritize the needs of vulnerable populations in terms of assets and access, and increase resiliency by addressing micro and macro shocks and stresses (Chambers & Conway, 1991).

Defining gender

In the 20th century, it was common in Western societies to dress newborn babies in ascribed colors – blue for boys and pink for girls. Even though this tradition is no longer followed as strictly as it once was, there remain socially prescribed ideas and beliefs about what it means to be a man and a woman. This is known as gender. Drolet and Heinonen (2012) define gender as "the social, behavioural and cultural attributes, expectations and forms associated with being a woman or a man" (p. 76). Others, similarly, refer to gender as the social norms, practices, opportunities, and institutions that determine men apart from women and how they relate to one another (Hannan, 2001; United Nations Department of Economic and Social Affairs, 2008). Gender is not biologically determined but rather it is socially constructed (Food and Agriculture Organization, 1997). Therefore, the sex categories of "male" and "female" should not be confused with gender categories of "man/masculine" and "woman/feminine" (Drolet & Heinonen, 2012; Whitehead, Talahite, & Moodley, 2013; World Health Organization, 2014). The Food and Agriculture Organization (1997) points out that as a principle, gender not only organizes societies but directs such processes as production, reproduction, consumption, and distribution. Gender has several correlating components. Gender identity refers to how a man or a woman understands himself or herself in regard to a "sex" context or a "gendered" context. Drolet and Heinonen (2012) assert that gender identity is a contested notion since many individuals relate to being on a "gender spectrum" not necessarily as a man or a woman but rather identifying as third gender, two-spirited, trans, transgender, transsexual, intersex, or cross-dresser. In addition, Sullivan (2005) notes that gender identity is not static but rather a dynamic concept since individuals may or may not conform to society's prescribed view of it. Gender roles are the social expectations of men's and women's behavior, attitudes, aspirations, and responsibilities in the household, in the community, and in the society. Drolet and Heinonen (2012) explain that "in some cultures, these roles are sharply defined and differentiated. Gender roles may restrict women and men in terms of certain tasks, jobs, opportunities or spaces" (p. 76). Gender roles are linked to gender relations in that they affect the relationship between women and men. Thus, gender relations describe the way in which men and women relate to and interact with one another based on social norms. The United Nations Department of Economic and Social Affairs (2008) state that the social system of gender relations can also be called gender order determining "what is accepted, encouraged and allowed for women and men" (p. 4). Connell (2009) states that gender relations are not only direct interactions between men and women but also are indirect interactions that occur through other sources such as the market and technologies (e.g., the media or Internet).

Gender roles and gender relations cannot be discussed without understanding gender equality, gender equity, and gender inequality. Gender equality refers to an equal power relation between women and men. Furthermore, gender equality exists when women and men are equally valued and have equal rights, responsibilities, and access to resources and opportunities (Drolet & Heinonen, 2012). Gender equality is not only a "women's issue" but rather it concerns both women and men as a human rights issue (Hannan, 2001; United Nations Department of Economic and Social Affairs, 2008). Gender equity differs from gender equality in that it recognizes that the needs and interests of women and men are different, and therefore, its aim is not to create equal opportunities but rather redistribute power and resources to benefit both genders and in the process transform society (Drolet & Heinonen, 2012). Gender inequality describes a structured power differential between women and men – typically in the form of men exerting power over women with respect to roles, responsibilities, opportunities, and resources. Women encounter many disadvantages and discrimination in a number of areas such as political systems, health services, education, legal systems, social institutions, and labor markets. An element of gender inequality is gender gaps in the labor market, which denote the disadvantages that women experience compared to men. The International Labour Organization (2012) states that women have historically experienced more disadvantages in the labor market compared to men, particularly in terms of unemployment, noting that before the 2007 financial crisis the gender gap in unemployment for a five-year period was on average 0.5 percentage points; whereas by 2011 the gap increased to 0.7 percentage points with female unemployment at 6.4% and male unemployment at 5.7%. The current projections show high unemployment rates for females to at least 2017, if not past (International Labour Organization, 2012).

To close the gender gap between women and men, not only in the labor market but in other areas (e.g., education, health services, political system, etc.), gender issues have to be part of the discussion at local, regional, and international levels with commitments from governments, international agencies, and civil society groups to implement policies and practices to dismantle oppressive social structures that contribute to inequalities and inequities, particularly those faced by women. This requires an intersectional approach recognizing that gender oppression is experienced differently from one woman to another due to such factors as race, ethnicity, class, disability, and sexual orientation (Dominelli, 2011; Sullivan, 2005). Additionally, gender mainstreaming is a strategy that "[brings] the perceptions, experience, knowledge and interests of women as well as men to bear on policy-making, planning and decision-making" to create structural change for gender equality (Hannan, 2001). The MDGs' third goal, which is to promote gender equality and empower women, demonstrates a concerted effort at the international level to achieve equitable change for women and men with respect to roles, responsibilities, and opportunities. A target of this goal is to eliminate gender disparity in primary and secondary education by 2005, and in all education levels by 2015 (United Nations, n.d.). According to the United Nations (n.d.), equality in primary education between girls and boys has been globally achieved; however, few countries have attained gender parity at all levels of education. Thus, further progress is required in order to empower women and achieve gender equality post-2015. United Nations Women (2013) proposes an integrated approach for the post-2015 development framework and SDGs to address gender equality, women's rights, and women's empowerment in three target areas, including: freedom from violence; capabilities and resources; and voice, participation, and leadership. Building upon the third goal of the MDGs, the Open Working Group has put forward sustainable development goal five, which is to "achieve gender equality and empower all women and girls" (United Nations Department of Economic and Social Affairs, 2014, p. 8). This goal includes six targets:

1   ending all forms of discrimination against women and girls;
2   eliminating all forms of violence against women and girls;
3   eliminating harmful social and cultural practices;
4   recognizing women's paid and non-paid work through public service, infrastructure, and social protection policies;
5   ensuring women's full participation in political, economic, and public life; and
6   ensuring universal access to sexual and reproductive health, and reproductive rights (United Nations Department of Economic and Social Affairs, 2014).

Meeting these six targets, to achieve gender equality and empowerment for women and girls, requires transformative change within households, communities, and societies around the world.

Defining poverty

As a social concern, there has not been a topic so extensively studied as poverty. Academics, policymakers, and practitioners, in a number of different fields such as economics, sociology, healthcare, social work, and development, have sought to understand its nature and those issues directly and indirectly related to it. In the last 50 years, in particularly, there has been a major push to comprehensively research poverty as well as design and implement policies and programs that not only reduce poverty but eliminate it. Poverty occurs in rural and urban areas in countries in the Global North and Global South, making it a worldwide phenomenon (Cobbinah, Black, & Thwaites, 2013; United Nations, 1995). Currently 2.2 billion people are either precariously close to becoming poor or are living in a state of poverty (United Nations Development Programme, 2014). In addition, one in eight people, worldwide, suffer from undernourishment (Food and

Agriculture Organization, World Food Programme, & International Fund for Agricultural Development, 2012). Most regions around the world continue to experience the effects of the 2007–08 economic crisis, including unemployment and job gaps (e.g., those outside of the labor market who are discouraged from the lack of employment opportunities). For example 31.8 million more people were unemployed in 2013 than prior to the financial crisis (International Labour Organization, 2014). Food insecurity, unemployment, and job gaps are just a few issues among a number of poverty-related dimensions. Despite an abundance of knowledge regarding poverty and issues related to it, there is no universal definition for the term (Akindola, 2009; Cobbinah et al., 2013; Misturelli & Heffernan, 2010; United Nations Economic and Social Council, 2001b). Poverty is commonly described as deprivation. This could be related to barriers to knowledge resulting in illiteracy; low quality of life from malnutrition, unsafe water, unsanitary conditions, and barriers to services; and finally vulnerability to morbidity and premature death (Sen, 1999; United Nations Development Programme, 1997).

Although there is little consensus concerning the meaning of poverty, there are several widely applied perspectives. The economic or income-based perspective has been a favorable approach for decades, viewing poverty in terms of economic well-being whereby an individual and/or household lacks financial means or has insufficient purchasing power for a minimum basket of goods and services (Akindola, 2009; Calvo, Das Gupta, Grootaert, Kanbur, Kwakwa, & Lusting, 2000; United Nations Economic and Social Council, 2001b; Wagle, 2002; White, 2009). Absolute poverty refers to an abject condition in which a person is unable to meet his or her basic needs such as food, shelter, clothing, safe water, sanitation, and education for a minimum standard required to survive (Cox & Pawar, 2006; United Nations, 1995; United Nations Development Programme, 1997; Wagle, 2002; White, 2009). Relative poverty indicates a minimum level of income and/or consumption that is compared to the national standard or societal norms (Sachs, 2005; Sen, 1979; Wagle, 2002; White, 2009). Chronic poverty differs from both absolute and relative notions in that it is not concerned with a minimum standard but rather looks at the duration and dynamics of poverty for individuals and households (Hulme & Shepherd, 2003). Cox and Pawar (2006) explain that chronic poverty is the condition whereby individuals are born into poverty and likely to die impoverished or through a life-altering situation they are no longer able to provide for themselves and family. Sen (1999) proposes that poverty is a matter of capability deprivation, which is not only affected by income but also by other factors that inhibit human capabilities. From the capability approach, poverty refers to the deficiency of capabilities to function and/or the lack of opportunity to function with respect to "being well nourished, being adequately clothed and sheltered and avoiding preventable morbidity, to more complex social achievements such as partaking in the life of the community" (United Nations Development Programme, 1997, p. 16). The feminization of poverty perspective draws attention to gender-related issues regarding poverty such as the disproportionate burden women and girls bear in relation to poverty (United Nations, 1995; United Nations Economic and Social Council, 2001b). Medeiros and Costa (2008) define the feminization of poverty as "a change in poverty levels that is biased against women or female-headed households" (p. 1). Understanding the linkages of poverty to potentially vulnerable groups, including, women, children, older people, people with disabilities, indigenous populations, and ethnic minority groups, is critical to grappling the complexities of poverty. The multidimensional perspective is an encompassing approach to poverty that considers multiple deprivations in addition to income insufficiency (Calvo et al., 2000; United Nations Development Programme, 1997). The United Nations's World Summit for Social Development report suggests the following:

> Poverty has various manifestations, including lack of income and productive resources sufficient to ensure sustainable livelihoods; hunger and malnutrition; ill health; limited or lack of access to education and other basic services; increased morbidity and mortality from illness; homelessness and inadequate housing; unsafe environments; and social discrimination and exclusion. It is also characterized by a lack of participation in decision-making and in civil, social and cultural life.
>
> (United Nations, 1995, p. 41)

With the multidimensional perspective, poverty has many dimensions that cannot be overlooked. Moreover, an intersectoral approach is necessary in order to address poverty-related dimensions in the context of the individual, community, region, or nation.

There are a number of measurements that communicate different statistical information on poverty. The most commonly used measurement is the poverty-line that indicates an income shortfall (Sen, 1979); in other words, those individuals and households that fall below the standardized cut-off for income or consumption (Calvo et al., 2000). Another measurement is the poverty headcount that calculates the percentage of the population below the poverty-line (White, 2009). The poverty gap is similar to the poverty headcount in that it is concerned with the poverty-line but the former calculates the average distance of the poor from the income cut-off (Calvo et al., 2000). Even though these measurements provide important information regarding poverty rates among populations and countries, they focus on economic well-being. Therefore, other types of tools are necessary to gain further insight into people's lived experience with poverty such as the United Nations Development Programme's Multidimensional Poverty Index (MPI) that identifies interrelated deprivations at the household level with human development indicators – health, education, and living standards, to show the average of those who are multidimensional poor and the deprivations that they have to contend with (United Nations Development Programme, n.d.).

Poverty may not have a universal definition, yet there is overwhelmingly global agreement that it must be eradicated. In 2000, international agencies, civil society groups, and governments from the Global South and Global North committed to the MDGs. The first goal, out of eight, is to eradicate extreme poverty and hunger by 2015. Although this goal has not been achieved to date, one of its targets has been met when in 2010 the global poverty rate of $1.25 per day fell to less than half the rate in 1990 with 700 million fewer people living in conditions of extreme poverty (United Nations, n.d.). There is global recognition that there is more work to be done in terms of ending poverty, which is why the Open Working Group has proposed that the first goal of the SDGs is to "end poverty in all its forms everywhere" (United Nations Department of Economic and Social Affairs, 2014, p. 5). This goal applies a multidimensional approach to eradicating poverty with targets such as implementing social protection systems and floors; ensuring equal access to economic resources and basic services; reducing environmental vulnerabilities, shocks, and stresses; and creating policies at all levels of government based on pro-poor and gender-sensitive strategies for development (United Nations Department of Economic and Social Affairs, 2014). Wagle (2009) states it well when he says "Human beings do not just want to survive, as the 'bare subsistence' or the minimum food calorie concepts suggest; they want to live qualitatively better lives with dignity" (p. 162). An integral part of any concept of poverty must champion a dignified and better quality of life for all people.

Conclusion

In this chapter a number of key concepts, terms, and definitions are presented to clarify the meanings and understandings, and their implications for social protection. Many of the concepts remind us of the integration between the social, economic, and environmental dimensions of well-being. This is evident in terms such as sustainable development, livelihoods and sustainable livelihoods, and poverty. Social development, itself, is widely understood to have linkages with economic development. According to Mkandawire (2004), "one factor accounting for the increasing recognition of the important role of social policy has been the persistence of poverty even in situations of economic success" (p. 8). The eradication of poverty requires a multidimensional approach that considers the interrelationship between the social, economic, and environmental spheres. Further progress is required in order to empower women and achieve gender equality post-2015. The chapters in this volume clearly elaborate the case that social policy can work together with economic policy to foster social development. New approaches in social protection contribute to the evolution of key terms and concepts based on practice and policy implementation.

References

Akindola, R.B. (2009). Towards a definition of poverty: Poor people's perspectives and implications for poverty reduction. *Journal of Developing Societies, 25,* 121–150.
Barker, R.L. (2003). *The social work dictionary* (5th ed.). Washington, DC: NASW Press.

Calvo, C.M., Das Gupta, M., Grootaert, C., Kanbur, R., Kwakwa, V., & Lustig, N. (2000). *World development report 2000/2001: Attacking poverty*. Washington, DC: World Bank. Retrieved from http://documents.worldbank.org/curated/en/2000/09/1740 8018/world-development-report-20002001-attacking-poverty.

Cetingok, M., & Rogge, M. (2006). Democratic models and social development. *Social Development Issues, 28*(3), 1–15.

Chambers, R., & Conway, G.R. (1991). *Sustainable rural livelihoods: Practical concepts for the 21st century* (IDS Discussion Paper 296). Brighton: Institute of Development Studies. Retrieved from http://opendocs.ids.ac.uk/opendocs/bitstream/handle/123456 789/775/Dp296.pdf?sequence=1.

Cobbinah, P.B., Black, R., & Thwaites, R. (2013). Dynamics of poverty in developing countries: Review of poverty reduction approaches. *Journal of Sustainable Development, 6*, 25–35.

Connell, R.W. (2009) *Gender (Polity short introductions)*. Cambridge: Polity Press.

Conway, T., de Haan, A., & Norton, A. (Eds.) (2000). *Social protection: New directions of donor agencies*. London: Department for International Development. Retrieved from www.odi.org/sites/odi.org.uk/files/odi-assets/publications-opinion-files/2233.pdf.

Cox, D., & Pawar, M. (2006). *International social work: Issues, strategies, and programs*. Thousand Oaks: Sage.

Davies, M., Béné, C., Arnall, A., Tanner, T., Newsham, A., & Coirolo, C. (2013). Promoting resilient livelihoods through adaptive social protection: Lessons from 124 programmes in South Asia. *Development Policy Review, 31*, 27–58.

Devereux, S., & Sabates-Wheeler, R. (2004). *Transformative social protection* (IDS Working Paper 232). Brighton: Institute of Development Studies. Retrieved from www.ids.ac.uk/files/dmfile/Wp232.pdf.

Dominelli, L. (2011). Claiming women's place in the world: Social workers' roles in eradicating gender inequalities. In L.M. Healy & R.J. Link (Eds.), *Handbook of international social work: Human rights, development, and the global profession* (pp. 249–253). New York: Oxford University Press.

Drolet, J., & Heinonen, T. (2012). Gender concepts and controversies. In T. Heinonen & J. Drolet (Eds.), *International social development: Social work experiences and perspectives* (pp. 75–97). Halifax: Fernwood Publishing.

Elliott, D. (1993). Social work and social development: Towards an integrative model for social work practice. *International Social Work, 36*, 21–36.

Estes, R.J. (1993). Toward sustainable development: From theory to praxis. *Social Development Issues, 15*(3), 1–29.

Food and Agriculture Organization. (1997). *Gender: The key to sustainability and food security*. Rome: Food and Agriculture Organization. Retrieved from ftp://ftp.fao.org/docrep/fao/010/w4430e/w4430e00.pdf.

Food and Agriculture Organization, World Food Program, & International Fund for Agricultural Development. (2012). *The state of food insecurity in the world 2012: Economic growth is necessary but not sufficient to accelerate reduction of hunger and malnutrition*. Rome: FAO. Retrieved from www.fao.org/docrep/016/i3027e/i3027e.pdf.

Gentilini, U., & Were Omamo, S. (2011). Social protection 2.0: Exploring issues, evidence and debates in a globalizing world. *Food Policy, 36*, 329–340.

Global Agenda for Social Work and Social Development. (2014). First report: Promoting social and economic equalities. *International Social Work, 57*, 3–16.

Gray, M. (2006). The progress of social development in South Africa. *International Journal of Social Welfare, 15*(Suppl. 1), S53–S64.

Gray, M. (2010). Social development and the status quo: Professionalization and Third Way co-optation. *International Journal of Social Welfare, 19*, 463–470.

Grist, N. (2008). Positioning climate change in sustainable development discourse [Special issue]. *Journal of International Development, 20*, 783–803.

Hannan, C. (2001). *Gender mainstreaming: Strategy for promoting gender equality.* Retrieved from www.un.org/womenwatch/osagi/pdf/factsheet1.pdf.

Heltberg, R., Siegel, P.B., & Jorgensen, S.L. (2009). Addressing human vulnerability to climate change: Toward a "no-regrets" approach. *Global Environmental Change, 19*, 89–99.

Holden, E., Linnerud, K., & Banister, D. (2014). Sustainable development: Our common future revisited. *Global Environmental Change, 26*, 130–139.

Hulme, D., & Shepherd, A. (2003). Conceptualizing chronic poverty. *World Development, 31*, 403–423.

International Institute for Sustainable Development. (n.d.). *Sustainable livelihoods.* Retrieved from www.iisd.org/economics/poverty/livelihoods.asp.

International Institute for Sustainable Development. (2012). *Sustainable development timeline.* Retrieved from www.iisd.org/pdf/2012/sd_timeline_2012.pdf.

International Labour Organization. (2001). *Social security: A new consensus.* Geneva: International Labour Office. Retrieved from www.ilo.org/wcmsp5/groups/public/--ed_protect/--soc_sec/documents/publication/wcms_209311.pdf.

International Labour Organization. (2011). *Social protection floor for a fair and inclusive globalization.* Geneva: International Labour Office. Retrieved from www.ilo.org/wcmsp5/groups/public/--dgreports/--dcomm/--publ/documents/publication/wcms_165750.pdf.

International Labour Organization. (2012). *Global employment trends for women.* Geneva: International Labour Office. Retrieved from www.ilo.org/wcmsp5/groups/public/--dgreports/--dcomm/documents/publication/wcms_195447.pdf.

International Labour Organization. (2013, May 20). *Jobs and livelihoods in the post-2015 development agenda: Meaningful ways to set targets and monitor progress* (ILO Concept Note No. 2). Retrieved from www.ilo.org/wcmsp5/groups/public/--dgreports/--dcomm/documents/genericdocument/wcms_213309.pdf.

International Labour Organization (2014). *Global employment trends 2014: Risk of a jobless recovery?* Geneva: International Labour Office. Retrieved from http://ilo.org/wcmsp5/groups/public/--dgreports/--dcomm/--publ/documents/publication/wcms_233953.pdf.

International Labour Organization & World Health Organization. (2009). *The social protection floor: A joint crisis initiative of the UN chief executive board for co-coordination on the social protection floor.* Retrieved from www.un.org/en/ga/second/64/socialprotection.pdf.

Kates, R.W., Parris, T.M., & Leiserowitz, A.A. (2005). What is sustainable development? *Environment, 47*(3), 8–21.

Lawrence, D. (2012). Sustainable livelihoods: Strategizing to improve lives. In T. Heinonen & J. Drolet (Eds.), *International social development: Social work experiences and perspectives* (pp. 98–120). Fernwood: Winnipeg.

Lunt, N. (2009). The rise of a "social development" agenda in New Zealand. *International Journal of Social Welfare, 18*, 3–12.

Medeiros, M., & Costa, J. (2008, July). *What do we mean by "feminization of poverty"?* (No. 58). International Poverty Centre for Inclusive Growth. Retrieved from www.ipc-undp.org/pub/IPCOnePager58.pdf.

Midgley, J. (1995). *Social development: The developmental perspective in social welfare.* London: Sage Publications.

Midgley, J. (2008). Microenterprise, global poverty and social development. *International Social Work*, *51*, 467–479.

Midgley, J. (2010). Global debates and the future of social development. *Social Work Researcher Practitioner*, *22*(1), 8–23.

Midgley, J. (2012). Social protection and social policy: Key issues and debates. *Journal of Policy Practice*, *11*, 8–24.

Midgley, J. (2014). *Social development: Theory and practice*. London: SAGE Publications.

Midgley, J. & Conley, A. (Eds.). (2010). *Social work and social development: Theories and skills for developmental social work*. New York: Oxford University Press.

Misturelli, F., & Heffernan, C. (2010). The concept of poverty: A synchronic perspective. *Progress in Development Studies*, *10*(1), 35–58.

Mkandawire, T. (2004). Social policy in a development context: Introduction. In T. Mkandawire (Ed.), *Social policy in a development context* (pp. 1–33). New York: Palgrave Macmillan.

Mosher, C.R. (1979). Social development: A process. *Journal of Social Welfare*, *6*(1), 21–26.

Newman, L. (2006). Change, uncertainty, and futures of sustainable development. *Futures*, *38*(5), 633–637.

Omer, S. (1979). Social development. *International Social Work*, *22*(3), 11–26.

Ortiz, I. (2001). ADB's social protection framework. In T. Conway, A. de Haan, & A. Norton (Eds.), *Social protection: New directions of donor agencies* (pp. 40–63). London: Department for International Development. Retrieved from www.odi.org/sites/odi.org.uk/files/odi-assets/publications-opinion-files/2233.pdf.

Paiva, J.F.X. (1977). A conception of social development. *Social Service Review*, *51*(2), 327–336. Retrieved from www.jstor.org/stable/30015486.

Peeters, J. (2012). The place of social work in sustainable development: Towards eco-social practice. *International Journal of Social Welfare*, *21*(3), 287–298.

Remion, G. (1995). Bases, objectives and dimensions of social development. *Scandinavian Journal of Social Welfare*, *4*(4), 290–297.

Roelen, K., & Devereux, S. (2013, July). *Promoting inclusive social protection in the post-2015 framework* (IDS Policy Briefing 39). Brighton: Institute of Development Studies. Retrieved from www.ids.ac.uk/files/dmfile/PB39.pdf.

Rogers, P.P., Jalal, K.F., & Boyd, J.A. (2006). *An introduction to sustainable development*. Cambridge, MA: Harvard University Press.

Sabates-Wheeler, R., & Devereux, S. (2007). Social protection for transformation. *IDS Bulletin*, *38*(3), 23–28.

Sabates-Wheeler, R., & Devereux, S. (2011). *Transforming livelihoods for resilient futures: How to facilitate graduation in social protection programmes* (CPS Working Paper 023). Future Agricultures Consortium. Retrieved from www.ids.ac.uk/publication/transforming-livelihoods-for-resilient-futures-how-to-facilitate-graduation-in-social-protection-programmes.

Sachs, J.D. (2005). *The end of poverty: Economic possibilities for our time*. New York: The Penguin Press.

Scoones, I. (1998). *Sustainable rural livelihoods: A framework for analysis* (IDS Working Paper 72). Brighton: Institute of Development Studies. Retrieved from www.ids.ac.uk/publication/sustainable-rural-livelihoods-a-framework-for-analysis.

Sen, A. (1979). Issues in the measurement of poverty. *Scandinavian Journal of Economics*, *81*(2), 285–307.

Sen, A. (1999). *Development as freedom.* New York: Anchor Books.

Social protection, poverty reduction and pro-poor growth. (2008). *OECD DAC Journal on Development, 9*(4), 33–54.

Standing, G. (2007). Social protection. *Development in Practice, 17*(4/5), 511–522.

Sullivan, N.E. (2005). Gender issues. In F.J. Turner, *Encyclopedia of Canadian social work* (pp. 159–161). Waterloo: Wilfrid Laurier University Press.

Ting, W.F. (2013). Asset building and livelihood rebuilding in post-disaster Sichuan, China. *China Journal of Social Work, 6*(2), 190–207.

United Nations. (n.d.). *We can end poverty: Millennium development goals and beyond 2015.* Retrieved from www.un.org/millenniumgoals/gender.shtml.

United Nations. (1995). *Report of the world summit for social development* (A/Conf. 166.9). Retrieved from http://daccess-dds-ny.un.org/doc/UNDOC/GEN/N95/116/51/PDF/N9511651.pdf?OpenElement.

United Nations Children's Fund. (2012). *Integrated social protection systems: Enhancing equity for children (Social Protection Strategic Framework).* New York: UNICEF. Retrieved from www.unicef.org/socialprotection/framework/files/UNICEF_Social_Protection_Strategic_Framework_full_doc_std%281%29.pdf.

United Nations Conference on Sustainable Development (RIO+20). (2012a). *Current ideas on sustainable development goals and indicators* (Issue Brief No. 6). Rio de Janeiro: UNCSD. Retrieved from www.uncsd2012.org/content/documents/218Issues%20Brief%206%20-%20SDGs%20and%20Indicators_Final%20Final%20clean.pdf.

United Nations Conference on Sustainable Development (RIO+20). (2012b).*The future we want* (A/CONF.216/L.1). Retrieved from https://rio20.un.org/sites/rio20.un.org/files/a-conf.216l-1_english.pdf.pdf.

United Nations Department of Economic and Social Affairs, Division for the Advancement of Women. (2008, December). *Women 2000 and beyond: The role of men and boys in achieving gender equality.* Retrieved from www.un.org/womenwatch/daw/public/w2000/W2000%20Men%20and%20Boys%20E%20web.pdf.

United Nations Department of Economic and Social Affairs, Division for Sustainable Development. (2014, July 19). *Outcome document: Open working group on sustainable development goals.* Retrieved from http://sustainabledevelopment.un.org/content/documents/4518SDGs_FINAL_Proposal%20of%20OWG_19%20July%20at%201320hrsver3.pdf.

United Nations Development Group. (2013). *The global conversation begins: Emerging views for a new development agenda.* Retrieved from www.worldwewant2015.org/the-global-conversation-begins.

United Nations Development Programme. (n.d.). *The multidimensional poverty index (MPI).* Retrieved from http://hdr.undp.org/en/content/multidimensional-poverty-index-mpi.

United Nations Development Programme. (1997). *Human development report 1997.* New York: Oxford University Press. Retrieved from http://hdr.undp.org/sites/default/files/reports/258/hdr_1997_en_complete_nostats.pdf.

United Nations Development Programme. (2014). *Human development report 2014.* New York: Oxford University Press. Retrieved from http://hdr.undp.org/sites/default/files/hdr14-report-en-1.pdf.

United Nations Development Programme & International Recovery Platform. (2010). *Guidance note on recovery: Livelihood.* Retrieved from www.unisdr.org/files/16771_16771guidancenoteonrecoveryliveliho.pdf.

United Nations Economic and Social Council. (2001a). *Enhancing social protection and reducing vulnerability in a globalizing world: Report of the Secretary-General* (E/CN.5/2001.2). Retrieved from http://daccess-dds-ny.un.org/doc/UNDOC/GEN/N00/792/23/PDF/N0079223.pdf?OpenElement.

United Nations Economic and Social Council. (2001b). *Substantive issues arising in the implementation of the International Covenant on Economic, Social, and Cultural Rights: Poverty and International Covenant on Economic, Social, and Cultural Rights* (E/C.12/2001/10). New York: United Nations. Retrieved from www2.ohchr.org/english/bodies/cescr/docs/statements/E.C.12.2001.10Poverty-2001.pdf.

United Nations Women. (2013). *A transformative stand-alone goal on achieving gender equality, women's rights and women's empowerment: Imperatives and components.* New York: UN Women. Retrieved from www.unwomen.org/en/what-we-do/~/media/F4AA23E30D8248B09A3E61283807A677.ashx.

Wagle, U. (2002). Rethinking poverty: Definition and measurement. *International Social Science Journal, 54,* 155–165.

White, H. (2009). *Poverty, global.* Princeton: Princeton University Press.

Whitehead, S., Talahite, A., & Moodley, R. (2013). *Gender and identity: Key themes and new directions.* Don Mills: Oxford University Press.

World Commission on Environment and Development. (1987). *Our common future.* Oxford: Oxford University Press.

World Health Organization (2014). *Gender, women and health.* Retrieved from www.who.int/gender/whatisgender/en/.

Zaccai, E. (2012). Over two decades in pursuit of sustainable development: Influence, transformations, limits. *Environmental Development, 1*(1), 79–90.

6 Adaptive social protection

Climate change adaptation and disaster risk reduction

Haorui Wu and Julie Drolet

Adaptive social protection

Within contemporary society, there are many challenges to sustainable development such as environmental degradation, natural and (hu)man-made disasters, poverty, inequities, global health threats, conflict and humanitarian crises (United Nations, 2015d). The Sustainable Development Goals (SDGs), building on the Millennium Development Goals (MDGs), provide an important framework for development (United Nations Development Program [UNDP], 2015). The international community has been increasingly recognizing that "social protection systems have the potential to shield people from multiple risks and stresses associated with climate change and degraded ecosystems, and help them in coping with structural transitions to more sustainable development patterns" (International Labour Organization, 2014, p. 2). Researchers at the Institute of Development Studies and United Kingdom Department for International Development created the term "adaptive social protection" in order to demonstrate that social protection can be adapted to ensure its contribution toward growth and development that it is "climate-and-disaster-resilient" (Vincent & Cull, 2012, p. 4).

As the first step of social protection systems (Social Protection Floor, 2009b), the social protection floor is nationally defined as a set of "basic social security guarantees" (International Labour Organization, n.d., para. 1), a "pivotal component of the sustainable and resilient growth strategy" (International Labour Organization, 2011, para. 3), and a "tool to accelerate the achievement of the Millennium Development Goals and promote social justice" (International Labour Organization, 2011, para. 3). The United Nations System Chief Executives Board for Coordination (UNCEB) defines the social protection floor as an approach that "promotes access to essential social security transfers and social services in the areas of health, water and sanitation, education, food, housing, life and asset-savings information" (International Labour Organization, 2009, para. 7). Universal minimum income security, especially for vulnerable populations, and access to universal healthcare are the guarantees that comprise the two pillars of the social protection floor (Social Protection Floor, 2009a). Hence, protecting all people's human rights of health care and basic income should be the essential guarantees with regard to adaptive social protection.

According to the United Nations Research Institute for Social Development, social protection "is concerned with preventing, managing, and overcoming situations that adversely affect people's well-being" (CIC Insurance Group, 2012, p. 4). The Governance Social Development Humanitarian Conflict (GSDRC), a partnership of international research institutes, think-tanks and consultancy organizations with expertise in the fields of social development and humanitarian conflict, illustrates that "social protection is concerned with protecting and helping those who are poor and vulnerable, such as children, women, older people, people living with disabilities, the displaced, the unemployed, and the sick" (GSDRC, n.d., para. 1).

Devereux and Sabates-Wheeler state that social protection comprises:

> All public and private initiatives that provide income or consumption transfers to the poor, protect the vulnerable against livelihood risks and enhance the social status and rights of the marginalised; with the overall objective of reducing the economic and social vulnerability of poor, vulnerable and marginalised groups.
>
> (Devereux & Sabates-Wheeler, 2004, p. i)

Climate change is causing an increase in the frequency and intensity of natural disasters (National Aeronautics and Space Administration, n.d.). The United Nations Office for Disaster Risk Reduction (2015) reported that a 10-year study, which was conducted after the 2005 Indian Ocean Tsunami, indicated that 87% of disasters worldwide were climate-related (para. 1). Natural disasters can change people's lives and disrupt everyday functioning by causing deaths, destroying infrastructure and resources, and increasing vulnerability. The UN's Open Working Group (OWG) on Sustainable Development Goals (SDGs) argues that climate change and sustainable development are always interwoven (Sustainable Development Knowledge Platform, 2013). Natural disasters can put social development and sustainable lifestyles in jeopardy. Helping rebuild lives, both physically and socially, from climate change's devastating effects is the main task that all nations worldwide need to confront and address. Thus, in the context of climate change, adaptive social protection plays a significant role in protecting peoples' rights and contributing to social development.

As one of the government policies aimed at sustainable development, social protection mainly concentrates on reducing poverty and vulnerability, underpinning inclusive and sustainable development (CIC Insurance Group, 2012). In addition to these goals, in the context of climate change and disaster, adaptive social protection focuses on how to reduce vulnerability and enhance resiliency, including environmental degradation, pollution and other extreme environmental and climate-related events. Thus, adaptive social protection is built on the overlap of these three dimensions: social protection, climate change adaptation and disasters risk reduction (Davies, Oswald, Mitchell, & Tanner, 2008, p. 11).

Therefore, adaptive social protection discussed in this chapter consists of the following aspects:

1   from the decision-making perspective, it is one of the government policies based on the national social protection floor;
2   it is adopted in the context of climate change and disaster;
3   the target group is all people who are affected by climate change and disasters, especially the vulnerable populations in the developing countries;
4   in addition to these objectives of reducing poverty and promoting human development, adaptive social protection specifically aims to reduce vulnerability, enhance resilience, and achieve sustainable development.

In this chapter, adaptive social protection is discussed as a government policy grounded in national social protection floors to protect citizens' basic human rights. The chapter begins with a macro-level perspective on how international initiatives such as the Sustainable Development Goals and the Post-2015 Development Agenda advance basic human rights in the context of climate change adaptation and disaster risk reduction to foster long-term sustainable development. Furthermore, during this process, how do social workers, who are trained to help people to build their social capacity, contribute to adaptive social protection strategies? Lastly, from a macro level, how do various organizations and nations worldwide implement adaptive social protection initiatives at home and abroad, to guarantee people's basic human rights and assist in building resilience?

Climate change, disasters and vulnerability

"Global warming will increase the variability of weather and most likely result in more extreme weather events" (Hoppe, n.d., para. 1). The World Bank's *2014 World Development Report* estimated that by 2030, damages, in regard to health, food security and physical environment, resultant of climate change would cost between US$2 trillion and US$4 trillion (World Bank, 2014b). Climate change has a long-term impact on both the natural and built environment (United States Environmental Protection Agency, n.d.b). Visible evidence of climate change includes the dramatic increase in the number of extreme weather events, such as tornados, typhoons, floods, droughts, outcomes of which possibly culminate as hazards, disasters and catastrophes. Natural and (hu)man-made disasters have multiple impacts in various arenas: physical, social, psychosocial, demographic, economic and political, such as death, grief and loss, displacement, financial loss and political disruption (Lindell, 2013). The negative influence of climate change and disaster is experienced by all nations. It is well-documented that the most vulnerable people, particularly older people (seniors), children, persons with disabilities, the less educated, minorities and low-income population groups suffer most from climate change and disasters (United Nations, 2015b). The poor within all nations, especially poor communities in developing countries or the Global South, suffer the most (United Nations, 2015b).

The influence of extreme weather events has already become an international concern that deprives people of their basic human right to food, clean water and safe residential places. This comprises a significant part of the work of human rights and adaptive social protection systems. For example, climate change contributes to hunger because of lowered crop production, which greatly contributes to the worsening of poverty in developing countries (Block, n.d.). The affected poor are required to put more time and energy into their farmlands than ever before but obtain less yield (Oxfam Canada, n.d.). The U.S. Department of Health and Human Service illustrates that climate change increases the frequency of climate-related and environment-related diseases, such as asthma, respiratory allergies, waterborne diseases, which not only seriously threaten people's physical health condition, and weaken the international health care system, but also, and at least equally important, negatively affect their mental condition (Environmental Health Perspective and the National Institute of Environmental Health Sciences, 2010). According to Hoppe (n.d.), "developing countries do not have a history of large emissions of greenhouse gases and thus have not contributed significantly to the causes of climate change" (para. 2). This is a "deep injustice," which is worsening the gap between developed countries and developing countries (Oxfam Canada, n.d.). Juxtaposed with the vulnerability, and suffering and injustice imposed on certain groups of people, it is important to recognize that even the most vulnerable populations still have capacity to make changes at the local level to improve community resilience, which focuses on "what communities can do for themselves" and how communities can strengthen their capacities to deal with "disaster," "environmental shocks," "stresses" and/or "environmental change" (Twigg, 2009, p. 8).

Sudarshan (2010) argues that "coping with disasters, whether through prevention or mitigation, is clearly an important part of an overall social protection approach" (p. 170). All of the 2015 international agreements must be aimed at promoting human rights with the intent to build the resilience of vulnerable and marginalized people and communities (Drolet, Dominelli, Alston, Ersing, Mathbor, & Wu, 2015). Social protection initiatives contribute to realizing the universal human right to social security. Social protection facilitates access to fundamental services and income by reducing the risks of disaster, and further enhancing the affected people's resilience through the approaches of improving the quality of economic security, health and well-being (Drolet et al., 2015). Hence, the protection of human rights calls for new strategies in the context of climate change and disaster; this is adaptive social protection.

It is well known that greenhouse gases (GHGs) are the main contributors to global climate change (United States Environmental Protection agency, n.d.a). The United States and China made a joint announcement on November 12, 2014, committing to combating global climate change. Their mutual commitment stated that they would reduce their GHGs emissions by 28% (USA) and 20% (China) respectively until 2030 (The White House, 2014, para. 3). In the year 2014, both countries accumulatively contributed to 35.7% of the world GDP and were ranked as the top two on the 2014 International GDP Contribution Ranking

List (Gross domestic product, 2014, p. 1). Both of them were the two highest ranking in their GHGs emissions during that same year, contributing to a total of 38.12% of the global GHGs emissions (The Statistics Portal, 2014, para. 2). Hence, cooperation between these two superpowers was expected to "inject momentum into the global climate negotiations and inspire other countries to join in coming forward with ambitious actions as soon as possible, preferably by the first quarter of 2015" (The White House, 2014, para. 4).

Adaptive social protection and sustainable development

Climate change, one of the greatest challenges of our time, has an undermining effect on "the ability of all countries to achieve sustainable development" (United Nations, 2015e, para. 14). Based on the United Nations' Post-2015 Development Agenda on Sustainable Development and the Sendai Framework for Disaster Risk Reduction 2015–2030, this section addresses how the international sustainable development initiatives consider social protection within the context of climate change and disasters.

Scott and Horn-Phathanothai (2014) state that "historically, climate change and development have been addressed through separate tracks in the UN system" (para. 2). The term "sustainable development" was first used in 1987 in the Brundtland Report, "Our Common Future" (World Commission on Environment and Development, 1987). Since then, sustainable development incorporates three pillars of sustainability: the social, the economic and the environmental (United Nations Commission on Sustainable Development, 2007). Five years later, in June 1992, at the Earth Summit, the United Nations Conference on Environment and Development (UNCED) signed the intentional environment treaty, titled as the United Nations Framework Convention on Climate Change (UNFCCC) to stabilize greenhouse gases, the main causative agent of climate change and global warming (Stavins & Ji, 1992). The Rio + 20 in 2012, the United Nations Conference on Sustainable Development, called for effective social policies, including social protection floors, to address vulnerability in nations that have been affected by climate change and disasters, specifically those developing countries whose economies rely on the natural environment, to achieve sustainable development goals (United Nations Commission on Sustainable Development, 2012). The 2014 UN climate conference, referred to as the Conference of the Parties (COP 20/CMP 10) to the United Nations Framework Conventions on Climate Change (UNFCCC), held in Lima, Peru, garnered international cooperation to curb GHGs emissions (United Nations Framework Conventions on Climate Change [UNFCCC], 2014). Finally, the High-level Political Forum (HLPF), which is a newly formed intergovernmental platform offering high-level political leadership regarding achieving global sustainable development and a platform to link nations and organizations worldwide and to share international knowledge, experience and practices on social protection initiatives including inequity, climate change and disaster mitigation and adaptation, illustrates that climate change is "inextricably intertwined with all three dimensions of sustainable development" (Leong, 2014, para. 4).

Post-2015 Development Agenda

The United Nations' Post-2015 Development Agenda, aiming to further advance the global development framework, and succeeding the MDGs, calls for global partnership for effective development cooperation to achieve international sustainable development (Tritton, 2015). The United Nations' seventh session of the Open Working Group on Sustainable Development Goals reveals a strong agreement that "climate change should be integral to the post-2015 development framework" (Scott & Horn-Phathanothai, 2014, para. 1). The International Labour Organization, the United Nations' Open Working Group on Sustainable Development Goals, Oxfam International and the Post-2015 Women's Coalition proposed to involve social protection in the Post-2015 Development Agenda through the following approaches:

The International Labour Organization (2014) argues that social protection floors and social protection are recognized as part of 17 new SDGs, that should be included at the helm of the Post-2015 Development Agenda to achieve the eradication of vulnerability, poverty and inequity. On August 2, 2015, the 193 Member States of United Nations adopted the new agreement to constitute the new sustainable development agenda, aiming to "end poverty by 2030 and universally promote shared economic prosperity, social development and environmental protection" (United Nations, 2015a, para. 1). The United Nations' Open Working Group on Sustainable Development Goals indicates that all-inclusive social protection systems could contribute to the following SDGs (United Nations, 2015c):

Sustainable Development Goal 1: Ending poverty in all its forms everywhere, implement social protection systems and measures for all, and achieve substantial coverage of the poor and the vulnerable.

(United Nations, 2015c, para. 1)

Sustainable Development Goal 5: Achieve gender equity and empower all women and girls, on recognize and value unpaid care and domestic work through the provision of public services, infrastructure and social protection policies.

(United Nations, 2015c, para. 5)

Sustainable Development Goal 10: Reduce inequality within and among countries, on adopt fiscal, wage, and social protection policies to progressively achieve greater equality.

(United Nations, 2015c, para. 10; from Sustainable Development Goals, by United Nations Department of Economic and Social Affairs, © (2015) United Nations. Reprinted with the permission of the United Nations)

Winnie Byanyima (2014), the Executive Director of Oxfam International, holds that inequity and climate change, as two major injustices, "are threatening to undermine the efforts of millions of people to escape poverty and hunger" (para. 1). Inequity has limited or even deprived the poorest people access to the most basic resources, such as food, clean water, essential health services, which, if accessed, would assist them to improve the quality of their lives. There is a need to address inequity and climate change through the protection of human rights in the new set of the UN's SDGs (Post-2015 Development Agenda).

Furthermore, women's rights and social justice have received heated discussion in the Post-2015 Development Agenda (Post-2015 Women's Coalition, 2015b). The Post-2015 Women's Coalition (2015a) deems that the Post-2015 Development Agenda offers an opportunity for social justice organizations to address the issue of improving women's and marginalized populations' lives. It is well documented that women, children and people in vulnerable situations are the worst hit by climate change and disasters (United Nations, 2015b). Social workers make important contributions to advance women's rights and social justice during recovery and reconstruction, and work to foster resilience among individuals, households and communities (Drolet et al., 2015). Adaptive social protection contributes to strengthening the movement for gender equality, women's rights and women's empowerment in the context of climate change and disaster. With the fulfillment of basic human rights, women are positioned to work together to address the negative influence of climate change and disaster, in order to reduce poverty, decrease environmental degradation and achieve sustainable development goals.

Sendai Framework for Disaster Risk Reduction 2015–2030

The Sendai Framework for Disaster Risk Reduction 2015–2030, endorsed by the UN General Assembly at the third United Nations World Conference on Disaster Risk Reduction in Sendai, Japan, was considered the "first major agreement" of the post-2015 development agenda (The United Nations Office for Disaster Risk Reduction, 2015, para. 1). In the context of disaster risk reduction, the Sendai Framework illustrates that climate change is addressed as one of the critical drivers of disaster risk because in terms of the frequency and intensity of disasters, the majority of them are exacerbated by climate change, and have an extremely deleterious effect on the process of sustainable development (United Nations, 2015b).

The Sendai Framework for Disaster Risk Reduction 2015–2030 puts protection of human rights as the dominant priority for disaster risk reduction (United Nations, 2015b). At the national level, the design and implementation of government policies, plans and standards should involve the vulnerable population's voice. "Building resilience and reducing losses and damages should focus on people, their health and livelihoods, and regular follow-up" (United Nations, 2015b, p. 12). Furthermore, due to the increase of exposure of people and assets to disasters, which take place swifter than the process of vulnerability reduction, this unbalance has generated more risks and losses, which harmfully effect the economic, social, health, cultural and environment in all the phases of post-disaster reconstruction and recovery (United Nations, 2015b). Enhanced work to reduce exposure and vulnerability, which would protect basic human rights, should concentrate on addressing "underlying disaster drivers," such as "the consequences of poverty and inequity, climate change and variability" (United Nations, 2015b, p. 10). Protection of human rights and vulnerability eradication are mentioned in the following guiding principles C, D and H as follows:

> Principle (c): Managing the risk of disasters is aimed at protecting persons and their property, health, livelihoods and productive assets, as well as cultural and environmental assets, while promoting and protecting all human rights, including the right to development;
> Principle (d): Disaster risk reduction requires an all-of-society engagement and partnership. It also requires empowerment and inclusive, accessible and non-discriminatory participation, paying special attention to people disproportionately affected by disasters, especially the poorest. A gender, age, disability and cultural perspective should be integrated in all policies and practices, and women and youth leadership should be promoted. In this context, special attention should be paid to the improvement of organized voluntary work of citizens; and
> Principle (h): The development, strengthening and implementation of relevant policies, plans, practices and mechanisms need to aim at coherence, as appropriate, across sustainable development and growth, food security, health and safety, climate change and variability, environmental management and disaster risk reduction agendas. Disaster risk reduction is essential to achieve sustainable development.
>
> (United Nations, 2015b, p. 10; from Sendai Framework for Disaster Risk Reduction 2015–2030, by United Nations Office for Disaster Risk Reduction, © (2015) United Nations. Reprinted with the permission of the United Nations)

Meanwhile, Priority 3 and Priority 4 for action highlight the protection of basic human rights in pre-disaster preparedness and post-disaster reconstruction and recovery.

Priority 3 focuses on disaster risk reduction for resilience:

> Priority 3: Investing in disaster risk reduction for resilience: Public and private investment in disaster risk prevention and reduction through structural and non-structural measures are essential to enhance the economic, social, health and cultural resilience of persons, communities, countries and their assets, as well as the environment.
>
> (United Nations, 2015b, p. 18; from Sendai Framework for Disaster Risk Reduction 2015–2030, by United Nations Office for Disaster Risk Reduction, © (2015) United Nations. Reprinted with the permission of the United Nations)

At the national and local levels, in order to achieve Priority 3, the Strategy (c) and Strategy (j) concentrate on social service and livelihood enhancement:

> Strategy (c): To strengthen, as appropriate, disaster-resilient public and private investments, particularly through structural, non-structural and functional disaster risk prevention and reduction measures in critical facilities, in particular schools and hospitals and physical infrastructures; building better from the start to withstand hazards through proper design and construction, including the use of the principles of universal design and the standardization of building; retrofitting and rebuilding; nurturing a culture of maintenance; and taking into account economic, social, structural, technological and environmental impact assessments; and
>
> Strategy (j): To strengthen the design and implementation of inclusive policies and social safety-net mechanisms, including through community involvement, integrated with livelihood enhancement programs, and access to basic health-care services, including maternal, newborn and child health, sexual and reproductive health, food security and nutrition, housing and education, towards the eradication of poverty, to find durable solutions in the post-disaster phase and to empower and assist people disproportionately affected by disasters. (United Nations, 2015b, p. 19; from Sendai Framework for Disaster Risk Reduction 2015–2030, by United Nations Office for Disaster Risk Reduction, © (2015) United Nations. Reprinted with the permission of the United Nations)

At the global and regional levels, in order to achieve Priority 3, Strategy (g) concentrates on the development of social safety nets:

> Strategy (g): To promote and support the development of social safety nets as disaster risk reduction measures linked to and integrated with livelihood enhancement programs in order to ensure resilience to shocks at the household and community levels.
> (United Nations, 2015b, p. 20; from Sendai Framework for Disaster Risk Reduction 2015–2030, by United Nations Office for Disaster Risk Reduction, © (2015) United Nations. Reprinted with the permission of the United Nations)

Priority 4 focuses on enhancing disaster preparedness:

> Priority 4: Enhancing disaster preparedness for effective response and to "Build Back Better". In recovery, rehabilitation and reconstruction, empowering women and persons with disabilities to publicly lead and promote gender equitable and universally accessible response, recovery, rehabilitation and reconstruction approaches is key.
> (United Nations, 2015b, p. 21; from Sendai Framework for Disaster Risk Reduction 2015–2030, by United Nations Office for Disaster Risk Reduction, © (2015) United Nations. Reprinted with the permission of the United Nations)

At the national and local levels, in order to achieve Priority 4, Strategy (b) and Strategy (g) focus on involving all the affected people in the disaster preparedness and community social recovery planning:

> Strategy (b): To invest in, develop, maintain and strengthen people-centered multi-hazard, multispectral forecasting and early warning systems, disaster risk and emergency communications mechanisms, social technologies and hazard-monitoring telecommunications systems; develop such systems through a participatory process; tailor them to the needs of users, including social and cultural requirements, in particular gender; promote the application of simple and low-cost early warning equipment and facilities; and broaden release channels for natural disaster early warning information; and
> Strategy (g): To ensure the continuity of operations and planning, including social and economic recovery, and the provision of basic services in the post-disaster phase.
> (United Nations, 2015b, p. 21; from Sendai Framework for Disaster Risk Reduction 2015–2030, by United Nations Office for Disaster Risk Reduction, © (2015) United Nations. Reprinted with the permission of the United Nations)

As discussed in this chapter, protecting human rights plays a key role in the United Nations' and other government and non-government organizations' initiatives in the context of global climate change adaptation and disaster risk reduction. Adaptive social protection contributes to the "social, health and economic well-being of individuals, communities and countries" affected by climate change and disaster (United Nations, 2015b, p. 25). Since social workers are being called upon to protect people's human rights, and to engage with the natural environment, it is necessary to consider the role of social work in adaptive social protection by incorporating the environment in social work perspectives. This is being achieved through green social work (Dominelli, 2012), environmental social work (Zapf, 2012) and eco-social work practice approaches (Molyneux, 2010).

Social work and adaptive social protection

Climate change and disaster do not respect national boundaries and affluent countries have an obligation to help the disadvantaged everywhere (Hawkins, 2010). Environment crises and natural disasters can put social development and sustainable lifestyles in jeopardy. Social workers are being called upon to help rebuild lives due to the devastating effects of climate change (and related natural disasters) (Drolet, Wu, & Dennehy, in press). Social work aims to help individuals, families and communities improve the quality of their lives in a way that fosters empowerment, builds resilience and is respectful (Scottish Executive, 2006). Social workers' holistic perspectives equip them with the knowledge of how to best help individuals, families and communities cope with natural disasters (Norton, 2012). Through the knowledge of utilizing sustainability and social development approaches, social workers contribute to processes that aim to address prevention, adaptation and mitigation, which are concordant with the ultimate achievements of social protection (Scottish Executive, 2006).

Social development approaches enable social workers to effectively address prevention, and adaptation and mitigation measures in the context of climate change and disaster. Moreover, it is social workers' responsibility to directly work with vulnerable people (such as the most marginalized and oppressed individuals and communities) to improve the quality of their lives and protect their human rights, by assisting them to get access to social services and social support. Social workers make an important and unique contribution to the environmental movement in relation to their strong skill set of promoting equity, solidarity, human rights and the dignity and worth of all, which can be implemented on all levels of practice to promote sustainability (Norton, 2012). Hence, social workers should be at the forefront in the field of social protection, advocating in partnership with disenfranchised communities (Bent-Goodley, 2015).

Social workers are well equipped to provide professional support to governmental and non-governmental organizations in facilitating community participation for community development programs (Pandey, 1993). Social workers strive to give voice to the experiences of vulnerable and marginalized populations in both the community and government arenas and work for economic, social, and environmental justice in the context of social protection (Schmitz, Matyók, Sloan, & James, 2012). Through supporting community development and community organizing, social workers apply the practice of sustainable and social development at the community level (Schmitz et al., 2012) Moreover, social workers strive to integrate sustainability and social development principles and practices into the improvement of people's lives in a comprehensive manner, thus protecting the natural environment and its people from exploitation (Kennedy, Ashmore, Babister, & Kelman, 2008).

As demonstrated, in the context of climate change and disaster, social workers play a critical role in offering suggestions to government policy-makers regarding adaptive social protection, in their endeavor to assist vulnerable people to build back better lives and advance their resilience (Schmitz et al., 2012). The next section presents some examples of adaptive social protection initiatives to indicate how adaptive social protection assists vulnerable populations.

Adaptive social protection initiatives

The United Nations Research Institute for Social Development illustrates that, in the last decade, social protection "has emerged as a policy framework employed to address poverty and vulnerability in developing countries" (Barrientos, 2010, p. 1). Generally, social protection consists of the following three types, labor market interventions, social insurance, and social assistance (GSDRC, n.d.). Labor market interventions provide job opportunities for everyone, especially the vulnerable population (Barrientos, 2010). Social insurance relieves risks associated with illness, disability, injury, unemployment, aging, and so on (Actuarial Standards Board, 1998). This is commonly known as health insurance, unemployment insurance and pensions. Social assistance means to provide a transfer, either cash or in-kind resources, to vulnerable populations, including the poor, single parents, homeless, injured, disabled, or other groups, who are lacking in adequate support (Department for International Development, 2011). Social assistance may consist of these types: cash transfers, in-kind transfers, social pensions, public works programs and so on (GSDRC, n.d.). Other than these three types of social protection, other types, such as social care and support, especially for children (United Nations Children's Fund, 2011) and price support (Norton, Conway, & Foster, 2001) are also widely conducted. In the context of climate change and disaster, all of these types of social protection initiatives have been conducted in communities, towns, cities and countries. Various nations and organizations worldwide established their adaptive social protection policies according to their strengths and specific foci according to the unique local situation.

The World Bank's Safety Nets Program in Africa

The World Bank argues that "despite threats of economic, political or climatic crisis as well as risks of unemployment, disability or illness, people and families around the world are discovering new and improved ways to not only deal with these risks, but to access opportunities" (World Bank, 2001, para. 1). The World Bank focuses social protection in job market and labor strategies aiming to utilize economic strategies to offer people job opportunities to build their capacities (World Bank, 2012a). This strategy, guaranteeing the basic income of local residents, is still widely accepted in adaptive social protection (World Bank, 2014b). From the perspective of policies, the World Bank (2001) deems that social protection should include certain policies, regulations, plans and programs, which have been designed to reduce poverty and vulnerability by improving people's capacity to manage natural and (hu)man-made disasters as well as economic and social risks, such as climate change related disasters, environmental pollution, unemployment, sickness, disability and old age.

Due to the fact that the economy of the vast majority of African countries depends on land, natural resources and the environment, these countries are specifically vulnerable to climate change and natural disasters (New Partnership for African Development, 2013). Countries such as Cameroon, Ethiopia, Uganda and Kenya have experienced severe drought and climate related disease, which have worsened hunger and aggravated poverty and social inequity (UN Office for the Coordination of Humanitarian Affairs, 2011). The World Bank's Africa Social Protection Strategy 2012–2022 adopted a Safety Nets Program to reform local safety nets in order to address poverty and vulnerability (World Bank, 2012b). The Safety Nets are "a subset of broader social protection policies and programs along with social insurance and social legislation such as labour laws and safety standards that set minimum civic standards to safeguard the interests of individuals" (Monchuk, 2013, p. 16). Through the "non-contributory" and "contributory" cash and in-kind transfer programs, targeting the poor and vulnerable, the Safety Nets aim to "increase the consumption of basic commodities and essential services, either directly or through substitution effects" (Monchuk, 2013, p. 16).

For example, the Social Safety Net Project (2014–2016) in Cameroon, financed by World Bank's International Development Association, targets poor and vulnerable households in five rural regions; in total, 420,000 vulnerable people will benefit (World Bank, 2014a). In addition to receiving a bimonthly cash transfer, more importantly, the poor and vulnerable households receive:

1   education and training opportunities for work and improving their agricultural skills and nutrition knowledge;
2   paid employment for working on infrastructure maintenance and reforestation; and
3   60 days employment per year during the agricultural lean season (World Bank, 2014a, para. 3).

The cash transfer guarantees families' basic living requirements and needs. The job opportunities and training offer basic income and skill development to create more income resources. These two aspects protect basic human rights in the context of climate change and disaster. Moreover, the improved infrastructure system and recovered natural environment can better protect residents in the face of climate change and disaster. Carlo Del Ninno, World Bank task team leader for the Social Safety Nets Project, deems that this project meets the local families' basic living requirements, and contributes to building resilience and productive capacity in order to cope with drought and the effects of disasters (World Bank, 2014a).

Similar projects such as the Productive Safety Net Program in Ethiopia 2005–2009 (World Food Program, 2012), the Public Transfers and Social Safety Net in Swaziland (World Bank, 2012), and the National Safety Net Program in Kenya 2013–2018 (World Bank, 2015) aim to deliver social protection initiatives in the context of environmental concerns. "With 47.5 percent of people in Sub-Saharan Africa still living on less than $1.25 a day" and "with the number of shocks and natural disasters in a volatile new century increasing," social protection plays an important role in assisting with the process of redevelopment and resilience (World Bank, 2012b, para. 6). The various country case studies featured in this chapter have already strongly demonstrated that adaptive social protection policies funded by the World Bank in many African countries fulfilled poor families' basic living demands and stabilized incomes. These policies have not only improved local people's resilience in facing climate change and natural disasters, but have also effectively boosted the regional and national economic growth throughout the region. This has fundamentally contributed to the process of poverty and vulnerability reduction. Furthermore, the World Bank's strategy strengthens national and cross-national government capacity to "coordinate and implement integrated social protection programs" (World Bank, 2012b, para. 7), which serves as examples for other nations dealing with similar situations. Hence, adaptive social protection measures incorporate a holistic approach that "provides basic economic security" and "access to affordable social and health services, education and information" for people to build their capacities to improve their resilience in the context of climate change and disaster (Comprehensive social policies, 2013, para. 3)

Europe: 2020 strategy and Social Open Method of Coordination (OMC)

The European Union's social protection system is based on the Europe 2020 strategy and the Open Method of Coordination for Social Protection and Social Inclusion (Social OMC), and intends to "promote social cohesion and equality through adequate, accessible and financially sustainable social protection systems and social inclusion policies" (European Commission, n.d., para. 3). The European Commission (2012a) deems social protection as an integral part of the European Union's development policy. Social protection and climate change adaptation measures can be complementary "in order to reduce the vulnerability of poor people to the effects of climate change" (European Commission, 2012a, p. 12). Through cooperation among all European Union members, the European Union's adaptive social protection policy aims to "fund the setting-up and strengthening of social protection systems, including in situations which call for the development of systems that can be rapidly scaled up to address recurrent natural disasters" (European Commission, 2012a, p. 11).

According to 2013 European statistics, 122.6 million people (24.5% of the European Union's population) are at risk of poverty or social exclusion (Eurostat Statistics Explained, 2015, para. 3), as a result of three main causes: income poverty, being severely materially deprived and low work intensity (Eurostat Statistics Explained, 2015). The European Union's social protection systems prioritize the problem of unemployment (European Commission, 2012a). On the one hand, all Member States cooperate to increase working opportunities and address gender-related working issues by offering equal job opportunities to women (European Commission, 2012a). The adaptive social protection system facilitates labor markets and mobility by ensuring that the majority of workers, especially migrant workers, have access to social insurance (European Commission, 2012a). The European Union has also set up an agenda for adequate, safe and sustainable pensions to guarantee pension rights (European Commission, 2012b).

Australia and United Kingdom: cash and in-kind transfer

Australia is highly vulnerable to natural and climate-related disasters, and the Department of Foreign Affairs and Trade (DFAT) within the Australian government aims to build resilience through humanitarian assistance, disaster risk

Table 6.1 Developmental outcomes of cash transfer (DFID, 2011, p. 47)

Developmental outcomes of cash transfer
1   Reducing poverty, hunger and inequality
2   Human development
3   Addressing social inequities and empowering women
4   Coping with environmental stress and shocks
5   Economic development and inclusive growth
6   Facilitating social cohesion and state-building

reduction and social protection (Department of Foreign Affairs and Trade [DFAT], Australian government, 2015, para. 1). Through adaptive social protection initiatives, Australia has been pursuing various measures to build resilience (DFAT, 2014a). For example, in addition to addressing risks, vulnerability and poverty, the DFAT (2014b) provides cash or in-kind transfers to individuals, households and communities. This support is evident in national and international initiatives, for example, in developing countries such as Indonesia, the Philippines, Laos, Cambodia, Bangladesh and Kenya, which have been negatively affected by climate change and disaster (para. 7). Transfers include "cash and food transfer," "income generating asset" and "cash-for-work transfer" (DFAT, 2014b, para. 2), in order to fulfill the poor's basic living requirements so that they may be able to access work opportunities.

Similarly, the Department for International Development (DFID) in the United Kingdom facilitates social assistance, particularly cash transfer, which is "direct, regular and predictable non-contributory cash payments" in order to assist poor and vulnerable families to "raise and smooth incomes" (Department for International Development [DFID], 2011, p. i). DFID conducted international case-based research regarding the efficiency and importance of cash transfer as a productive adaptive social protection strategies. For example, from 2009 to 2015, DFID conducted the Expanding Social Protection (ESP) program in Uganda to help the government of Uganda to establish the national social protection system (DFID, n.d., p. 1). This program created the national cash transfer system to provide regular and reliable cash transfer to the most vulnerable households in the 14 poorest regions in Uganda (DFID, n.d., p. 1). With basic income security, households' basic requirements such as nutrition, health and education were fulfilled. The developmental outcome of cash transfers is summarized in Table 6.1.

China: adaptive social protection and reconstruction after the Wenchuan earthquake

Many nations worldwide confront the challenges of post-disaster reconstruction and recovery in the face of climate change and related natural disasters. Recent studies underline that the various dimensions of disaster recovery (physical, social, cultural, economic and political) (Reiss, 2012) interweave with one another to influence recovery outcomes (Hoffman & Oliver-Smith, 2002). When faced with post-disaster reconstruction and recovery, most countries give priority to physical reconstruction rather than social recovery (Kamel & Loukaitou-Sideris, 2004; Oliver-Smith, 2005). Physical recovery aims to repair, construct and reconstruct all buildings and infrastructural systems damaged and destroyed in a disaster. The quality of the physical reconstruction will be dramatically influenced by economic and political recovery as well as the inclusion of cultural and other social dimensions (Reiss, 2012). All governments must pay attention to the opportunities available in social protection initiatives in the disaster reconstruction and recovery process in order to fulfill social demands (Wu, 2014). Adaptive social protection is an approach to achieve social recovery in post-disaster contexts, and can potentially improve the local residents' ability to adapt to climate change and advance communities' resilience (Davies et al., 2008).

The Wenchuan earthquake that took place in Sichuan, China, on May 12, 2008, ranked among the top 10 largest and deadliest earthquakes until 2014 (The United States Geological Survey, 2014). After the Wenchuan earthquake, the Chinese central government invested approximately one trillion Chinese yuan (about US$150 billion) in the post-earthquake reconstruction and recovery, including infrastructure, housing, education, health and all dimensions of local inhabitants' daily life (Chen & Booth, 2011, p. 229). This investment represents 25% of the total fiscal stimulus package of China (four trillion Chinese yuan) and most of the funds were spent on infrastructure and related construction (Jia & Liu, 2010, as cited in United Nations, 2011, p. 88). It is important to note that this fiscal stimulus package took place in the aftermath of the global economic crisis, when many industrialized countries invested in social protection and social development initiatives, and served to effectively maintain aggregate demand and growth in the recovery period (Jia & Liu, 2010, as cited in United Nations, 2011, p. 88).

China utilized the approach of stimulating the development of infrastructure and related construction to boost the economy and improve the quality of disaster survivors' physical living environment (Garrett, 2010). The worst hit areas and second worst hit areas were rural areas. Most farmers were relocated to urban residential communities because of the geological hazards in the original communities. The majority of relocated earthquake survivors lost their livelihoods based in agriculture. In this context, the massive infrastructure and related construction projects presented new employment opportunities, which, to some extent, relieved the economic impact of the post-disaster unemployment situation. Furthermore, the government applied very strict high-seismic standards to all newly built structures, especially residential, schools, hospitals, and other public service buildings, in order to assist the earthquake survivors in the event of potential future earthquakes (Zhao, Taucer, & Lu, 2010). This also offered an opportunity to improve the quality of these public service buildings. According to Beranl (2012), about 108 billion Chinese yuan (about US$17 billion) was spent on updating "medical and sanitation facilities and social management," "social welfare houses, elderly homes, community service centers, village activity centers, etc." (para. 14), which, to some extent, guarantee the quality of local social service.

It is important to consider the geographic context of the reconstruction and recovery projects, as almost all the worst hit areas were located in rural areas. By the end of 2008, the Chinese government adopted the New Rural Cooperative Medical Schemes in the rural areas, and extended universal health coverage, directing the provision of coverage for 91.5% of the rural population (International Labour Organization, 2010, p. 12). In the year 2008, the government made available a free pension for the earthquake survivors who had lost their children in the earthquake (Wu, 2014). Since 2009, the new rural pension system has been activated (Gao, Su, & Gao, 2012). Most of the earthquake survivors obtained cash and in-kind transfers, such as food, water, other daily necessities, and building materials, for three months after the earthquake (The State Council, the People's Republic of China, 2008, para. 4). Special social protection benefits were afforded to those who experienced significant losses in the earthquake such as orphans, people living with disabilities, and older people without children. These special groups could access extended social insurance, financial and other related aids (The State Council, the People's Republic of China, 2008). In China social workers provided counseling to affected individuals and families, especially school children. Other types of assistance, such as education and training programs for re-employment as well as consulting services, were also provided by different levels of government and other related organizations in the quake-hit areas to help the earthquake survivors to build back better (Gupta, Velasquez, Nag, Panda, Kuberan, Hari, & Suryono, 2010; Wu, 2014).

The post-Wenchuan earthquake reconstruction can be considered an adaptive social protection initiative, which provided important support in the post-disaster recovery period. After the fulfillment of the survivors' basic living requirements, the government policy offered work opportunities that served the physical reconstruction process, to improve the quality of the built environment. The outcomes of physical reconstruction supported and guaranteed the physical foundation of social service and other social support resources, which, to some extent, advanced the households', communities' and regions' resilience toward both disaster preparedness and recovery.

Conclusion

Building on social protection, climate change adaptation and disaster risk reduction, this chapter presents adaptive social protection as a government policy grounded in national social protection floors. Adaptive social protection aims to protect local inhabitants' basic human rights in the context of climate change and disaster, which has already been highlighted in the United Nations' Sustainable Development Goals and the Post-2015 Development Agenda. Social workers bring knowledge and skills in building social capacity, protecting people's human rights, supporting social justice in rebuilding post-disaster, and fostering resilience in post-disaster reconstruction and recovery. These knowledge and skills also endow social workers with unique contributions in the development and implementation of adaptive social protection strategies.

Adaptive social protection plays an essential role in protecting vulnerable people against current and potential risks caused by climate change and disaster (Davies et al., 2008). Through cash or in-kind transfers, it is possible to meet the basic living requirements of those affected by the impacts of climate change and natural disasters. Adaptive social protection initiatives can provide employment opportunities to those affected by climate change and natural disasters by providing an income and involving affected individuals in the rehabilitation of their physical environment. During this process, social capital is rebuilt and even strengthened. This is the main achievement of adaptive social protection – the strengthening of vulnerable populations' resilience.

In May 2016, the United Nations Secretary General, Mr. Ban Ki-moon will initiate the World Humanitarian Summit in Istanbul, Turkey, on how to better meet the demands of those who are affected by conflicts and disasters (World Humanitarian Summit, 2015). Building on the knowledge and innovative transformation through eight regional consultations, the summit will focus on the improvement of humanitarian action to reduce vulnerability and manage risk by serving the needs of people in conflict (World Humanitarian Summit, 2015). Adaptive social protection could serve as a bridge between humanitarian action and sustainable development in order to build resilience in the context of climate change and disasters.

References

Actuarial Standards Board. (1998). *Social insurance: Actuarial standard of practice no. 32.* Retrieved from www.actuarialstandardsboard.org/wp-content/uploads/2014/07/asop032_062.pdf.

Barrientos, A. (2010). *Social protection and poverty.* UNRISD flagship report: Combating poverty and inequality. Retrieved from www.unrisd.org/80256B3C005BCCF9/(httpPublications)/973B0F57CA78D834C12576DB003BE255?OpenDocument.

Bent-Goodley, T.B. (2015). The art and science of social work revisited: Relevance for a changing world. *Social Work, 60*(3), 189–190.

Beranl, V.A. (2012, May 11). Four years on: What China got right when rebuilding after the Sichuan earthquake. The World Bank. Retrieved from http://blogs.worldbank.org/eastasiapacific/four-years-on-what-china-got-right-when-rebuilding-after-the-sichuan-earthquake.

Block, B. (n.d.). Climate change will worsen hunger, study says. Worldwatch Institute. Retrieved from www.worldwatch.org/node/6271.

Byanyima, W. (2014, July 1). Overcoming inequality and climate change key to ending poverty. *Post2015.org What comes after MDGs.* Retrieved from http://post2015.org/2014/07/01/overcoming-inequality-and-climate-change-key-to-ending-poverty/.

Chen, Y., & Booth, D.C. (2011). *The Wenchuan earthquake of 2008: Anatomy of a disaster.* Beijing: Science & Springer.

CIC Insurance Group. (2012). *Enabling social protection: The role of co-operatives.* Retrieved from http://social.un.org/coopsyear/documents/KuriaEnablingsocialprotection AddisAbaba.pdf.

Comprehensive social policies. (2013). National Institute for Health and Welfare. Retrieved from www.thl.fi/en/web/thlfi-en/topics/information-packages/global-social-policy/comprehensive-social-policies.

Davies, M., Oswald, K., Mitchell, T., & Tanner, T. (2008). *Climate change adaptation, disaster risk reduction and social protection.* Center for Social Protection Climate Change and Development Centre, Institute of Development Studies, University of Sussex, Brighton, UK. Retrieved from www.ids.ac.uk/files/IDS_Adaptive_Social_Protection_Briefing_Note_11_December_2008.pdf.

Department for International Development (DFID). (n.d.). *Expanding social protection in Uganda.* Retrieved from iati.dfid.gov.uk/iati_documents/4202091.doc.

Department for International Development (DFID). (2011). *Cash transfers literature review, policy division 2011.* London: Department for International. Retrieved from http://r4d.dfid.gov.uk/PDF/Articles/cash-transfers-literature-review.pdf.

Department of Foreign Affairs and Trade. (2014a). *Australia's aid program.* Retrieved from http://dfat.gov.au/aid/Pages/australias-aid-program.aspx.

Department of Foreign Affairs and Trade. (2014b). *Overview of Australia's assistance for social protection.* Retrieved from http://dfat.gov.au/aid/topics/investment-priorities/building-resilience/social-protection/Pages/social-protection.aspx.

Department of Foreign Affairs and Trade, Australian Government. (2015). *Building resilience: Humanitarian assistance, disaster risk reduction and social protection.* Retrieved from http://dfat.gov.au/aid/topics/investment-priorities/building-resilience/Pages/building-resilience.aspx.

Devereux, S., & Sabates-Wheeler, R. (2004). *Transformative social protection* (IDS Working Paper 232). Brighton: IDS.

Dominelli, L. (2012). *Green social work: From environmental crises to environmental justice.* Cambridge, MA: Polity Press.

Drolet, J., Dominelli, L., Alston, M., Ersing, R., Mathbor, G., & Wu, H. (2015). Women rebuilding lives post-disaster: Innovative community practices for building resilience and promoting sustainable development. *Gender and Development, 23*(3), 433–448.

Drolet, J., Wu, H., & Dennehy, A. (in press). Social development and sustainability: Social work in the post-2015 sustainable development framework. In J. McKinnon & M. Alston (Eds.), *Ecological social work: Towards sustainability.* Hampshire: Palgrave.

Environmental Health Perspective and the National Institute of Environmental Health Sciences. (2010). *A human health perspective on climate change.* Retrieved from www.niehs.nih.gov/health/materials/a_human_health_perspective_on_climate_change_full_report_508.pdf.

European Commission. (n.d.). *Social protection.* Retrieved from http://ec.europa.eu/social/main.jsp?catId=1063&langId=en.

European Commission. (2012a). *Communication from the commission to the European Parliament, the Council, the European Economic and Social Committee and the Committee of the Regions. Social Protection in European Union Development Cooperation.* Retrieved from http://eur-lex.europa.eu/LexUriServ/LexUriServ.do?uri=COM:2012:0446:FIN:EN:PDF.

European Commission. (2012b, February 16). EU sets out plans for adequate, safe and sustainable pensions. *News @ European Commission.* Retrieved from http://ec.europa.eu/social/main.jsp?langId=en&catId=89&newsId=1194&furtherNews=yes.

Eurostat Statistics Explained. (2015). *People at risk of poverty or social exclusion.* Retrieved from http://ec.europa.eu/eurostat/statistics-explained/index.php/People_at_risk_of_poverty_or_social_exclusioEu.

Gao, Y., Su, B., & Gao, F. (2012). New rural pension system of China: Is it possible? An exploratory study of Feidong County, Anhui Province. *Journal of Cambridge Studies*, *7*, 122–132.

Garrett, G. (2010). G2 in G20: China, the United States and the world after the global financial crisis. *Global Policy*, *1*, 29–39.

Gross domestic product. (2014). *Databank @ World Bank*. Retrieved from http://databank. worldbank.org/data/download/GDP.pdf.

GSDRC. (n.d.). *Social protection*. Retrieved from www.gsdrc.org/go/topic-guides/social-protection/what-is-social-protection.

Gupta, M., Velasquez, G., Nag, S., Panda, A., Kuberan, R., Hari, K., & Suryono, R. (2010). *Building back better for next time*. European Union (EU); United Nations Office for Disaster Risk Reduction Regional Office for Asia and Pacific (UNISDR AP).

Hawkins, C. (2010). Sustainability, human rights, and environmental justice: Critical connections for contemporary social work. *Critical Social Work*, *11*, 68–81.

Hoffman, S.M., & Oliver-Smith, A. (Eds.). (2002). *Catastrophe & culture: The anthropology of disaster*. Santa Fe: School of American Research Press.

Hoppe, P. (n.d.). *Proposal: Developing countries are most affected by climate change and need the support of the industrialized countries to adapt to the unavoidable risks*. Retrieved from www.global-economic-symposium.org/knowledgebase/the-global-environment/managing-adaption-to-climate-change-in-the-developing-world/proposals/developing-countries-are-most-affected-by-climate-change-and-need-the-support-of-the-industrialized-countries-to-adapt-to-the-unavoidable-risks.

International Labour Organization. (n.d.). *Social protection floor (SOCPRO)*. Retrieved from www.ilo.org/secsoc/areas-of-work/policy-development-and-applied-research/social-protection-floor/lang-en/index.htm.

International Labour Organization. (2009). *Social protection*. Retrieved from www.ilo.org/global/about-the-ilo/decent-work-agenda/social-protection/lang-en/index.htm.

International Labour Organization. (2010). *Employment and social protection policies from crisis to recovery and beyond: Review of experience*. Retrieved from www.ilo.org/public/libdoc/jobcrisis/download/g20_report_employment_and_social_protection_policies.pdf.

International Labour Organization. (2011). *Social protection floor*. Retrieved from www.ilo.org/public/english/protection/spfag/socialfloor/index.htm.

International Labour Organization. (2014). *Social protection floors in the post-2015 agenda: Targets and indicators*. Retrieved from www.socialprotectionfloor-gateway.org/files/post-2015_and_SPF.pdf.

Kamel, N.M.O., & Loukaitou-Sideris, A. (2004). Residential assistance and recovery following the Northridge earthquake. *Urban Study*, *41*, 533–562.

Kennedy, J., Ashmore, J., Babister, E., & Kelman, I. (2008). The meaning of "Build Back Better": Evidence from post-tsunami Aceh and Sri Lanka. *Journal of Contingencies & Crisis Management*, *16*, 24–36.

Leong, A. (2014). The high-level political forum and climate change. *Post2015.org What comes after MDGs*. Retrieved from http://post2015.org/2014/06/26/the-high-level-political-forum-and-climate-change/.

Lindell, M.K. (2013). Recovery and reconstruction after disaster. *Encyclopedia of Natural Hazards*, *8*, 12–824.

Monchuk, V. (2013). *Reducing poverty and investing in people: The new role of safety nets in Africa*. Washington, DC: World Bank Publications.

Molyneux, R. (2010). The practical realities of eco-social work: A review of the literature. *Critical Social Work*, *11*, 61–69.

National Aeronautics and Space Administration. (n.d.). The impact of climate change on natural disasters. *Earth Observatory*. Retrieved from http://earthobservatory.nasa.gov/Features/RisingCost/rising_cost5.php.

New Partnership for African Development (NEPAD). (2013). *African agriculture, transformation and outlook*. NEPAD. Retrieved from www.un.org/africarenewal/sites/www.un.org.africarenewal/files/Agriculture%20in%20Africa.pdf.

Norton, A., Conway, T., & Foster, M. (2001). *Social protection concepts and approaches: Implications for policy and practice in international development*. Working Paper 143, London: Overseas Development Institute.

Norton, C.L. (2012). Social work and the environment: An eco-social approach. *International Journal of Social Welfare, 21*, 299–308.

Oliver-Smith, A. (2005). Communities after catastrophe: Reconstructing the material, reconstituting the social. In S.E. Hyland (Ed.), *Community building in the twenty-first century* (pp. 25–44). Santa Fe: School of American Research Press.

Oxfam Canada. (n.d.). *Climate change*. Retrieved from http://oxfam.ca/our-work/climate-change?gclid=CjwKEAjwitKtBRCt3uOYsY2v7FASJACJU5XsizQxyfdlLPWrLXJuYsppm4lkd0a5lt3oB4KDGAQoPRoCXQTw_wcB.

Pandey, S. (1993). Women, environment, and sustainable development. *International Social Work, 41*, 339–355. Retrieved from http://isw.sagepub.com.ezproxy.lib.ucalgary.ca/content/41/3/339.

Post-2015 Women's Coalition. (2015a). *Feminist sustainable development: A transformative alternative for gender equality, development and peace*. Retrieved from www.post2015women.com/wp-content/uploads/2015/04/Post2015WomensCoalition-VisionStatement_FINAL.pdf.

Post-2015 Women's Coalition. (2015b). The post 2015 development agenda: What's at stake for the world's women? Post-2015 Women's Coalition. Retrieved from www.post2015women.com.

Reiss, S.P. (2012). *The field programming environment: A friendly integrated environment for learning and development* (Vol. 298). New York: Springer Science & Business Media.

Schmitz, C.L., Matyók, T., Sloan, L.M., & James, C. (2012). The relationship between social work and environmental sustainability: Implications for interdisciplinary practice. *International Journal of Social Welfare, 21*, 278–286.

Scott, A., & Horn-Phathanothai, L. (2014, January 21). 5 propositions for tackling climate change in the post-2015 development agenda. Independent Research Forum 2015. Retrieved from www.irf2015.org/5-propositions-tackling-climate-change-post-2015-development-agenda.

Scottish Executive. (2006). Report of the 21st century social work review: Changing lives. Scottish Executive. Retrieved from www.gov.scot/resource/doc/91931/0021949.pdf.

Social Protection Floor. (2009a). *About the social protection floor*. Retrieved from www.socialprotectionfloor-gateway.org/4.htm.

Social Protection Floor. (2009b). *Social protection floors*. Retrieved from www.socialprotectionfloor-gateway.org.

The State Council, the People's Republic of China. (2008). *The notice regarding aids for Wenchuan earthquake survivors*. Retrieved from www.gov.cn/gongbao/content/2008/content_1035807.htm.

The Statistics Portal. (2014). *The largest producers of CO2 emissions worldwide in 2014, based on their share of global CO2 emissions*. Retrieved from www.statista.com/statistics/271748/the-largest-emitters-of-co2-in-the-world/.

Stavins, R., & Ji, Z. (1992). *International cooperation: Agreements & instruments.* Retrieved from http://report.mitigation2014.org/drafts/final-draft-postplenary/ipcc_wg3_ar5_final-draft_postplenary_chapter13.pdf.

Sudarshan, R.M. (2010). Reading the signposts: Social protection for home-based women workers in South Asia. In S. Cook & N. Kabeer (Eds.), *Social protection as development policy* (pp. 165–189). New Delhi: Routledge.

Sustainable Development Knowledge Platform. (2013). *Open working group proposal for sustainable development goals.* Retrieved from http://sustainabledevelopment.un.org/focussdgs.html.

Tritton, B. (2015, July 2). Will the post-2015 agenda support country ownership of sustainable development processes? *Post2015.org What comes after MDGs.* Retrieved from http://post2015.org/2015/07/02/will-the-post-2015-agenda-support-country-ownership-of-sustainable-development-processes/.

Twigg, J. (2009). *Characteristics of a disaster-resilient community: A guidance note for government and civil society organizations working on disaster risk reduction initiatives at community level.* Retrieved from www.abuhrc.org/research/dsm/Pages/project_view.aspx?project=13.

UN Office for the Coordination of Humanitarian Affairs. (2011, June 10). *Eastern Africa drought humanitarian report No. 3.* Retrieved from http://reliefweb.int/report/burundi/eastern-africa-drought-humanitarian-report-no-3.

United Nations. (2011). *The global social crisis: Report on the world social situation 2011.* Retrieved from www.un.org/esa/socdev/rwss/docs/2011/rwss2011.pdf.

United Nations. (2015a, August 2). Consensus reached on new sustainable development agenda to be adopted by world leaders in September. *2015 Time for Global Action.* Retrieved from www.un.org/sustainabledevelopment/blog/2015/08/transforming-our-world-document-adoption/.

United Nations. (2015b). *Sendai framework for disaster risk reduction 2015–2030.* Retrieved from www.preventionweb.net/files/43291_sendaiframeworkfordrren.pdf.

United Nations. (2015c). Sustainable development goals. *2015 Time for Global Action.* Retrieved from www.un.org/sustainabledevelopment/sustainable-development-goals/.

United Nations. (2015d). *Sustainable development knowledge platform.* Retrieved from https://sustainabledevelopment.un.org/index.html.

United Nations. (2015e). *Transforming our world: The 2030 agenda for sustainable development.* Retrieved from https://sustainabledevelopment.un.org/post2015/transformingourworld.

United Nations Children's Fund (UNICEF). (2011). *Children protection from violence, exploitation and abuse.* Retrieved from www.unicef.org/protection/57929_58004.html.

United Nations Commission on Sustainable Development. (2007). *Sustainable development in action: Farming sustainable development, the Brundtland report-20 years on.* Retrieved from www.un.org/esa/sustdev/csd/csd15/media/backgrounder_brundtland.pdf.

United Nations Commission on Sustainable Development. (2012). *The future we want.* Retrieved from http://daccess-dds-ny.un.org/doc/UNDOC/GEN/N11/476/10/PDF/N1147610.pdf?OpenElement.

United Nations Development Program. (2015). *Post-2015 sustainable development agenda.* Retrieved from www.undp.org/content/undp/en/home/mdgoverview/post-2015-development-agenda.html.

United Nations Framework Conventions on Climate Change. (2014). *Lima climate change conference – December 2014.* Retrieved from http://unfccc.int/meetings/lima_dec_2014/meeting/8141/php/view/seors.php.

United Nations Office for Disaster Risk Reduction. (2015, March 6). *Ten-year review finds 87% of disasters climate-related.* Retrieved from www.unisdr.org/archive/42862.

United States Environmental Protection Agency. (n.d.a). *Climate change.* Retrieved from www.epa.gov/climatechange/.

United States Environmental Protection Agency. (n.d.b). *Climate change impacts and adapting to change.* Retrieved from www.epa.gov/climatechange/impacts-adaptation/index.html.

United States Geological Survey. (2014). *Largest and deadliest earthquakes by year.* Retrieved from http://earthquake.usgs.gov/earthquakes/eqarchives/year/byyear.php.

Vincent, K., & Cull, T. (2012). *Adaptive social protection: Making concepts a reality – guidance notes for practitioners.* Retrieved from www.ids.ac.uk/files/dmfile/ASPGuidance Notes_FINAL.pdf.

White House. (2014, November 11). U.S.-China joint announcement on climate change. The White House Office of the Press Secretary. Retrieved on February 27, 2015, from www.whitehouse.gov/the-press-office/2014/11/11/us-china-joint-announcement-climate-change.

World Bank. (2001). *Social protection sector strategy paper: From safety net to springboard.* Washington, DC. Retrieved from www-wds.worldbank.org/external/default/WDSContentServer/WDSP/IB/2001/01/26/000094946_01011705303891/Rendered/PDF/multi_page.pdf.

World Bank. (2012). *Swaziland: Using public transfers to reduce extreme poverty.* Washington, DC: World Bank Group. Retrieved from http://documents.worldbank.org/curated/en/2012/11/18622692/swaziland-using-public-transfers-reduce-extreme-poverty.

World Bank. (2012a). *Resilience, equity and opportunity: Social protection & labor strategy 2012–2022.* Retrieved from http://web.worldbank.org/WBSITE/EXTERNAL/TOPICS/EXTSOCIALPROTECTION/0,,contentMDK:23043115~pagePK:210058~piPK:210062~theSitePK:282637,00.html.

World Bank. (2012b, December 18). A ten-year strategy to support the development of social protection systems in Sub-Saharan Africa. *The World Bank News.* Retrieved from www.worldbank.org/en/news/feature/2012/12/18/a-ten-year- strategy-to-support-the-development-of-social-protection-systems-in-sub-saharan-africa.

World Bank. (2014a, April 2). World Bank to help build Safety Net System aimed at reducing poverty and vulnerability in Cameroon. *The World Bank News.* Retrieved from www.worldbank.org/en/news/press-release/2014/04/02/world-bank-to-help-build-safety-net-system-aimed-at-reducing-poverty-and-vulnerability-in-cameroon.

World Bank. (2014b). *World development report 2014: Risk and opportunity managing risk for development.* Retrieved from http://siteresources.worldbank.org/EXTNWDR 2013/Resources/8258024-1352909193861/8936935-1356011448215/8986901-138004 6989056/WDR-2014_Complete_Report.pdf.

World Bank. (2015). *Kenya – National Safety Net program for results: P131305 – implementation status results report, Sequence 04.* Washington, DC: World Bank Group. Retrieved from http://documents.worldbank.org/curated/en/2015/06/24693352/kenya-national-safety-net-program-results-p131305-implementation-status-results-report-sequence-04.

World Commission on Environment and Development. (1987). *Our common future.* Oxford: Oxford University Press.

World Food Program. (2012). *Productive safety net program in Ethiopia.* Retrieved from www.wfp.org/sites/default/files/PSNP%20Factsheet.pdf.

World Humanitarian Summit. (2015). *About the world humanitarian summit.* Retrieved from www.worldhumanitariansummit.org/whs_about?utm_source=About&utm_medium= banner&utm_campaign=WHS_FrontPage&utm_content=Banner+Click.

Wu, H. (2014). *Post-Wenchuan earthquake rural reconstruction and recovery, in Sichuan China: Memory, civic participation and government intervention* (Doctoral Dissertation). Retrieved from http://circle.ubc.ca/handle/2429/50340.

Zapf, M.K. (2012). Social work and the environment: Understanding people and place. *Critical Social Work, 11,* 30–46.

Zhao, B., Taucer, F., & Lu, X. (2010). Lesson learned from Wenchuan earthquake of 12 May 2008. European Union. Retrieved from https://ec.europa.eu/jrc/sites/default/files/jrc_20100618_shanghai_expo_earthquake.pdf.

7 Social protection and the fight against poverty

Valter Martins

Introduction

Since the 1970s, when there was a restructuring of national economies on a global scale, especially in the Global West, nation states have adopted a set of social policies and strategies to confront poverty. Despite an expansion of socially produced wealth, generational poverty remains entrenched, expressions of poverty appear and the grave problem of hunger persists in many regions of the world. Generational poverty refers to the reproduction of poverty from generation to generation of poor families, given that the children of poor families reproduce the traits of poverty experienced by their parents and thus successively. Although compensatory policies can help relieve the situation of family poverty, they do not break this cycle. Our analyses about income transfer policies in Brazil show that when the second generation of users of the compensatory policies become adults they turn to the same benefits that their parents received to guarantee basic needs for the survival of the nuclear family (Martins, 2008). We also have the manifestations of poverty associated with wide-scale unemployment, precarious employment and informal employment as well as the growth of AIDS and the absence of treatment for its victims. All of these factors have triggered concerns about the importance of overcoming poverty and inequality, which are policy goals in various developing countries, particularly those that have historically suffered from the deepest expressions of inequality, and which have still not consolidated strong social protection systems for confronting poverty and inequality and the scars they leave on people.

There is no single definition of poverty that is universally accepted, but there are indications of how to identify it. The most recurrent are related to the poverty of earnings, or of income (PNUD, 2003). Income poverty is expressed in long-lasting conditions related to a lack of financial income, although understanding this factor is limited by technical measurements that do not consider specific social, cultural and historic contexts. For Lister (2005) the definition should distinguish between the state of poverty and of non-poverty, and it should recognize humiliation, indignity and the denial of human rights. It is notorious and consensual among the academic community and a wide variety of political institutions (Silva, 2010) that poverty is the result of deep inequality, marked by a profound concentration of wealth, and by the lack of access to basic healthcare, social assistance, decent food, housing, education, information, work and decent income, and to political participation. Poverty is a structural phenomenon in contemporary society, which has a complex, relative and multidimensional nature, and cannot be considered as a mere insufficiency of income (Silva, 2010).

In this context, and over the years, social work practice has worked to confront expressions of poverty in all countries that suffer from it. The work conducted by social workers aims to protect the vulnerable populations exposed to social risks by providing services to support children, women, the elderly, families and refugees from wars, and by operating programs and projects at various levels in the implementation of social protection policies. Meanwhile, the elimination of poverty is the motivation of any committed social work professional.

According to Lister (2005) the concept of poverty should be broad to allow recognition of non-material aspects related to how poor people are seen and treated in daily interactions with institutions. Therefore, poverty cannot be understood solely as a disadvantaged economic condition, but "also as a shameful and corrosive social relationship" (Lister, 2005, p. 8). A study conducted by Yazbek (2010) found that poverty is expressed in the trajectories of exploitation, oppression, the absence of housing or in discomfort because of precarious or unhealthy conditions, in unemployment, in poor health, ignorance, despair, in the suffering expressed in speech, in silence, in language, and in language that goes beyond discourse.

In concrete terms, an anti-poverty policy in any country should combine and emphasize investment in education, skills, healthcare, public services, housing, and improving benefits and specialized services for women, children and the elderly. These policies should address many levels and dimensions after the identification of the causes and expressions of poverty in each country.

Practices to fight poverty and other misfortunes of natural and social life are present in all human societies. All societies have some mechanism of social protection for their most vulnerable members (Giovanni, 1998), whether in a simple manner, provided through non-specialized and multi-functional institutions such as the family, or through sophisticated organizations as in the models developed by nation states. Different forms of social protection have thus emerged and developed over time and space in societies through mechanisms for combating or preventing the expressions of poverty. Social protection thus involves the forms, which may be more or less institutionalized, which societies establish to protect part or all of their members. These configurations are derived from certain vicissitudes of natural or social life, expressed in old-age, disease, misfortune and need.

The social and historic development of methods for fighting and preventing poverty led to the establishment of what Bobbio (1999) calls second-generation rights, or social rights. These rights begin with a focus on the individual and the right to education, employment and to live in safety. As societies develop, these social rights have progressed, incorporating an increasing number of people and establishing themselves as legal forms for social protection recognized by states.

To understand poverty and the ways to confront it by means of social protection, it is necessary to consider the specificities and cultural context of societies and human groups. Studies have accumulated an important foundation based on research that contribute to understanding the mechanisms of social protection in the fight against poverty.

Development of social protection

Historically, the first experiences of social protection were provided by families, churches and other associations (Castel, 1998). The family does so by expressing ties of solidarity and affection through a kinship group; the church through its organizations and dogmas; and other religious-based associations through concepts of charity and philanthropy. The consolidation of social protection began to take on broader dimensions with the rise and development of capitalism, with the intensification of nascent social inequalities that accompanied the transformation of the urban environment as a consequence of industrialization.

Industrialization created a strong demand for a large number of workers, and technological growth stimulated the concentration of labor in urban areas. This industrial urbanization generated demand for goods and profits for industrialists and led to an intense demographic transformation. In a short period of time, a broad group of workers were absorbed by industry. Throughout the 18th and 19th centuries these workers were central elements of a new urban industrial scene. The industrializing process began in England and soon spread through Western Europe and North America, and produced a set of new social characteristics and relations at an enormous social cost. In the first industrial regions, groups of workers were subjected to long shifts at very low pay. The meager wages forced entire families to work on the assembly lines, where women and children conducted the same tasks as adult men without any regulations or suitable facilities for safety or hygiene. The new standard of living in this industrial age degraded the health and shortened the life expectancy of workers. This contributed to the establishment of new forms of poverty. Some of these characteristics that marked the beginning of industrialization still persist or have been revised. A new type of pauperism arose which is not expressed by natural disasters, but in a new form of organizing and responding to survival needs in cities expanding with industrialization. Technology imposes various transformations and demands on workers, and these demands are revised at each moment that the means of production are innovated. The labor force suffers a true metamorphosis and its degradation comes to be determined by the conditions of production, with the deterioration of the lives of workers. For each new need generated or new machine developed, workers must respond by working longer hours or with an intensification of production, so that the form of production comes to be determined by the velocity at which technologies can be operated. Long and exhausting work shifts, low pay, precarious work unprotected by labor law such as domestic work and child labor are some of the characteristics that are more visible in developing countries.

The long-term organization of workers led to the formation of a working class that began to organize unions, proletarian parties and associations, and gave rise to workers' movements in liberal democracies. These workers' movements led to struggles and demands for better working conditions and social protection. The workers' main demands focused on guarantees against the leading risks such as disease, old age without savings, and work accidents. These demands entered the public debate, workers associated the poverty in which they lived with the form of organization and emergence of capitalist society. It is important to remember that the poverty found in the new urban centers as a result of the industrial process was substantially different from the indigence caused by natural disasters that compromised food production and generated hunger.

Inequalities were gradually recognized, and the state came to use its power to regulate social rights for workers with measures that limited the workday and created public health services. Mechanisms to help families were established, either by state support for religious projects or by creating specific institutions. Thus began the institutionalization of demands for social protection in the realm of the states, configuring the emergence of social policy in industrialized societies (Yazbek, 2012).

Social protection first focused on a wide variety of biological and social factors needed to sustain life, which were specifically recognized by social policy. Traditionally, the literature on social policy tends to see this rise in a dualistic manner (Pereira, 2013). Social policy is often understood as a concession from the state, or as a result of the struggle of workers. This dualistic perspective leads to the mistaken thinking that there are two natures of social policy that compete with each other. The first understands the state as an evil entity that has long served its own interests or only those of specific social segments. This understanding of the state portrays the medieval state, whose interests were exclusively those of the successors to absolute power. It may portray states that did not adopt democratic statutes that allowed a conflict of ideas, projects and positions. Meanwhile, the second concept of the state understands that social policy emanates from workers' movements and is the legitimate route capable of conquering protective laws that go beyond the interests of exploitation.

To understand social policy, it is necessary to go beyond the traditional dualistic approach. Social policy is an expression of relations and conflicts, it is the expression of humans in their totality and particularity. Humans compose the state and civil society, and there is no state and civil society without humanity as a whole. What is society if not a product of the reciprocal action of people, people who are free by law and able to choose one or another form of society. The state is a universal legal and political community, through which people are connected, with rights and responsibilities toward the state, while the state has rights and responsibilities in relation to the people.

While there are social policies that arose from the struggle of workers as well as social policies that are the initiative of the state, nevertheless, this is not to say that there is a dichotomy between one and the other. This thinking results in a trend toward fragmentation of humanity, with emphases given by supporters of one institution or another.

Although human needs expand and reproduce infinitely along with human progress, there are fundamental rights, which are constitutionally guaranteed, such as human dignity that must be guaranteed to any person (Dimoulis & Martins, 2007). The human inequalities change according to the understandings and needs of each historic epoch and with the correlation of political forces. Social rights, like the basic rights, are also forms of consensus, or of what Bobbio (1999) denominates the general consensus about legitimacy, involving a historic foundation of consensus, and therefore, one that is not absolute.

The consensus around social rights, or second-generation rights, represents a set of fundamental values that are specific to a certain community or nation. Social policies represent forms of historic consensus. They are not born by chance, they are not born exclusively from the isolated will of one group or another, but are born from the historic needs that arise from the concrete reality experienced by humans. The right to work, education and healthcare are expressed by social policies that are social rights, and it is understood that in a politically developed society no one should die of hunger. In the 20th century deep economic and social transformations established new relations between states and societies, culminating in concern and establishing guarantees of citizenship made viable by the concept of protections supported by welfare states.

Development of social protection to combat expressions of poverty

The transformations that took place during the 20th century, with the recognition of the value of labor and of the organization of wage society in the realm of nation states, created various models of social protection that were established after World War II. Social welfare states in Europe provided conditional guarantees against a variety of risks of a biological and social nature, such as protection against unemployment, accidents, illness and old age, thus establishing pensions, various social services and insurance. A set of social services and benefits of universal scope were inaugurated, promoted by the state to guarantee a certain harmony between the advance of market forces and relative social stability, providing society with social benefits that provide individuals the security that they will be able to maintain a basic material base and standard of living, and can thus face the destructive effects of an exclusionary mode of production (Martins, 2011).

Misha (2000) affirms that what characterizes the origin of the welfare state is a political consensus about the concepts proposed by Keynes (1996) and Beveridge (1942), without which we would not now have the social protection systems in their various contemporary expressions and experiences. In England in 1942, William Beveridge published *The Social Insurance and Allied Services Report*, which expressed the principles upon which social security policies should be enacted through cooperation between the state and the individual, with the state assuring the services and contributions. Meanwhile, John Maynard

Keynes (1996) applied an economic component to the policies by affirming the state's capacity to control demand in a market economy to assure a high level of economic activity and full male employment, by encouraging the development of the coal industry, railroads, highways and the manufacturing of raw materials. A junction was established of two great initiatives by on one hand creating new jobs, and on the other, by offering protection to workers and to the unemployed or retired. William Beveridge's social security program proposed actions that would combat the risks of unemployment, aging and labor accidents in a market economy with a strong incidence of salaried work. Each one of these concepts led to a mechanism, an intervention in the economy and the provision of services, which were designed to complement the market economy. In other words, the conjunction of these components, in an operation of social engineering, would fulfill the function of giving social legitimation to the market society (Mishra, 2000). The inscription of the needs of urban workers on the political agenda of states was gradually changing and accompanying the new needs of workers for social services. New demands were incorporated such as paid maternity leave and pensions for death and/or illness. Nevertheless, the recognition of these new rights was not automatic, it was a product of political consensus between workers, the state and owners focused on recognizing the concrete need to maintain the lives of the working class and their children (Martins, 2011). By the second half of the 20th century in the Western world, these developments would lead to the establishment of an advanced social model based on a type of property unknown until then: social property. According to Castel (1998), if the survival of workers who are not owners had previously depended essentially on the sale of labor power, this condition was overcome with the consolidation of social property as a form of support for the existence of individuals. This property allows individuals to enjoy the rights of citizenship in an egalitarian manner, and is of a public nature. Castel (1998) mentions retirement as an example, because the right to retirement cannot be sold; when this right is established, it is up to the state to guarantee it. Retirement functions as a minimum form of property that guarantees security.

This was the response conceived by the states of law, to guarantee that all people would have the ability to assure their own existence (Corujo, 2006). As European countries consolidated their social welfare states, the concept of social property was established in the process of confronting the expressions of poverty. This is how most developed countries helped their property-less citizens, who did not have economic resources, to meet their basic needs and alleviate poverty. Thus, the states became decisively involved with the protection of citizens through the recognition of social rights. The welfare state was extended to proposals involving measures with three purposes: achieving full male employment, reducing the inequalities generated by the labor market and socializing the risks inherent to this market. These mechanisms for combating the expressions of poverty and misfortune came to influence developing countries in the creation of social protection measures.

The consequence was nothing less than the birth of the wage society based on male labor, in which a part of the population gains citizenship under labor laws, that is, by means of recognition of rights to retirement pay, pensions, paid vacation and health and maternity leave for women inserted in the labor market, which previously did not exist without the guarantee of labor laws. This supposes a decisive transformation of the social structure by focusing attention on risks created by life in society. It substituted the system in which only property owners were able to confront situations of needs, for a new system in which policies were established to provide access to protection for the majority of the population: social property supported by social rights.

As the social welfare state developed, protections were expanded to reduce risks. The state took on the role of reducer of risks through the construction of a legal status (the recognition of rights) initially based on salaried work. For instance, the healthcare services created and financed by funds that workers pay into, and managed by the state, gradually marked the recognition of the rights of those who have a labor contract. The creation of these services, in addition to responding to protections against risks linked to poor health, also represented freeing real income from healthcare spending.

The role of the state as a provider of well-being decisively influenced the configuration of social policy, which was understood as government measures for managing inequalities, assuring to each sphere of the social structure a certain role in the satisfaction of the needs of individuals (Adelantado, Nogueira, & Rambla, 2000). Therefore, the social structure particular to capitalist societies, the group of institutions, rules and resources that attribute unequal living conditions to individuals and the inherent inequalities are affected by the intervention of various institutions. Thus, the satisfaction of social needs can be realized by the state, the market or the family (Esping-Andersen, 2000).

For a number of years welfare states allowed the execution of two objectives, in a reasonably satisfactory way. First, the management of macroeconomic policy that generated stability and avoided the cyclical crises of production and employment as occurred before World War II. Second, a redistribution of income that facilitated the improvement of living conditions of the more unfortunate members of society, in the case of workers with insufficient income (Castells & Bosch, 1998).

This redistribution, the consecration of solidarity, as a key principle, is of decisive importance, especially in relation to those aspects of state organization most linked to satisfaction of individual needs linked to the risks of social life. The protective action of the state is presented as a right to redistribution (Dupeyroux, 1998), offered through a set of mechanisms for redistribution of income in favor of the ill, disabled, elderly, families with children, the unemployed and the poor (Euzéby, 2004).

Economic recession and the reconfiguration of the mechanisms of social protection

In the early 1970s, the cyclical crises of the productive system came to decisively compromise the more consolidated protection systems. The effort to break the pact between capital, labor and the state was based on criticisms of the developmentalist model of the "Golden Age" (Hobsbawm, 2011, p. 158), especially in the form of state intervention, on social policies and on the power that worker associations have to pressure the state and capital for a more equitable share of the profits resulting from production. The revival of liberal ideas and reforms, which became known as neoliberalism, supported the stimulation of free competition, an increase in productivity through the implementation of technologies, and an accelerated search for economic growth, triggering a new historic era, with a strong impact on states, workers and social protection. The crisis that hit developed and developing capitalist countries in the 1970s reconfigured the form of conducting politics and how the state responded to the demands for social protection.

The control of geopolitics by international economic regulatory agencies and the dominance of financial globalization associated with neoliberalism appeared as responses to the crisis, proposing formulas for restoring national economies with a package of deep reforms. The reform package guided countries like Chile, Brazil, Argentina and Mexico to cut public investments in social protection policies and services, and transfer to the market a significant portion of healthcare and social security services. Services and benefits were transferred to non-governmental organizations, without being recognized as rights, and their supply was restricted by highly selective and focused means testing. This same phenomenon has taken place in recent years in the countries of Mediterranean Europe, especially in Greece, Portugal and to a lesser degree Spain.

Thus, after 1973, the world lost many of it references and slipped into the instability of crisis. The curiosity of the crisis of the 1970s was that the global economy became less stable despite the fact that those elements established by the "control of computerized inventory, better communication and faster transportation that sustained the economy, were in fact stronger than ever which reduced the importance of the volatile 'stock cycle' of the old 'mass production'" (Hobsbawm, 2011, p. 394). The new information technology of the 1970s, which allowed the creation of methods capable of eliminating the stocks associated to the previous cycle by applying the Just-in-Time method of supply, thus provided "a much greater capacity to vary production from one moment to another, to confront the demands for change" (Hobsbawm, 2011, p. 394). These events contribute to the reduction of work and to the reduction of funds that financed social protection policies in the countries that were incorporating the new logic.

It is worth pointing out elements that triggered the crisis, from the liberal perspective, which I will present in two blocks. First, the structural problems of a model in which the state intervenes in the market and acts as its guarantor, and that is made concrete in three manifestations. On the one hand, it led to the end of what was called the Keynesian Consensus (Hobsbawm, 2011) and the imposition of orthodox economic precepts that proposed minimum state intervention. On the other, Friedman (1982) argued that social policies have grave negative effects because they increase taxes and harm private initiative; while social protections discourage their beneficiaries from working thus creating dependency and rigidity in labor markets by guaranteeing a minimum wage and unemployment benefits. Finally, there were criticisms of the failures of the state and the inefficiency of the public sector, which contrasts with the efficient action of the private sector; which justifies the privatization not only of the state-owned companies, but also of many public services (Bresser-Pereira & Grau, 1999).

The second block of the causes that explain the crisis of the welfare state are related to important historic changes in various fields. First of all, economic plans with very significant alterations were made as the consequence of two factors: one was the consolidation in the more developed countries of a post-industrial or informational economy (Castel, 1997) based on the realization of services instead of the production of goods; and on the other, the consolidation of the dynamic and growing global integration of open markets for labor, goods, services, technologies and capital, that is, financial globalization, accompanied by accusations that social policies are impediments to international competitiveness.These transformations led to a scenario of growing insecurity to the degree that as financial globalization grows, society exalts individualism in a context dominated by economic liberalism, in which state actions, the collective good and solidarity are all given secondary importance (Esping-Andersen, 2000).

The crisis of the welfare state questions the distribution of responsibilities; it now involves reducing the size of the state to fundamentally reinforce the action of the market when dealing with social risks. Based on strongly individualistic concepts, the detractors of government affirm that public social protection measures must be substantially reduced (or even disappear completely), because that is the only way to revive the weakening economy and the best way to hold individuals responsible for their conditions.

Bob Jessop (1999) labels this new phase adopted by the state as the Schumpeterian Workfare State, in which the focus is shifted to the promotion of innovation in products, organizational processes and markets, to achieve structural competitiveness of open economies, based on economic mechanisms that give priority to the supply and not the demand side, in contrast to the Keynesian welfare state. Therefore, based on the ideas of Schumpeterian workfare, we have the reduction of state coverage that strengthens the private sector. This allows identifying important transformations in the following planes: in the services offered by the market, in labor contracts, in union activities and in the collective defense of workers' interests, as they struggle to maintain historically acquired rights (Corujo, 2006).

The right to social protection is expressed by a set of public and private measures aimed at meeting the social needs of citizens and differentiated in two blocks: public social protection and private social protection. The needs of citizens began to be met by a combination of measures: social security systems, which in many countries are the exclusive responsibility of the state, with its regulation and laws solely the responsibility of the state. While in many other countries it may be complemented by private insurance. Healthcare services involve a broader range of heterogeneous solutions. Many countries have private health insurance programs, while others use public mechanisms with the participation of the private sector in laboratory and diagnostic services and others, for example, guarantee free public services. There are other countries that have public healthcare facilities, but which charge for care. Meanwhile, many countries have social assistance programs that are not based on contributions, providing other forms of social protection found in a wide variety of mechanisms, objectives and modalities that vary by country. Born from charitable organization in some countries, social assistance programs not based on the contributions of beneficiaries became consolidated in public policy in many social protection statutes, and are provided in many ways, ranging from public programs executed by state agencies, public programs executed by private companies, public systems based on conditionalities, and private systems.

Finally, there is unemployment insurance. This is a social protection mechanism provided by states to reduce risk in situations of unemployment when a worker and his or her family lose income and experience a deterioration of well-being. Among the most common modalities are: monthly pay for a certain number of months for formal workers with a labor contract, grants for training or retraining, or even compulsory savings programs, under which a percentage of monthly salary is deducted. At the end of the contract or in a situation of unemployment the amount, plus interest, is returned to the worker.

Thus, from the 1970s until the 1990s deep fissures appeared in the social protection mechanisms and programs of nation states. In many Latin American countries, under military dictatorships after their democracies were silenced in a series of military coups, the social protection systems were weakened, with the rise of highly meritocratic systems in the field of labor and clientelistic politics. These years were difficult for developing countries, not only because of the absence of sovereignty and democracy. Unemployment grew widely, while expressions of poverty multiplied, leaving many countries in grave situations, particularly those that sustained their social policies with resources from taxing labor. Over the years of developing social protection in Latin America, especially after 1960, with the installment of military dictatorships, the measures were essentially guided by social security systems. The systems introduced in the region after World War II consist in supports for aging, illness, pensions and some elements of health insurance, as took place with the models of the healthcare systems in Brazil, Argentina and Chile, before the constitutional reforms in which receiving care in the public healthcare system required the user to have a formal contractual labor tie, or when unemployed or not able to work, the tie must be established as a dependent of a person with a labor contract. The coverage was limited to formal workers, since receipt of social security in Latin America has always been dependent on work, the main criteria for access was having formal employment, and even so many professional categories did not have access to these guarantees. Moreover, a very limited fraction of the population was formally employed. Most people without a formal labor contract and without access to more solid social protection mechanisms depended on residual food supply programs (Ferreira & Robalino, 2010). Since then the use of means

testing to determine if an individual or a family is eligible to access public benefits has become more demanding in the inspection of families with the expansion
of policies to fight poverty in Latin America, establishing a strong character of
selectivity for social protection.

Risks of unemployment and gender inequality

Formal labor relations have suffered important changes since the 1960s, and
with them came similar changes in the forms of social protection, the concept of
citizenship and social rights. The economic crisis in the capitalist economies in
the 1970s created a sharp reduction in the size of the formal labor market, which
was somewhat unexpected by workers, given the expansion of production lines.
This created an awareness of the vulnerability and instability in the maintenance
and creation of new fields of employment in the industrialized or industrializing
countries, based on strategic and structural alliances of neocolonial exploitation,
which argued for the advance of new technologies and a new morphology of
work as a necessary step for development. Jobs came to require greater skills for
operating new technologies, while the number of jobs was reduced through the
use of automation, robotics and information technology in production.

The crisis radically modified industrial organization. The large industrial
regimes, which were iconic expressions of power and progress, were quickly
converted into archaeological relics, crushed by a new business dynamic in
which to reduce costs, and operations were transferred to emerging countries,
often causing a severe precarization of material living conditions as well as
environmental degradation.

The global division of labor, and above all, the rules that govern and articulate the relations of exchange between countries, varied deeply and became lib-
eralized and globalized as called for by the new rhetoric being promoted. All this
meant that the sense of stability that is one of the central resources of the civic
imaginary of developed and democratic countries, was set adrift, instilling a new
sense of crisis and vulnerability, as well as the need for adjustments, as if each
day there was a discursive tonic that gave rise to a new psychic landscape. The
adjustments deeply affected industrialized workers and regions, and a new type
of unemployment appeared, not caused by the conjuncture, but by deeper structural forces. Some of the most solid and vital concepts, such as progress, stability
and security inherited or influenced by the Keynesian period, quickly became
volatile, which led to a regime of uncertainty and instability. The intellectual
debate (Silva, 2010), especially in France, sought to understand the new dynamic
and began to speak of the end of the society of labor, and the rise of the society
of risk or of the fluid society, creating a new metaphorical mark that gave
meaning to new forms of insecurity.

In Europe, the increased precariousness experienced after the financial crises
of 2008, now affects segments of workers who had previously achieved stability,
re-establishing a mass vulnerability that had been overcome in the period of the
hegemony of the social welfare policies, characterizing a dynamic that is no

longer marginal and comes to be the center of this phase of capitalist develop-ment. Meanwhile, in Latin America, the poverty has deep and historic roots that have long ravished the continent, still associated with weak, residual and poorly developed social protection systems in some sectors and countries, which creates deep marks of generational poverty. Hunger and poverty are manifest on an exponential scale in the Global South, where many countries are unable to guar-antee democratic and basic social institutions to care for their populations and have a total absence of social protection policies (Harvey, 2007).

There are common elements found in all these regions, yet on different scales, involving the articulation and inseparability between the precarious forms in which social life has been produced. They are expressed in the restructuring of labor markets and of the role of the state, in the lack of social protections, in weak democratic institutions, and the corrosion of historically achieved social rights, in the tireless search for the wealth of some at the cost of others. These are global processes that financial globalization appears to deepen throughout the world. This scenery establishes challenges to understanding the various situ-ations of poverty and how social protection systems have articulated with the labor market to overcome, through the establishment and application of social rights, these situations that are no longer exclusive to certain geographic regions of the planet.

Before the international financial crisis the International Labour Organization (2008) presented a global panorama of labor from 1990 to 2007 that warned of a still fragile and precarious world of labor marked by a deficit of decent work. After the crisis, the degradation of working conditions increased the risks and the vulnerability, especially for the most poor who do not have access to or have been laid off from formal work posts.

According to the International Labour Organization's World of Work Report (ILO, 2008) there there was an increase in income inequality, an increase in indebtedness of workers and their families, growth in atypical employment (char-acterized by temporary contracts or informal and unregistered work, which does not provide labor or social rights, with lower salaries and precarious working con-ditions), which, according to the report, may have contributed to the weakening of labor's negotiating power, especially that of less qualified workers.

Beyond problems with employment, extreme poverty remains an ongoing dis-aster. The United Nation's Human Development Report of 2014 indicates that more than 1.2 billion people continue to live in a situation of poverty (PNUD, 2014, p. 74). This means that 22% of the world's population survives on less than US$1.25 per day (PNUD, 2014, p. 74). If we consider a poverty level of US$2.5 dollars per day per person, a shocking 50% of the world's population, or 2.7 billion people, live in poverty (PNUD, 2014, p. 74).

People living in extreme poverty require alternative forms of social protection not linked to employment because those living in extreme poverty do not have access to the formal labor market. Women suffer various types of disadvantages and discrimination in the realms of healthcare, education and employment. Throughout the world, the Human Development Index (HDI) for females is on average 8% lower than the HDI for men. The Gender Inequality Index in 149 countries demonstrates national actions in the field of reproductive health, empowerment and participation in the labor market are marked by gender inequality (PNUD, 2014). Unlike HDI, a higher value on the Gender Inequality Index indicates poor performance (PNUD, 2014). The indicators vary between an average of 0.0317 for Europe and Central Asia and 0.575 for Sub-Saharan Africa (PNUD, 2014, p. 181). UN data show that Slovenia exceeds all countries, with an index of 0.021 – an exception in the world, while Yemen has the highest rate of 0.733 (PNUD, 2014, p. 40).

Insufficient and precarious reproductive healthcare services constitute one of the main reasons for gender inequality, particularly in developing countries. In Sub-Saharan Africa maternal mortality is 474 per 100,000 births (PNUD, 2014, p. 40). Maternal deaths have grave consequences for newborns and their older siblings, because children grow up without a maternal figure, and in many cases the older siblings take responsibility for caring for the younger ones. Pregnancy in adolescence is another problem. In Sub-Saharan Africa there are 110 births per 1,000 adolescents aged between 15 and 19 (PNUD, 2014, p. 41). The high rate of pregnancy in adolescence demonstrates the inefficiency of the healthcare services for adolescent women and the lack of family planning, and compromises the opportunities of adolescent mothers to study and enter the labor market. This indicator confirms that in countries or regions with low social protection, the expressions of poverty are more rigid and are transmitted across generations. This scenario has presented challenges to the establishment of what is known as social protection and how it needs to be acknowledged as an inalienable citizenship right in all parts of the world.

Social protection in Latin American and the Caribbean

The establishment of social protection systems in Latin America and the Caribbean is traditionally associated with the fight against poverty. Initiated in some countries of the region in the early 20th century, they are characterized by residual systems sustained mostly by contributions from workers, their employers and government.

The social protection mechanisms in Latin America and the Caribbean never came close to the better known forms of social payments of the European social welfare states. Their configuration as rights supported by the states reflects the late democratic formation of the continent and the fragile formal labor market found in the main countries of the continent, like those found in Brazil, Argentina, Peru and Colombia, as well as the poorest countries such as Haiti, Honduras, Paraguay and Bolivia. Without exception, until the mid 1980s, social policies and social protection programs on the continent were based on means testing, the documentation of contributions, or formal employment. This situation changed with the end of the military dictatorships and the establishment of democracies in the region, allowing elected governments under pressure from social movements to attain gains in the drafting of social rights linked to healthcare, the provision of social services, pensions and reform of laws regarding care for the vulnerable such as children, adolescents and the elderly living in situations of risk.

Nevertheless, it appears that the continent went against international trends. At the same time as the more developed economies of the world entered the crisis of the 1980s, forcing a reconfiguration on a global scale of production and employment systems and also of spending on social protection, contradictorily countries in Latin America and the Caribbean, at the peak of the international crisis, sought to build social protection systems for the entire population, breaking with means testing, direct contributions or programs linked to formal employment, and many have new constitutions that guarantee forms of social protection. Nevertheless, Chile has experimented with privatizing adjustments in its social policies, transferring to the private sector services of healthcare, education and social security, and even funeral insurance. Others, such as Brazil, established laws and regulations that led to a deep reorientation, with the re-establishment of means testing so that if a family or society is unable to provide basic needs, the state assumes the risks even if it only offers a fragile social net. Other countries with budget difficulties advanced little in the construction of their systems, such as Paraguay, Haiti, Bolivia, Honduras and others.

It is perceived that the problem of poverty and the absence of strong social protection mechanisms reveal the region's historic condition at the periphery of the world associated with low economic growth, which leads to a constant lack of protection. This situation, compounded by low or poor quality education, deficits of learning, malnutrition, hunger, absence of basic sanitation, pensions and of participation leads to the generational reproduction of poverty, given that the children of poor families have a strong likelihood of reproducing their parents' condition, and are not able to access quality jobs or protection systems that could help them break away from the clutches of poverty, leading to its systematic reproduction. What appears to give an identity to the Latin American people is not cultural traits or equality, to the contrary, it is the inequality among the populations in all the countries that is the identity of this region.

This trait presents us with an important point of convergence between social workers and the locations where they work, given that their actions and efforts are focused on the expressions of poverty and inequality. Although they do not have the capacity to qualitatively alter the scenario, they influence certain realities and promote initiatives for significant portions of the population, allowing these groups to achieve slightly better standards of living. Nevertheless, social work in the region is traditionally related to the administration of situations of non-work. That is, social work focuses on those expressions of poverty in which people do not have access to formal employment. Social workers in Latin America and the Caribbean mostly attend to people who live on the streets, in the peripheries of large cities and get by with small jobs in the informal sector or with various forms of assistance. Social workers serve adolescents who commit crimes, the unprotected elderly, those without income, as well as women and children who are victims of domestic and/or sexual violence. They also attend to the disabled who are unable to work and to victims of disasters increasingly caused by extreme weather events. More recently social workers respond to the recognition of the rights of indigenous people and those of Afro-descendent communities in countries like Brazil, Bolivia, Venezuela and Ecuador. In addition, they work with sexually diverse populations. Social workers play a key role in operationalizing the social and citizenship rights of individuals, family and community members. This is evident in common efforts in the provision of social services, health and education.

In parallel to the attempts to establish social protection systems, in the 1990s, the continent experienced a period of deep paradigmatic transformations. On the one hand the young democracies organized and established political institutions, while an economic crisis shook the countries, especially those that had a strong industrial base such as Mexico, Brazil and Argentina, which all nearly collapsed in the decade because of their high international debts. The adoption of liberal trade policies triggered a brief increase in exports and imports, but imports grew more than exports, and the trade imbalance led to a drop in economic activity and job creation. The direct consequences of reduced employment in the region led to an increase in informal, unregulated labor, that lacked the benefits of social protection, and an intensification of work even when protected. This movement led to a reduced number of people protected by social security programs, forcing governments to expand public spending in the social sphere. Social spending between 1990 and 2003 increased from 10% of GNP to 13.8% (Mattei, 2009, p. 2).

In 2005 the Economic Commission for Latin America and the Caribbean (ECLAC) identified families with per capita income of less than US$2 per day to characterize situations of poverty or indigence on the continent (Coelho, Tapajos, & Rodrigues, 2010, p. 286). Although ECLAC affirmed that social spending continued to grow, the resources allocated to fighting poverty seem to have been insufficient to attend to the vast number of poor on the continent, given that in 2002 there were 221 million people who were classified as poor, which represents 44% of the total population (ECLAC, 2005, p. 101). Of this total, nearly 96 million people were in a situation of extreme poverty, that is, they lived with US$1 or less per day (ECLAC, 2005, p. 101). Most of the poor were living in urban regions lacking in urban planning and with poor infrastructure.

The social protection systems organized in Latin America during this period were characterized in a comparative study conducted by Dixon (2000; 2010) that shows three important forms of social policies and their funding sources. The first is funded under the government budget and is aimed at the entire population or designated categories and their dependents. It is designed to reduce or prevent poverty, and provide social compensations. These programs are characterized by means testing to determine eligibility. The second, also financed by the government budget as well as contributions from employers and employees, is aimed at workers in specific or formal categories and their dependents, and has the prime objective of poverty prevention. These policies are characterized by user contributions. The third group, financed by individual contributions, is aimed at the insured, and is designed to prevent poverty with eligibility based on payment of the most recent contributions.

These policies involve various operational strategies: employer contributions, mandatory contracting of private plans, mandatory personal plans, social assistance, social contributions and mandatory public funds – National Social Security Funds (Dixon, 2000; 2010). Nevertheless, there are gaps of implementation between the systems, in terms of coverage programs, eligibility for benefits and the generosity of benefits and in the forms of administrating and financing the programs. These gaps can be significant in countries that suffer from serious economic disequilibrium.

The various countries of the region have different types of coverage. Some countries opt for universalization of some policies yet not of all, with coverage restricted through the exclusion of specific segments of the population for ideological, political or economic reasons. Some countries establish restrictions based on criteria related to need, or to budget provisions, or previous salaries. In the field of healthcare we find the provision of benefits that include medical, hospital and paramedical care, in different modalities, those covered by systems for the contributors and their dependents, those countries that restrict the availability, or the range of healthcare benefits provided by the system (Dixon, 2000). There are also countries that provide incentives to encourage or train users to enter the labor market to reduce dependence (Dixon, 2000).

Income transfer programs and the reconfiguration of social protection

The Latin America and the Caribbean region continues to face huge challenges. Compounding the fragility of social and economic policies, basic citizenship rights are still weak in the region and access to broad quality public services limited. The rapid growth of cities has been a major challenge for local governments. In 1950, the region had only eight cities with more than one million inhabitants (ONU-Habitat, 2012, p. 32). In 2012, there were 56 (ONU-Habitat, 2012, p. 32). This exponential growth has led to urban problems that aggravate poverty and inequality. Informal and precarious housing (in improvised settlements and "favelas"), lack of basic services, insufficient public transportation, problems with private transportation, and the scarcity of community facilities and public spaces are some of the factors that aggravate poverty. All these problems are compounded by the absence of political will and by the weak government institutions responsible for social protection mechanisms (ECLAC, 2012).

Although the number of social workers has increased in public agencies and non-governmental organizations that enact social policies in these regions, there is still an insufficient number of personnel, instruments and resources to attend to all the people who require social programs and policies. Nevertheless, the greater challenge for social work in this context is the fragility of the social policies and the focalization and selectivity of programs that exclude many poor people from accessing resources that could promote a decent life. In many cases, the benefits and services are not sufficient for conducting long-term work to improve a family's situation of poverty. Many actions have been occurring in large cities and their surroundings to improve housing conditions and provide urban infrastructure and services. This initial work to permanently organize the population and provide information and education has been conducted by social workers and some of the experiences have demonstrated good results.

To strengthen efforts to overcome poverty and inequality, the United Nations presented the post-2015 development agenda, which includes the Sustainable Development Goals (SDGs) to guide global development. Once again the document emphasizes attaining dignity for all, and is entitled *The Road to Dignity by 2030: Ending Poverty, Transforming All Lives and Protecting the Planet*. The document presents 17 objectives and 169 goals related to sustainable development that compose the agenda for the United Nations and the signatory countries (United Nations, 2014, pp. 5–14). The objectives focus on overcoming hunger and improving indicators of healthcare, education, gender equality and on the promotion of economic sustainability with inclusionary growth, employment and infrastructure, as well as environmental sustainability.

The concern for confronting growing poverty gained a definitive space on national agendas with the implementation of actions in various countries in Latin America and the Caribbean (see Table 7.1). These include the Zero Hunger program in Brazil, the Family in Action program in Colombia, the Family Program in Argentina, the National Food Plan in Uruguay, the Workers' Food

Table 7.1 Cash transfer programs in Latin America and the Caribbean

Country	Program
Honduras	Family Grant Program (1990)
Mexico	Opportunities (1997)
Ecuador	Human Development Grant (1998)
Colombia	Families in Action (2000)
Jamaica	Program of Advancement through Health and Education PATH (2001)
Chile	Solidary Chile (2001)
Brazil	Family Grant (2003)
El Salvador	Solidarity Network, The Solidarity Rural Communities Program, The Solidarity Urban Communities Program, (2005–2009)
Peru	The All Together Network (National Program of Direct Support for the Most Poor (2005)
Paraguay	The Hug Program, Program Tekoporã and Program Ñpytyvô (2005)
Dominican Republic	Solidarity Program (2005)
Panamá	Opportunities Network (2006)
Costa Rica	We Move Forward (2006)
Trinidad and Tobago	Target Conditional Cash Transfer (2007)
Uruguay	The New Regime for Family Grants Program (2008)
Bolivia	The Juana Azudy Mother-Child Grant Program (2009)
Argentina	The Universal Grant per Child for Social Protection (2009)
Guatemala	My Insurance Grant (2012)

Plan in Venezuela and the Opportunities Program in Mexico. All of the countries in the region gradually came to develop social policies to fight hunger.

In addition to the more specific initiatives to face the problem of hunger, since the 1990s, many countries established income transfer programs, aimed at population groups experiencing greater social vulnerability, and based on means testing, to verify the degree of poverty with the institution of mandatory conditions for the beneficiary families so that they overcome the condition of extreme poverty.

The income transfer programs established in Latin America and the Caribbean since the 1990s focus on dispersed, small-scale programs that have little impact on the extent of poverty (Silva, 2014). After 1995, these programs took on new scope and dimensions, so that social protections in the region were redesigned and income transfer programs became the main mechanisms for confronting poverty. Organized in this way, social protection is redimensioned by encompassing systems that are incapable of confronting the structural determinations that generate the poverty, because, in general, they are limited to immediate relief of the traits of poverty without confronting the structural causes.

Social protection ranges from a universal proposal based on the right to citizenship and sustainability to a concept focused on people with immediate needs. The right is substituted by a more rational strategy. By focusing resources and political and professional efforts on the most vulnerable or poorest, rights come to be restricted to a few, and lose their universal character. The fight against inequality, specific to classic models of social protection, is not embodied in this model.

Although the income transfer programs compose an important part of family income, it is apparent that income from work continues to be the primary source of livelihoods for families, obtained by the participation of family members in the labor market (Lavinas, 2014). This demonstrates how the disparity between income from labor and the concentration of wealth remains unequal in Latin America. The transfer of income by means of these programs is still quite low. Most of the beneficiaries of income transfer programs are those most affected by poverty: children and adolescents, women, indigenous peoples, older people, disabled, those who have been left homeless or were expelled from their territories and others.

Gender inequality

Gender inequality continues to be a considerable problem in the region that can compound the effects of poverty. Women suffer from inequality and discrimination. Women assume most of the workload in the family, including non-paid domestic work and child care, while they also work outside the home, often at informal jobs that are poorly paid. This situation is traditionally aggravated by the conditions and location where most women in poverty live, often in distant regions of the urban peripheries, which forces them to spend long hours traveling from home to work and back. The rapidly growing urban centers of Latin

America suffer from poor quality or absent basic services, while many women are unable to access public services because their daily work shift coincides with the hours that services are offered. Many women are also victims of domestic, psychological, physical and sexual violence (Bott, Guedes, Goodwin, & Mendonza, 2013).

In 2005, there were 563 million people living in Latin America and the Caribbean (Costa, Horta, & Roldan, 2007, p. 56), and in 2012 there was an estimated population of 593 million people, including 291 million men and 301 million women (United Nations, 2013). The higher number of women, combined with the historic context of their disadvantaged position in the region, means that there is a higher rate of poverty among women, and of families composed solely of mothers and children.

According to data provided by 14 countries, 6.7% of the employed Latin American population works in the care provision sector, and three-quarters of these are employed in domestic services (ECLAC, 2012, p. 128). Women occupy 94% of the jobs associated with this sector, 71% in domestic services and 23% in educational and healthcare services (ECLAC, 2012, p. 128). The remaining 6% are men employed in domestic services or other jobs in the care sector (ECLAC, 2012, p. 128).

The scarce or weak regulation of domestic labor in all countries of the region, low salaries, low access to social protection, discrimination and precarious working conditions places many domestic workers in a deeper state of poverty, a situation that is aggravated in families where women are the heads of household, and even more seriously when older or ill people are in the family. Although it is difficult to precisely measure the portion of the population that lives with some type of disability, it is estimated that at least 12% of the Latin American and Caribbean population live with some type of disability, or approximately 66 million people (ECLAC, 2012, p. 185).

The disadvantged position of women, who are victims of oppressive relations and who usually earn less than men, even when performing the same job, is indicated by the fact that they occupy a greater proportion of jobs in the informal sector, where millions of women struggle daily for survival and sell their labor as domestic servants, temporary house cleaners or in other sectors of the informal economy, such as collectors of recyclable material. Many women are also subject to sexual exploitation.

This situation is present from small cities to the larger and more developed ones, mainly in the latter, where poor women are dually victimized because they are invisible to residual social policies that are poorly institutionalized, by urban and police violence and by suffering caused from gender discrimination. Meanwhile, in rural areas, women often continue to be treated as the property of men or husbands (Lisboa, 2003). In the remote interiors of countries in which agriculture is still an important source of subsistence for many families, archaic family structures are found, in which women exercise the role of reproducers to provide new laborers in the fields. Women must also assume all the responsibility for preparing food and other domestic chores, while still dividing their time with work in the fields. This situation is aggravated by their total submission to orders from men, not only those from their husbands, but also of older male children. These traits also submit younger women to submission, under which they do not have authorization to study or work outside the domestic circle, and they may not marry as they wish.

An important characteristic to be emphasized is the role that income transfer programs have promoted in the lives of women. Although the amount of money provided is low, it is often sufficient to allow many women to break historic marks of hunger and disadvantaged status. It may allow them to separate from violent companions on whom they are no longer dependent for meeting domestic expenses, breaking with histories of domestic, physical and psychological violence. In addition, women who sustain maternity alone are able to establish better rates of development for their children with the assistance of income transfers. This situation alone presents important advances, even if the broader social protection model is not universal. Without the income transfer programs, these women would be unprotected and left on their own to face the risk of living in society. Nevertheless, it is important to highlight that social protection based on rights allows continuity and diversity in services and attention, allowing focusing on more than the most immediate needs.

In relation to criticisms, the central complaint about the transition of social protection systems is that the concept of the sovereignty of the citizen has been exchanged for the concept of the sovereignty of the consumer. This phenomenon, which developed with the implementation of economic adjustment policies and enhanced by these income transfer programs, has imposed a new paradigm in social protection. The nature of social protection programs has changed substantially, even if the class extracts that are aided by the income transfer programs cannot be considered consumers. Although the families acquire a certain power to consume and take on debt, in general, the history of poverty in which these families are immersed has never allowed them to consume the minimum that a person needs for their physical development, including good quality food, with proteins and vitamins, which are essential for proper physical and mental development, as well as home appliances, cultural goods, or others of any kind.

Economic indicators point to a range of possibilities in the continent. In 2011, regional production grew 4.3% while per capita GNP grew 3.2% (ECLAC, 2012, p. 17). While this was lower than growth in 2010, the region is showing signs of recovering from the crisis of 2009 (ECLAC, 2012, p. 17). The ECLAC indicates that employment rates rose in the region every year since 2002, with the exception of 2009, because of the global crisis. Average unemployment in 2010 in the region was 7.3% (ECLAC, 2012, p. 17). This average rate is the lowest for the region since the 1990s when Latin America was plunged into a deep crisis. Nearly all of the countries of the region now have unemployment below 8% (ECLAC, 2012, p. 17).

This general economic growth has helped reduce poverty, and despite weak real growth in real wages with an increase of focused programs, there has been a real and expressive reduction of the population that lives in poverty. In 1998, the region had 192 million people living in indigence and poverty (Kliksberg, 2002), while in 2012, there were 167 million people living in situations of indigence or poverty (ECLAC, 2014). This represents 28.8% of the population in the region (ECLAC, 2014). Meanwhile, the policies for fighting situations of indigence were not efficient if the years 2011 and 2012 are compared, the number of 66 million people living in situation of indigence remained stable in the two years (ECLAC, 2012, p. 18). This is also caused by the low public investments in diversification of benefits and basic social protection services. Despite positive indicators in relation to the growth of salaries and reduction of poverty on the continent, other social protection policies, such as citizenship rights, have been de-emphasized or transferred to the private sector, as has been occurring with healthcare that is increasingly treated as a commodity.

Poverty in Latin America continues its declining trend, even if at a slower pace than in recent years, while the historic traits of generational poverty are perpetuated. Even with the reduction in poverty rates and an expanding formal labor market, many countries on the continent still have unacceptable levels. For this reason, the creation of a social protection floor for the continent is essential to assist governments to develop policies that can overcome the expressions of poverty. Despite the reductions of poverty on the continent, there has been little change in income inequality. One of the historic marks of the region is the high concentrations of wealth in the hands of a few. The statistics available for 18 countries show that the wealthiest 10% of the population in Latin America received 32% of the total income while the poorest 40% received only 15% (ECLAC, 2012, p. 22). The situation presented is largely due to the good economic performance in the region in recent years. The real growth in GNP in most nations has allowed improved rates of redistribution of income through salaries and also the implementation of social protection measures for a wider portion of the population, even if still limited.

The growth of GNP also permitted governments in the region to invest more resouces in social policies and programs, broadening the labor market for social workers with the creation and expansion of new services. This took place in Brazil with the creation of the Single Social Assistance System in 2005, which increased the hiring of professionals in the field of social services. In 2013, for instance, 294,000 people were employed in the field (Martins, 2015, p. 66), with social workers being the key public employee in the sector – 40% of those hired were social workers (Martins, 2015, p. 66). The growth of government resources allowed the expansion of income transfer programs in nearly all the countries, making them more generous. In these programs, the social workers assist families with registration, accompany them and provide guidance about what families must do. They help place children and adolescents in schools and encourage the use of basic healthcare services and vaccines. They also work in groups with women who are victims of violence for overcoming male oppression and the marks of poverty (Martins, 2015).

Among other dimensions of the work of social workers, they are found inserted in healthcare systems, where they facilitate and provide information about procedures for accessing services, and provide treatment for very poor families who do not have the means to acquire medication and purchase food. The concern with the aging population in Latin America has also raised the need for new services led by social workers such as protecting the homeless or older people who suffer poor treatment or those who are not able to meet their basic needs because of a lack of income, enabling access to non-contributory social benefits. Improvements and expansions have been seen in healthcare and in elementary, high school and college education, there are more people participating in social security programs, while social policies not based on contributions have expanded along with conditional income transfers and benefits for specific age groups from childhood to the elderly. Although the continent is still far from achieving the standards of the systems proposed by Beveridge (1942) and Keynes (1996) for Europe after World War II, the region is heading toward a concrete reduction of poverty.

Conclusion

The rise and development of social protection mechanisms to fight poverty and inequality have provided millions of people throughout the world access to better living conditions. Social protection expresses attentions that are real responses to needs for survival, to fragility and to the victimization of the human condition.

The great challenge today is to think of and disseminate increasingly broader mechanisms for social protection that offer solidarity to citizens, regardless of geographic region or country. Social protection encompasses basic rights to survival, the preservation of life and the guarantee of human rights. Although there is no universally accepted and clear concept of social protection, it converges on the protection of workers and families and cannot only be reduced to fighting poverty, but must incorporate social risks and vulnerabilities.

Social protection should be constructed by strong institutions, with multisectoral offerings that crystalize state intervention in the induction of continuing development of countries by supplying services for citizenship, healthcare, education, nutrition and a wide variety of protections, and that incorporate management tools that respond to the particular characteristics of the demands of people in each context. Nevertheless, there is still much to be done to overcome the fragilities or absence of protection in various countries to construct more egalitarian societies.

References

Adelantado, J., Nogueira, J., & Rambla, X. (2000). El marco de análises: las relaciones complejas entre estrutura social y políticas sociais [Analyses within the complex relationships between social and political structure]. *Cambios en el Estado del Bienestar.* Barcelona: Icaria.

Beveridge, W. (1942). *Social insurance and allied services.* London: Published by His Majesty's Stationery Office.

Bobbio, N. (1999). *A era dos direitos* [The era of rights] (10th ed.). Rio de Janeiro: Campus.

Bott, S., Guedes, A., Goodwin, M., & Mendonza, J.A. (2013). *Violencia contra la mujer en América Latina y el Caribe: Análisis comparativo de datos poblacionales de 12 países* [Violence against women in Latin America and the Caribbean: Comparative analysis of population data from 12 countries]. Washington, DC: Organización Panamerica de la Salud.

Bresser-Pereira, L.C., & Grau, N.C. (1999). *O Público Não-Estatal na Reforma do Estado* [The public non-state in state reform]. Rio de Janeiro: Fundação Getúlio Vargas.

Castel, M. (1997). *La era de la información. Economia Sociedad y Cultura – Vol. II El poder de la identidad* [The age of information: Economics society and culture – Vol. II The power of identity]. Madrid: Alienza.

Castel, R. (1998). *Las metamorfosis de la cuestión social. Una crónica del salariado* [The metamorphosis of the social question: A chronicle of wage labor]. Buenos Aires: Paidós.

Castells, A., & Bosch, N. (1998). El futuro Del Estado Del Bienestar: algunas líneas de reflexión [The future of the welfare state: Some reflections]. In A. Castells & N. Bosch, *El futuro Del bienestar* (pp. 17–100). Madrid: Civitas.

Coelho, M.F., Tapajos, L.S., & Rodrigues, M. (2010). *Políticas sociais para o desenvolvimento: superar a pobreza e promover a inclusão* [Social policies for development: Overcoming poverty and promote social inclusion]. Brasília: Ministério do Desenvolvimento Social e Combate à Fome & UNESCO.

Corujo, B.S. (2006). *Introducción al derecho de la protección social* [Introduction of the right to social protection]. Valencia: Tirant Lo Blanch.

Costa, C.D., Horta, C.R., & Roldan, M.I. (2007). Novas formas de exploração do trabalho e inflexões do modelo de desenvolvimento: precarização do trabalho e migração no século XXI [New forms of labor exploitation and inflections of the development model: Labor precariousness and migration in the twenty-first century]. *Revita de Políticas Públicas, 11*, 55–79.

Dimoulis, D., & Martins, L. (2007). *Teoria Geral dos Direitos Fundamentais* [General theory of fundamental rights]. São Paulo: RT.

Dixon, J. (2000). Sistemas de seguridade social na América Latina: uma avaliação ordinal [Social security systems in Latin America: An ordinal assessment]. *Opinião Pública, 6*, 263–281.

Dixon, J. (2010). Comparative social welfare: The existential humanist perspective and challenge. *Journal of Comparative Social Welfere, 26*, 177–187.

Dupeyroux, J.J. (1998). *Droit de la sécurité sociale* [Social security law]. Paris: Dallos.

ECLAC. (2005). *Hambrey cohesión social: como revertir la relación entre inequidad y desnutrición en América Latina y Caribe.* Santiago de Chile: Comissión Económica para América Latina y el Caribe Press.

ECLAC. (2012). *Social panorama of Latin America 2012.* Santiago de Chile: United Nations Press.

ECLAC. (2014, October 13). *Poverty continues to fall in Latin America, but still affects 167 million people.* Retrieved from www.cepal.org/en/pressreleases/poverty-continues-fall-latin-america-still-affects-167-million-people.

Esping-Andersen, G. (2000). *Fundamentos sociales de las economias postindustriales* [Social foundations of postindustrial economies]. Barcelona: Ariel.

Euzéby, A. (2004). Protección social: valores que hay que defender [Social protection: Values to be defended]. *Revista Internacional de Seguridad Social, 57*, 125–138.

Ferreira, F.H., & Robalino, D. (2010). Social protection in Latin America: Achievements and limitations. *Policy research working paper 5305* (pp. 1–41). Washington, DC: World Bank.

Friedman, M. (1982). *Capitalism and freedom.* Chigago: The University of Chicago.

Giovanni, G.D. (1998). Sistemas de Proteção Social: uma introdução conceitual [Systems of social protection: A conceptual introduction]. In M.A. Oliveira (Ed.), *Reforma do Estado & Políticas de Emprego no Brasil* [State Reform & Employment Policies in Brazil] (pp. 4–21). Campinas: Universidade Estadual de Campinas.

Harvey, D. (2007). *A condição pós-moderna: uma pesquisa sobre as origens da mudança cultural* [The postmodern condition: A search of the origins of cultural change]. São Paulo: Loyola.

Hobsbawm, E. (2011). *Era dos extremos: o breve século XX 1914–1991* [Age of extremes: The short twentieth century 1914–1991]. São Paulo: Companhia das Letras.

International Institute for Labour Studies. (2008). *World of work report 2008: Income inequalities in the age of financial globalization – ILO.* Geneva: ILO.

Jessop, B. (1999). *Crisis del Estado de bienestar: hacia una nueva teoría del Estado y sus consecuencias sociales* [Welfare state crisis: Towards a new theory of the state and its social consequences]. Santa Fé de Bogotá: Siglo del Hombre.

Keynes, J.M. (1996). *A teoria geral do emprego, do juro e da moeda* [The general theory of employment, interest and money]. São Paulo: Nova Cultual.

Kliksberg, B. (2002). *América Latina: uma região de risco, pobreza, desigualdade e institucionalidade social. Série desenvolvimento social 1* [Latin America: A risk region, poverty, inequality and social institutions. Social development series 1]. Brasília: UNESCO.

Lavinas, L. (2014). Políticas Sociales en América Latina en el Siglo XXI [Social policies in Latin America in the XXI Century]. Los programas de transferencias monetáras condicionadas [The conditional transfer programs monetáras]. *Desarrollo Económico, 54,* 45–74.

Lisboa, T.K. (2003). *Gênero, Classe, Etnia – Trajetórias de Vida de Mulheres Migrantes* [Gender, Class, Ethnicity: Trajectories of Women Migrants' Life]. Florianópolis: UFSC & Argos.

Lister, R. (2005). *Poverty and social justice: Recognition and respect.* Third Bevan Foundation Annual Lecture. Tredegar: The Bevan Foundation.

Martins, V. (2008). *O processo de implementação e gestão do Programa Bolsa Família em Florianópolis* [The process of implementation and management of the Bolsa Família in Florianopolis]. Florianópolis: Universidade Federal de Santa Catarina, Centro Sócio-Econômico. Programa de Pós-Graduação em Serviço Social.

Martins, V. (2011). O modelo de proteção social brasileiro: notas para a compreensão do desenvolvimento da seguridade social [The model of Brazilian social protection: Notes for understanding the social security development]. *Brazilian Journal of Public Policy, 1,* 137–158.

Martins, V. (2015). *O trabalho do assistente social no fio da navalha: a cena das aparências e a performatividade* [The work of the social worker on the edge: The scene of appearances and performativity]. São Paulo: Pontifícia Universidade Católica de São Paulo.

Mattei, L. (2009). *Pobreza na América Latina: heterogeneidade e diferenças intra-regionais. Texto para discussão nº 1* [Poverty in Latin America: Heterogeneity and intra-regional differences. Discussion paper no. 1]. Florianópolis: Instituto de Estudos latino-americanos.

Mishra, R. (2000). El estado de bienestar en transición: Estado Unidos, Canadá, Australia y Nueva Zelanda en la década de los noventa [The welfare state in transition: United States, Canada, Australia and New Zealand in the nineties]. In R.M. Llorente (Ed.), *El estado del bienestar en el cambio de siglo: una perspectiva comparada* (pp. 109–139). Madrid: Alianza.

ONU-Habitat. (2012). *Estado de las ciudades de América Latina y el Caribe 2012: Rumbo a una nueva transición urbana* [State of the cities of Latin America and the Caribbean 2012: Towards a new urban transition]. Nairob: Programa de las Naciones Unidas para los Asentamientos Humanos.

Pereira, P. (2013). Contemporary social protection: cui prodest? *Serviço Social & Sociedade, 116,* 636–651.

PNUD (2003). *Relatório do Desenvolvimento Humano 2003 – Objectivos de Desenvolvimento do Milénio: Um pacto entre nações para eliminar a pobreza humana* [Human development report 2003 – Millennium Development Goals: A compact among nations to end human poverty]. Programa das Nações Unidas para o Desenvolvimento, Lisboa: Programa das Nações Unidas para o Desenvolvimento (PNUD).

PNUD (2014). *Relatório do Desenvolvimento Humano 2014 – Sustentar o Progresso Humano: Reduzir as Vulnerabilidades e Reforçar a Resiliência* [Human development report 2014 – Sustaining human progress: Reducing vulnerabilities and strengthening resilience]. New York: Programa das Nações Unidas para o Desenvolvimento (PNUD).

Silva, M.O. (2010). Poverty, inequality and public policies: Characterizing and analyzing the Brazilian reality. *Katálysis, 13,* 155–163.

Silva, M.O. (2014). Panorama geral dos programas de transferência de renda na América Latina e Caribe [Overview of cash transfer programs in Latin America and the Caribbean]. *Revista de Políticas Públicas, 18,* 299–306.

United Nations. (2013). *2013 world hunger and poverty facts.* Retrieved from www. worldhunger.org/articles/Learn/world hunger facts.

United Nations. (2014). *The road to dignity by 2030: Ending poverty, transforming all lives and protecting the planet.* Geneva: United Nations.

Yazbek, M.C. (2010). Serviço Social e pobreza [Social services and poverty]. *Katálysis, 13,* 153–154.

Yazbek, M.C. (2012). Pobreza no Brasil contemporâneo e formas de seu enfrentamento [Poverty in contemporary Brazil and ways of solving them]. *Serviço Social & Sociedade, 110,* 288–322.

8 The Bolsa Família program in the context of social protection in Brazil

A debate on central issues: focus and impact on poverty

Maria Ozanira da Silva e Silva

Introduction

Historically, the beginnings of the establishment of a social protection system in Brazil go back to the 1930s. This was a time of significant social and economic transformations, when the development of the country was marked by the transition from an agro-exporting model of development to an urban-industrial one. The political dynamics of the country began to include the participation of an emerging working class. As a result, there was an increasing demand for the satisfaction of collective needs that emerged as a consequence of the process of industrialization and urbanization that was underway.

Thus, the Brazilian social protection system started to develop and expand from the 1930s onwards. This process was intensified in the 1970s, in the context of the military dictatorship's authoritarianism, in which social programs and services possibly took on the function of minimizing the strong repression against the working class and the popular sectors in general. In this context social protection had the role of contributing to the reproduction of the workforce and the legitimization of the emergency regime.

The 1980s were marked by the expansion of social movements in the field of labor, with the emergence of national central labor unions and neighborhood movements demanding the extension of social rights and the redemption of the social debt that resulted from the wage squeeze and high income concentration during the period of the military dictatorship. A new social movement and an authentic trade union movement arose in the context of the political reorganization of Brazilian society, focused on direct political action against the instituted repression. The struggles in the area of production, reproduction and party politics around the demands for political participation and the extension and universalization of social rights were united, culminating in the Federal Constitution of 1988. The latter significantly broadened social rights in an attempt to overcome the so-called regulated citizenship (Santos, 1987), which was restricted to the employees who worked in the formal sector of the economy and were regularly registered. It prioritized the criterion of actual need instead of the exclusiveness of the criterion of merit as a guideline for social protection policies in Brazil.

The Federal Constitution of 1988 established the social security system, made up of the health policy, the social welfare and the policy of social assistance, which amounted to a significant accomplishment in the field of social protection. This made it possible for social assistance to be regarded as a policy based on rights, rather than a practice based on favors, and to make everyone, even those excluded from the labor market, into Brazilian citizens.

It is in this context that, from 1991 onwards, the debate about income transfer programs became part of the Brazilian public agenda. The first programs of this kind were created at the municipal level in 1995, and they were followed by experiments implemented in several Brazilian states. Income transfer programs underwent a significant expansion at the national level from 2001 onwards, with the establishment of federal programs.

Thus, from the second half of the 1990s onwards the income transfer programs became central to the Brazilian social protection system. In this context, the Bolsa Família (Family Stipend) became the most important one due to its geographic coverage and the number of families assisted by it. In addition to it, other programs were developed, such as the Benefício de Prestação Continuada (Continuous Benefit), targeting senior citizens (older than 65) and persons with a disability who are unable to work and live in households whose per capita income is less than one-quarter of the minimum wage, as well as the Previdência Social Rural (Rural Social Security), which is a special retirement regime created by the Federal Constitution in 1988 and designed for people who work in family-based agriculture and are eligible even without having previously contributed to Social Security. Both programs transfer a monthly amount of one minimum wage (R$788.00 in 2015, about US$228.40)[1] to the beneficiaries (Ministry of Social Development and Fight against Hunger, 2015, p. 1).

In this chapter I describe the Bolsa Família and characterize it in the context of the reality of Brazil's social protection system and the social work perspectives. The chapter discusses the program's capacity to target the poor families in Brazil and to indicate its impacts on the reduction of poverty and inequality among the Brazilian population. At the same time that these impacts are regarded as indicators of the potential of the Bolsa Família as a program designed to fight poverty and to promote social inclusion in Brazil; the structural limits of the program that reduce its capacity to bring about deeper changes in the living conditions of the families assisted by it are also pointed out. The chapter is based on a study developed with the support of Fundação Coordenação de Aperfeiçoamento de Pessoal de Nível Superior (CAPES) and Conselho Nacional de Desenvolvimento Científico e Tecnológico (CNPq), which are Brazilian government agencies that promote the training of human resources and research, and by Fundação de Amparo à Pesquisa e Desenvolvimento Científico e Tecnológico do Maranhão (FAPEMA), a state agency that supports research projects in the state of Maranhão/Brazil.

Social work perspectives on social protection and its role in the Bolsa Família program

Positioning social work in the context of the Brazilian social protection system brings us back to the 1930s, when society underwent profound economic and political transformations. As shown in the introduction, in the economy a new format of development began to be structured, going from the agro-export model to the urban-industrial model. Two movements resulting from this process can be considered as main determinants of the rise and development of social work in Brazil. On the one hand, there is the advent and great expansion of the number of factory workers, and on the other an intense urbanization process with the displacement of significant population groups from the rural area to the city, seeking inclusion in an expanding labor market. The new workers begin to present new demands to meet emerging needs for housing, health and education. In this context, the first higher education school of social work was established in 1936, in São Paulo.

Initially marked by the Catholic tradition, social work became an institution and was legitimized as a profession, in Brazil, with the creation of large state-run institutions for assistance and social security, responsible for expanding social policies. In the new conjuncture, there is no longer any space for social and charity agents to cover the emerging demands, which, due to their complexity, begin to require the action of social workers. Therefore, the doctrinaire and religious origins became more technical during the process of institutionalizing the profession, and their field of legitimization passed from religion to the state.

From the beginning of the development of social work until the 1950s, history shows that the profession is institutionalized and consolidated, basically, responding to the bourgeois interest of society, acting as one of the supporting factors for the advance of industrialization by developing social policy actions that greatly contributed to forming the working class in Brazil. At the same time, these professionals were the legitimate representatives of the state in controlling the emerging working class. However, when they inserted themselves into social relations, and thus, into the sphere of contradiction of social classes, groups of social workers also constructed professional responses to the workers' demands. At the same time, the effort to organize these professionals to seek the construction of a new professional identity and new bases to legitimize social work among the lower classes gained significance, developing attempts at experiences connecting professional action to the processes of the struggle for changes (Silva, 2011). This professional perspective was favored by the strong political movement to form a national-popular consciousness developed from the second half of the 1950s until the beginning of the 1960s. This was a time of political effervescence in Brazil, with the emergence of a broad social reform movement led by the rural and urban population, by students and people from the shantytowns (favelados). The movement was asphyxiated by the military coup of 1964, which instituted a situation of repression and salary squeezing, increasing poverty and creating greater social inequalities, which prevailed until 1985.

Twenty years of military dictatorship in Brazil left deep marks on social work, holding back the emerging critical line and expanding the inclusion of those professionals into state agencies and institutions, with a significant expansion of the labor market. The social policies were broadened and compensated to attenuate the effects of repression and salary squeezing. The reality of the expansion of poverty and increased social inequality gives the practice of social work in Brazil, initially, a modernizing tendency which seeks the social advance of the profession aiming to perform a modern professional action efficiently. For this, the social worker's professional training is guided by an attempt at efficiency and modernization of the profession. Planning, coordination and administration begin to play an essential role for social workers who seek to act at the macro level of society, participating in interprofessional teams (Silva, 2011). However, in the space of social contradiction, Brazilian society initiates a process of political articulation beginning at the end of the 1970s with the rise of what began to be called new social movement and new trade union movement. In this context, the Marxist perspective begins to present itself to the Brazilian social work system, allowing the return and expansion of the critical professional practice and contributing to develop the professional practice beyond the state institutions, with a significant immersion into the social and trade union movements. A process began in the 1980s, of what was then called the Professional Project of Rupture, rendered clearly explicit the professional commitment to the lower classes of Brazilian society (Silva, 2011). This project is currently still hegemonic in the Brazilian social work system, even in the context of the introduction of the neoliberal project in the 1990s, whose hallmark was to diminish the state intervention in social protection. It is a juncture in Brazil in which the struggle for the expansion and universalization of social rights was even incorporated into the Federal Constitution of 1988, which institutes social security, giving rise to social policies and programs focusing on poverty and extreme poverty. It is also, in this context, that the policy of social assistance is structured and advances, culminating in creating the Sistema Único de Assistência Social (SUAS – Unified System of Social Assistance), whose main challenge is to overcome the practice of favors and clientelism which marked the history of social assistance in Brazil and changed it to a legal perspective, while maintaining poor populations as the focus of its intervention. In the same context, within the sphere of the Brazilian system of social protection, the conditional income transfer programs become prevalent. The main program is the Bolsa Família (Family Stipend), the subject of discussion in this chapter (Silva, Yazbek, & Giovanni, 2012). In this context there has been a significant growth of the undergraduate and graduate programs in the field of social work. Currently there are 48 social work undergraduate courses at public higher education institutions 527 at private institutions and 233 distance education courses (www.abepss.og.br). At the postgraduate level there are 33 programs offering 16 PhD courses and 33 master's courses (www.capes.gov.br). There are also approximately 120,000 social workers registered in the professional councils, who are to serve the also growing expansion of the work market for social workers (www.abepss.og.br).

Although social work professional activity has taken place historically in three spaces: within the sphere of the state; in non-governmental organizations; and in a direct relationship of support and assistance to the popular social movements and labor unions, in the recent situation the space of the state has expanded significantly. It is raising demands on the work of social workers in the development of socio-educational actions and also to work with poor families in a decentralized practice developed throughout the 5,570 Brazilian municipalities.

Outstanding in the field of professional intervention of social workers is what they do in the Bolsa Família implemented in all Brazilian municipalities. These social work professionals develop attributions ranging from program management to setting up teams with the participation of the human service professional developing different activities, such as carrying out socio-educational work, especially with mothers who are given preference in taking over the legal representation of the beneficiary families. They are also needed to follow up the conditions established by the program, which requires children and youths to enroll and attend school and participation in basic health protection actions, such as vaccination, prenatal care for pregnant women in the beneficiary families. If the conditions are not met, they must identify reasons why this has happened and follow up these families, generally the most vulnerable, so that they are not excluded from the program.

In brief, the practice of social work in Brazil is focused on working with the poor or most vulnerable populations in society. Social work professional action includes advocating for people's rights, in the sense of contributing to construct a more just, more democratic and more egalitarian society. It also includes an element of social control to address the required compliance inherent in the Bolsa Família program. However, we will only attain this with professional competence, resistance to any form of neglect regarding the well-being of the population, and with the professional and political commitment to really building, with all Brazilian workers, the society that we want and need, from a perspective of the right of all citizens to decent living conditions.

Characterization of the Bolsa Família program in the Brazilian context

Brazil is the largest country in Latin America, with a territory of about 8,547,403 km², divided into five regions with 26 states and 5,570 municipalities plus the Federal District (Instituto Brasileiro de Geografia e Estatística [IBGE], 2011, p. 6). According to the 2010 Census, its population was 190,732,694 (IBGE, 2011, p. 6). The recorded fertility rate was 1.86 (IBGE, 2011, p. 76). The number of households identified was 67.6 million, with 3.3 residents on average per household. The age structure of the population continues to exhibit a trend toward aging, as 11.3% of the population are 60 years old or more (IBGE, 2011, p. 2). The country is marked by great economic and social inequalities and cultural diversity, although Portuguese is the official language spoken throughout the national territory.

The most recent household survey, Pesquisa Nacional por Amostra de Domicílios (PNAD – National Household Sample Survey) in 2012 showed advances in several economic and social indicators, such as the increase of the number of regularly registered employees from 58.8% in 2008 to 74.6% in 2012, with a signed work card in the private sector; a continuous rise of the actual labor-based monthly income of 2.2% between 2008 and 2009 (IBGE, 2013, p. 86). The mean monthly income of the permanent private households in 2012 was R$2,721.00 [US$788.69], with a real gain of 6.5% compared to 2011 (IBGE, 2013, p. 59). There was a greater rise in the Northeast region (9.1%), but it maintained the lowest value compared to the other regions (R$1,851.00 [US$536.52]) (IBGE, 2013, p. 59). The income concentration measured by the Gini Index – which when it is closer to zero, indicates less inequality in the income distribution – kept on decreasing, from 0.535 in 2004 to 0.500 in 2012 (IBGE, 2013, p. 59). Furthermore, child labor also decreased: there were 3.5 million people aged five to 17 working in 2012, representing 8.3% of the population in this age group, whereas in 2008 there were 4.5 million and in 2004 5.3 million (IBGE, 2013, p. 40). In 2012 the 3.5 million children and adolescents aged five to 17 years worked 27.6 hours a week, with a concentration of 60.2% of the population aged five to 13 in agricultural activities, and the per capita monthly income per household of working children and adolescents from five to 17 was R$512.00 [US$148.40] (IBGE, 2013, p. 40). Unemployment has also been decreasing. In 2012 it was 6.1%, 7.6% in the Northeast and 4.1% in the South (IBGE, 2013, p. 120).

As to the level of schooling, the illiteracy rate for people aged 15 or older, although declining, is still high: it decreased from 11.5% in 2004 to 8.7% in 2012, and a great variation has been recorded in the regions of the country: in 2004 there were 22.5% of illiterates in the Northeast region, the poorest, diminishing to 17.4% in 2012, and in the South region, the richest, the population without schooling in 2004 was 6.3%, diminishing to 4.4% in 2012 (IBGE, 2013, p. 55). Also in 2012, the PNAD recorded 11.9% of the Brazilian population aged 25 years or more as not having schooling and with less than one year of schooling (IBGE, 2013, p. 55). There were 33.5% with incomplete basic education; 9.8% with complete basic education; 4% with incomplete secondary education; 25.2% with complete secondary education; 3.5% with incomplete higher education and 12.0% with complete higher education (total of 14.2 million people) (IBGE, 2013, p. 56). As to the mean number of years of schooling, among people aged 10 years or over an increase of two years was recorded from 2011 to 2012, so that 60.9 million people had at least 11 years of schooling, 28.0% of whom lived in the Northeast region, the poorest, and 41.4% lived in the South region, the richest (IBGE, 2013, p. 55). The rate of schooling in 2012 was 98.2% of the children aged 6 to 14 years and 84.2% of the adolescents aged 15 to 17 years attending school. The School Census performed in 2010 indicated that 51.5 million students were enrolled in basic education – which goes from the day care center to preschool and elementary school to secondary school – and that 85.5% of them were attending the public school system. Even though this shows major improvements in education, it is still a fragile field of Brazilian reality and deserves further attention (IBGE, 2013, p. 55).

Considering the population's living conditions, the aforementioned household survey showed an increase in access to services such as water supply from 72.3% of the households in 2004 to 85.4% in 2012; public garbage collection was performed in 75.5% of the households in 2004 and in 85.3% in 2009; the electrical energy supply network covered 85.3% of the households in 2004 and 99.5% in 2009; the sewage collection network or number of septic tanks connected to it covered 49.6% of the households in 2004 and 57.1% in 2012, with a great difference between the regions: only 13.0% in the North region and 84.1% in the South regions, the richest (IBGE, 2013, p. 108). Likewise, an increase in access to durable goods was also identified: in 2012 96.7% of the households had refrigerators; 55.1% had clothes washing machines; 97.2% had a television; 98.7% had a stove; 91.2% had a land line or mobile telephone; at least one resident of 42.4% of the households had a car and 20.0% had a motorbike for personal use. There was also a significant increase in the percentage of households that had a computer (46.4% in 2012) and Internet access (40.3%) (IBGE, 2013, p. 101).

Finally, it should be stressed that the Brazilian population, as in other countries, is aging (above 60 years), and consequently the number of young people is diminishing. Thus, in the period between 2004 and 2012 PNAD indicates that in 2004 42.8% of the population consisted of people up to the age of 24 years and that this percentage fell to 39.6% in 2012 (IBGE, 2013, p. 46).

In the above context, the Bolsa Família is the broadest income transfer program in Brazil, covering all 5,570 Brazilian municipalities (MDS, 2015, p. 1). According to data taken from the site MDS (2015, p. 1) on July 2015, 13,827,369 families were assisted. This means about 41,482,107 people, considering that an average family consists of three persons. In budgetary terms, taken from site MDS (2015, p. 1) in July 2015, an amount of R$2,311,298,975.00 [US$669,941,731.88] was used just to pay the benefits. This is a program that performs a direct money transfer to poor and extremely poor families, and it occupies a central position in the current Brazilian social protection system. It was instituted by Provisory Measure number 132 of October 20, 2003, transformed into Law number 10,836 of January 9, 2004, and regulated by Decree number 5,209 of September 17, 2004 (MDS, 2015, p. 1).

As a mechanism to unify the income transfer programs, the Bolsa Família was created to rectify problems identified in the operational implementation of the scattered ensemble of these programs that were then being developed since 1995, such as: superposition and competition between programs regarding their objectives and target public; need for planning and general coordination of these programs and expanding the target public (Report from the Transition Government Administration regarding the Social Programs, 2002).

In the context of the Plano Brasil sem Miséria (Brazil Without Poverty Plan), created in 2011, as the main strategy of President Dilma Rousseff's administration, the Bolsa Família must aim to raise the 16.2 million Brazilians who live on a per capita monthly income of less than R$70.00 [US$20.28] out of a situation of extreme poverty (MDS, 2015, p. 1). The Bolsa Família is one of the three program axes that are part of the Plan: guaranteed income, inclusion in production and access to public utilities: water, electricity, health, education and housing. Ever since its inception, the Bolsa Família has undergone a significant geographic expansion, covering a growing number of families. In 2013, when the program reached 10 years of implementation, it assisted more than 14 million of families with an annual budget of around 26 billion reais [US$7,536,231,884.05] (MDS, 2015, p. 1).

The Bolsa Família offers monetary benefits transferred monthly to the beneficiary families, and the values and composition of the benefits present a significant variation, constituting four types of benefits: Benefício Básico (Basic Benefit), to the amount of R$77.00 [US$22.31], given only to extremely poor families with a per capita income equal to or less than R$77.00 [US$22.31]; Benefício Variável (Variable Benefit), to the amount of R$35.00 [US$10.14] granted because the family has children aged from 0 to 15 years, pregnant and/or breastfeeding women (Benefício Variável Gestante (BVG) – Variable Benefit for Pregnant Women, Benefício Variável Nutriz (BVN) – Benefit for Breastfeeding Women), limited to five benefits per family; Benefício Variável Jovem (BVJ – Variable Benefit for Youth), to the amount of R$42.00 [US$12.17], given if in the family there are youths aged 16 and 17 years and limited to two young people per family who are attending school; and Benefício para Superação da Extrema Pobreza (BSP – Benefit to Overcome Extreme Poverty), with an amount corresponding to what is needed for all families who are beneficiaries of the Bolsa Família to surpass the monthly income of R$77.00 [US$22.31] per person (MDS, 2015, p. 2). In this way, the amounts of the benefits vary according to the characteristics of each family, considering the monthly family per capita income, the number of children and adolescents aged up to 17, pregnant women, breastfeeding women and members of the family. The minimum monetary value of the Bolsa Família for each family is R$35.00 [US$10.14] and the median benefit in July 2015 was R$167,15 [US$48.44] (MDS, 2015, p. 1).

From April 2011 onwards, President Dilma Rousseff, beginning a policy designed to strengthen and expand the Bolsa Família, ordered an average readjustment of 19.4% in the amount of the aid, and the correction in the 15-year range reached up to 45% (MDS, 2015, p. 1). This readjustment was justified as a measure to fight extreme poverty in Brazil, which is the main priority of the Administration, announced by President Roussseff and consolidated in the Plano Brasil sem Miséria. The program comprises three main axes: income transfer, conditionalities, and complementary programs. The first aims at promoting immediate poverty relief. The conditionalities are defined by the Ministério do Desenvolvimento Social e Combate à Fome (MDS – Ministry of Social Development and Fight against Hunger), the national managing agency of the Bolsa Família, as commitments taken on by the families and the government for the beneficiaries to be covered by services of education, health and social welfare, as a reinforcement to access basic social rights, while the complementary programs aim at increasing the families' ability to overcome their vulnerable situation. The families can use the money received freely and may remain in the program if they fulfill the eligibility criteria. They must comply with the conditions, which consist of enrolling children and adolescents aged six to 17 years in school; at least 85% regular attendance at school of children aged six to 15 years and 75% for youths 16 to 17 years old; children aged 0 to seven years must come to the outpatient clinics to be vaccinated, weighed, measured and to undergo basic health checkups, and the attendance of pregnant women for routine exams is also considered a conditionality in the field of health (MDS, 2015, p. 1).

Besides money transfers aimed at improving nutrition and basic living conditions of the family group, the Bolsa Família considers it necessary to include the adult members of the benefitting families in complementary actions offered by the three levels of government. The complementary programs articulated with the Bolsa Família at the federal level are as follows: Programa Brasil Alfabetizado (Literate Brazil Program) to teach literacy to people 15 years old and over; ProJovem (ProYouth) to reintegrate young people aged 15–29 in the process of education and social and professional qualification; Projeto de Promoção do Desenvolvimento Local e Economia Solidária (Project for the Promotion of Local Development and Solidarity Economy) for access to work and income for excluded communities and population groups; Programa Nacional de Agricultura Familiar (National Program of Family Agriculture) and microcredit programs of Banco do Nordeste for access to work and income, aimed at family farmers; Programa Nacional Biodiesel (National Biodiesel Program) for access to work and income, also aimed at family farmers; and Programa Luz para Todos (Light for All Program) to expand electricity in rural areas. Besides, the families are covered by other programs, such as: social tariff for electricity; courses for literacy, education of youths and adults and professional training; actions to generate work and income and improve housing conditions, besides exemption from fees to take federal exams to become civil servants.

The Bolsa Família aims to provide financial transfers as a direct benefit articulated with other structural programs at the three levels of the government, with special attention to the services in the fields of education, health and labor, to provide conditions for the economic and social inclusion of the adult members of the beneficiary families. It is implemented in a decentralized manner by the municipalities, with the financial support of the federal government. This process begins with the signing of the Letter of Agreement or Term of Accession, by which the municipality commits itself to instituting a local control committee or council made up of representatives of society and to appointing the municipal management agency for the program. In order to carry out the implementation process, a set of responsibilities shared by the Union, states, municipalities and society is established.

The Bolsa Família beneficiaries and their families

In this section, the socioeconomic profile of the beneficiary families of the Bolsa Família is outlined, in an attempt to answer three basic questions: Who are the beneficiary families? Who is legally responsible for the family assisted by the Bolsa Família? Who are the beneficiary members of these families and how do they live? To answer these questions, the main sources of data are drawn from the studies carried out in 2006 and 2009 by the Secretaria Nacional de Renda e Cidadania (National Office for Income and Citizenship) from the MDS referred to in the Cadastro Único (CadÚnico – Single Register). The CadÚnico is a mechanism for the registration of the families with a per capita income of up to half the minimum wage (MDS, 2010). It was developed by the federal government, but is under decentralized implementation in the 5,570 Brazilian municipalities and in the federal district. It is under the responsibility of the municipal administrators and the federal district's governor. This registration serves as a reference for the development of social protection programs in Brazil.

Who are the program's beneficiary families?

In July 2015 a total of 14,086,199 families were beneficiaries of the Bolsa Família. These families consisted on average of 3.6 persons and most of them lived in the Northeast region of the country (50.2%), the poorest, followed by the Southeast region, the most developed, with 25.4%, so that the two regions together made up three-fourths of the program's families (Camargo, Curralero, Licio, & Mostafa, 2013, p. 162).

Concerning the family income profile, before receiving the Bolsa Família most of the families lived in a state of extreme poverty (72.4%); for example, with a family per capita income of up to R$70.00 [US$20.28]. Only 20.5% had an income between R$70.00 [US$20.28] and R$140.00 [US$40.57], which places them on the poverty line established by the program. It was found that 7.1% obtained a family per capita income between R$140.00 [US$40.57] and R$339.00 [US$98.26], thus above the criterion for inclusion in the Bolsa Família, which is allowed by Ministerial Administrative Ruling n. 617 of August 11, 2010, which ensures that the family can stay in it for a minimum period of two years, as long as the family per capita income remains below half a minimum wage, R$382.00 [US$110.72] in 2014 (Camargo et al., 2013, pp. 163–164).

The smallest participation rate of extremely poor families is in the South region (54.0%), the most developed, while in the Northeast, the poorest region, are 82.2% of the extremely poor families (Camargo et al., 2013, p. 164).

It should be underscored that the five regions into which the Brazilian territory is divided are marked by contrasts and differences. The South, the Southeast and part off the Midwest regions are more developed, and the North and the Northeast regions are the least developed, and thus have the largest concentration of poor. This diversity can be understood looking at the economic and social formation of each region. The South and Southeast region received a large number of foreigners from various countries, including Japan, Italy and Germany. Immigrants from Japan and Italy settled mainly in São Paulo during the industrialization process in the 1920s. In the South region, there was a significant number of German and Italian immigrants who contributed to the production and industrialization of agriculture and livestock. Another important element was the concentration of federal and local public policies to support the development of the South, Southeast and Center West regions, where the federal capital, Brasilia, was built. The North region, with a large geographical area, isolated from the rest of the country and inhabited by a significant number of indigenous peoples, only began to receive more attention from the federal government in 1966, when the Superintendencia de Desenvolvimento da Amazonia (SUDAM – Superintendency for the Development of the Amazon) was established to attract tax incentives. The most important development was the creation of the Zona Franca de Manaus (Manaus Tax-Free Zone). The Northeast region, inhabited by a significant number of Africans, was also the subject of attention from the federal government beginning in 1959, when the Superintendência para o Desenvolvimento do Nordeste (SUDENE – Superintendency for the Development of the Northeast) was created to overcome the low

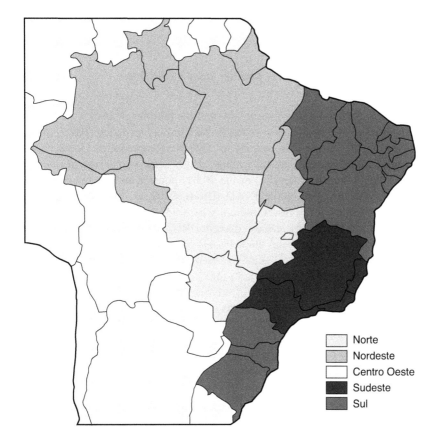

Figure 8.1 Map of regions in Brazil.

Note
By Valeu Cara. Retrieved from http://valeucara.blogspot.com.br/2012/12/mapa-do-brasil-vetorizado. html. Used under Creative Commons Attribution-Share Alike 3.0 Unported license (CC BY-SA 3.0) (http://creativecommons.org/licenses/by-sa/3.0/deed.en).

economic and social development of the region, worsened by recurrent droughts. Both federal institutions, SUDAM and SUDENE, were closed down in 2001, the justification for this being irregularities and corruption in the projects developed and inefficiency. They were respectively replaced by the Agência de Desenvolvimento da Amazonia (ADA – Agency for the Development of the Amazon) and Agência de Desenvolvimento do Nordeste (ADENE – Agency for the Development of the Northeast). However, both SUDAM and SUDENE were reinstated in 2007, and they are controlled externally, with the mission of promoting inclusive and sustainable development, and integrating the regional productive economy of the regions into the national and international economy.

Considering the family arrangements of the Bolsa Família beneficiaries, most are one-parent families headed by women (42.2%), followed by couples with children (37.6%). Further, the lowest mean age of people responsible for the families occurs in the female one-parent arrangements, 35.1 years, and the highest percentages of one-person families and couples without children are in the Northeast region (Camargo et al., 2013, p. 164).

Who is legally responsible for the families aided by the Bolsa Família?

The vast majority of the legal representatives of the families in 2013 were female (93.1%), which is in compliance with the Bolsa Família legislation (IBGE, 2013, p. 46). The legally responsible persons in 2009 were represented by 68.1% of black or mulatto (also called pardo) women, which is the percentage of married women or female heads of families of the 20.0% poorest households in Brazil, according to data from the 2008 PNAD (IBGE, 2009, p. 46). Once again an exception was found in the South region, where 75.0% of the persons legally responsible claimed to be of European descent (IBGE, 2009, p. 46).

The data from CadÚnico and 2008 PNAD are also close in relation to the educational level of the persons legally responsible for the families assisted by the Bolsa Família: in 2009, according to the CadÚnico, 78.3% of them had finished elementary school, and 81.5% of the married women or female heads of families of the 20.0% poorest households in Brazil were in the same situation, according to the 2008 PNAD (IBGE, 2009, p. 53). Yet the percentage of legally responsible persons without school education, according to the CadÚnico in 2009, was lower than the number identified by the 2008 PNAD (12.5% and 18.8%, respectively) (IBGE, 2009, p. 53). This ratio is inverted in relation to the unfinished elementary school education: 82.5% and 53.1%, respectively. As expected, the highest percentage of illiterate people was found in the Northeast region: 21.8% in 2006 and 17.0% in 2009 (IBGE, 2009, p. 53). This is very important for social work professionals to consider in the education actions.

Updating the information about the level of education of the people responsible for the family, the study by Camargo et al. (2013, p. 166) indicates that slightly over half (52.1%) declared that they had incomplete basic education, and 12.1% had no education whatsoever, for example they were illiterate. The latter are concentrated in the Northeast region, with 16.0% of people responsible for families lacking education. The low level of education determines the insertion of these people into the labor market, to a high degree leading them to informal, unstable jobs, with low wages.

This situation demonstrates that social protection aims to support and to place greater priority on the most vulnerable populations in Brazil. However, the Brazilian social protection system has been marked by punctual and compensatory actions, and does not reach the point of constituting a social welfare state that would privilege universal actions as measures of rights. An example is the narrow focalization of the Bolsa Família on the poorest population.

Regarding the insertion of those people legally responsible for the beneficiary families in the labor market, the study carried out by the MDS in 2006 found that more than half of them (51.4% in the whole country) did not work, so that the money transfer from the program was the main or the only source of income for these families (MDS, 2007, p. 5). The highest rate of insertion in the labor market was found in the rural area, with 15.3% of the total number of workers; 8.6% of them were self-employed workers without any connection to social security and 4.9% were wage-earners, but without a regular register (MDS, 2007, p. 10). Thus, the persons legally responsible for the families covered by the program did not have any kind of social protection.

The study conducted by the MDS (2010), based on micro-data from the CadÚnico, did not contain updated data about the work of the persons legally responsible for the beneficiary families of the Bolsa Família. It only reaffirmed that most of them did not work and that those who worked did so predominantly in agricultural activities. It also highlighted the great difficulty that these people face in entering the formal labor market due to their low educational level and their lack of professional qualification. To offer a good education and increase the professional qualifications of the poor population must be a priority of the Brazilian social protection system to address this situation.

Who are the beneficiaries of the Bolsa Família?

In March 2013, there were 49,637,552 beneficiaries of the Bolsa Família, that is 26% of the Brazilian population based on the 2010 Census, which recorded a total number of 190,755,799 Brazilians in the country (IBGE, 2011, p. 3).

According to data from the 2006 and 2009 CadÚnico, the beneficiaries of the Bolsa Família throughout the country were predominantly women: 53.0% in 2006 and 54.0% in 2009 (MDS, 2007, p. 10). The same situation was identified in the five Brazilian regions, and this data corresponds to the data revealed by the 2008 PNAD, which pointed out that 51.6% of the 46 million people who lived in the 20% poorest households in Brazil were women (MDS, 2007, p. 10). It is worth mentioning, though, that according to data from the 2006 and 2009 CadÚnico and the 2008 PNAD regarding the poorest one-fifth of the population, the highest concentration of males was found in the rural areas (MDS, 2007, p. 10; 2010, p. 5).

Concerning the age of the beneficiary population all over the country in 2009, the majority was below 20 years of age (54.6%), and children and teenagers aged up to 17 accounted for little more than half of the beneficiaries (50.6%) (IBGE, 2009, p. 46). These data are in accordance with the criteria of eligibility for the Bolsa Família, which privileges families with children and teenagers up to the age of 17. Data from the 2008 PNAD ratified the heavy presence of youth in the age group distribution of the people who belong to the poorest one-fifth of the population (IBGE, 2009, p. 46). Camargo et al. (2013, p. 172) also reaffirm these data, recording that the beneficiaries of the Bolsa Família present an essentially young profile: almost half (48.8%) are up to 17 years old, over one-quarter (28.0%) are in the age group from seven to 15 years, and the age group of up to six years comprises 15.1% of the beneficiaries.

Looking at the people aged 50 or older in 2009, they were the smallest beneficiary age group of the Bolsa Família, namely about 6.8%, while according to the 2008 PNAD they constituted 8.5% of the poorest one-fifth of the population (IBGE, 2009, p. 46). In the age group between 20 and 49, the percentages registered in two sources of information were close, namely around 40.0% (IBGE, 2009, p. 46).

In regional terms, the above situation related to the age groups is replicated. However, we find the highest concentration of young people covered by the program in 2009 in the North region, whereas the highest percentage of old people aided by the Bolsa Família was found in the Northeast.

When looking at the distribution of Bolsa Família beneficiaries in terms of race and color of skin, those who identified themselves as blacks or mulattos (or pardos) represented 64.6% of the total number of beneficiaries in 2006 and 71.1% in 2009 (IBGE, 2009, p. 47). Similar figures were found by the 2008 PNAD, according to which 68.4% of the black people belonged to the poorest one-fifth of the population (IBGE, 2009, p. 47). It is worth mentioning that, according to the 2008 PNAD and the CadÚnico, it was in the North and Northeast that poverty was mostly associated with the ethnic group, and in these regions we also find the highest concentrations of beneficiaries of African descent (87.9% in 2008 and 82.9%, in 2009, respectively). Conversely, in the South region the percentage of beneficiaries of European descent was higher (76.7%) (IBGE, 2009, p. 47).

Considering the skin color of Bolsa Família beneficiaries, the study by Camargo et al. (2013, p. 172) reaffirms the data presented by previous studies, indicating that most of the beneficiaries are pardo (66.7%), followed by white (24.8%) and black (7.0%), and that the regions that concentrate the highest proportion of blacks or pardos (88.4% and 83.5%, respectively) are the Northeast and North regions, while the South region has a population that is mainly of European origin and presents the lowest percentage of blacks or pardos (25.0%), with 73.4% of white beneficiaries. These numbers show the diversity of races in Brazil as result of immigration. At the same time, the poor and racialized groups experience various forms of social exclusion, mainly in relation to education and work.

As far as the indigenous population is concerned, its share among the beneficiaries of the Bolsa Família was less than 1.0% in 2009 (Camargo et al., 2013, p. 174). Only in the North region did their share reach 2.3%. In the state of Roraima, however, the indigenous population accounted for 11.3% of the program's beneficiaries. This situation reflects the reservation systems of indigenous land and reserves in the North region, particularly in Roraima. Camargo et al. (2013, p. 172) reaffirm that the presence of the indigenous population is 2.5% in the North region and 2.7% in the Midwest, with percentages that are much higher than the national percentage (0.8%). Consequently, due to the small number and isolation of Indigenous populations, it has only been in recent years, when organization and pressure from these populations occurred, that greater attention has been given to their social protection. Regarding this aspect, the regulation of their landownership and the direction given to education and health policies should be mentioned, although it is not yet sufficient, and sometimes does not take into account the cultural reality of Indigenous peoples.

As to school attendance, the data from the 2009 CadÚnico revealed, according to the information given by those responsible for the family units, that 8.1% of the children aged 0 to three and 60.1% of the children in the age group of four to six attended daycare or pre-school facilities (MDS, 2010, p. 6). The national percentages of both age groups is surpassed in the Northeast region, where they account for respectively 9.1% and 67.1%, possibly because this is the poorest region in Brazil and therefore the concentration of families assisted by the Bolsa Família is the highest (MDS, 2010, p. 6). As expected, in the age groups of seven to 14 and 15 to 17, where the condition of school attendance is compulsory for families to receive assistance by the Bolsa Família, the national average was 94.0% and 90.8% respectively, and a similar scenario was found in all regions of the country in this respect (MDS, 2010, p. 7). More significant data are that that 97.5% of the total number of the program's beneficiaries were enrolled at public schools, regardless of the age group, which indicates that the Bolsa Família is well focused on poor families (MDS, 2010, p. 7). Complementing the information on school attendance, it was found that in 2009, in the whole country, 33.9% of the beneficiaries between seven and 14 years of age and 55.1% of those aged 15 to 17 were lagging behind by at least two years in terms of the grade they should be attending in terms of their age (MDS, 2010, p. 7). The children and adolescents in the North and Northeast regions, which are the poorest ones in Brazil, were lagging even further behind.

Camargo et al. (2013) confirm the low level of education of the Bolsa Família beneficiaries. Thus, they reveal that more than half the people 25 years of age or older (53.5%) have incomplete basic education and 15.5% declare themselves illiterate, with no education whatsoever (Camargo et al., 2013, p. 172). These data, however, present a significant regional diversity, considering the different levels of development of the Brazilian regions. There is a higher level of illiteracy in the Northeast, the poorest region, which has 20.3% of uneducated beneficiaries, which means twice that found in the Midwest (11.2%), Southeast (8.8%) and South (8.5%) regions (Camargo et al., 2013, p. 172). This situation is a result of the diversity of development in the Brazilian regions, already mentioned previously in this chapter, and because the Bolsa Família itself was directed at the poor and extremely poor population that is concentrated in the North and Northeast region.

Where and how do the Bolsa Família beneficiaries live?

The results of the aforementioned MDS studies (of 2006 and 2009) indicate that the Northeastern region is the one with the highest percentage of families assisted by the Bolsa Família and the Midwest is the region with the lowest. Regarding the location of the assisted households, most of them are concentrated in urban areas, which is a trend found in all regions, although it was more significant in the Midwest. In 2009 the Northeastern region had 61.4% of the beneficiary households located in urban areas, but it was also the region that presented the highest percentage of households in rural areas (38.6%) (MDS, 2007, p. 12; 2010, p. 6). This reality is compatible with the high rate of urbanization in the country and the rate of urban poverty.

As far as the type of household is concerned, most families that are beneficiaries of the Bolsa Família lived in houses (91.8% in 2006 and 92.6% in 2009), followed by families that only inhabited rooms (5.2% in 2006 and 5.9% in 2009). This situation is found in all regions of the country. The number of families living in apartments or other types of housing was low (0.8% in 2006 and 0.7% in 2009) (MDS, 2007, p. 12; 2010, p. 7). To have one's own household in Brazil means to have security to live, so this is a strong belief and value practiced by the whole population.

Regarding the conditions of occupation of households throughout the country, which is a trend found in all regions, most of the beneficiary families lived in their own houses (in 2006, 62.7% and in 2009, 61.6% of the total number of households), followed by the families that lived in housing lent to the family by some friend or some person of his family (20.2% in 2006 and 22.8% in 2009) and in rented ones (11.2% in 2006 and 13.1% in 2009). The fact that in 2009 84.4% of the houses assisted by the program were owned by the families or given to them had a positive consequence for their budget (MDS, 2007, p. 12; 2010, p. 7). This means that when individuals or families own their own house, or live in a house that has been provided for their use (84.4%), there is no need to use income to pay rent. For this reason, the majority of the Bolsa Família beneficiary families can apply their low income to meeting other vital needs.

The number of people per household is shown by two indicators: the average number of people in each household and the average number of rooms in the house. As to the first indicator, in the whole of Brazil there were 3.97 people per household in 2009 (MDS, 2010, p. 6). The highest concentration of dwellers per house was found in the Northern region (4.3 people), while the other regions had the national average. The number of rooms per house was 4.03 throughout Brazil in 2009 (MDS, 2010, p. 6). The Northeastern region had the highest figures, with 4.27 rooms per house on average, and the Northern region had the smallest houses, since on average the assisted households had about 3.26 rooms (MDS, 2010, p. 6). In the Northeast, despite the fact that 74.3% of the assisted families lived in masonry houses, there was a high occurrence of precarious buildings using adobe or mud, particularly in the states of Maranhão and Piauí (respectively, in 2009, 51.6% and 47.8% of the families assisted by the program) (MDS, 2010, p. 6). These states are among the poorest ones in Brazil.

More recently, the study by Camargo et al. (2013, p. 167) identified a major regional difference in the type of housing construction, recording a high proportion of coated masonry homes in the Southeast (76.5%), Northeast (66.3%) and Midwest (66.5%) regions. On the other hand, the North region presented only 36.6% (Camargo et al., 2013, p. 167). However, considering the use of inadequate materials to build the houses, the study referred to emphasized that in the North and Northeast, the poorest regions, coated and non-coated lath and plaster or mud were used, with used lumber, straw and other materials in, respectively, 24.5% and 20.1% of the houses (Camargo et al., 2013, p. 167). These percentages are much higher than the national percentage for the Bolsa Família, recorded for the same situation, which is of 15.4% (Camargo et al., 2013, p. 167).

To have one's own house is very important for the Brazilian population who consider that having one's own place to live provides greater security in life. Many of the poor aspire to build their own home, and social work can play an important role in this respect to meet their housing needs by working together to keep costs low.

Regarding the energy supply with an appropriate meter it was found that there was a high incidence in the households assisted by the program (75.7% of the total in 2006 and 83.6% in 2009) (MDS, 2010, p. 5). In the year 2009 6.3% of the households still did not have a measuring device and 10.1% did not have energy supply (MDS, 2010, p. 5). In this respect, the region in the worst situation was the North, where, in 2009, only 66.8% of the families had access to energy supply with a measuring device (MDS, 2010, p. 5). This region also showed the highest percentage of households assisted by the Bolsa Família without energy supply (21.9% in 2009) (MDS, 2007, p. 11). On the other hand, the highest number of households with access to energy supply and a measuring device was found in the South and Southeast (91.2% and 91.1% respectively in 2009) (MDS, 2007, p. 11; 2010, p. 5).

As to water supply, in 2006 64.0% of the assisted families in the whole country had access to it, and this rate went up to 65.7% in 2009 (MDS, 2010, p. 5). This supply was concentrated in the urban areas, with 82.9% of the beneficiary families in that same year (MDS, 2010, p. 5). Again, the poorest regions, namely, the North and the Northeast, were in the worst situation, as less than half of the beneficiaries had access to water supply, while the richer regions, the Southeast (78.7%), South (76.5%) and Midwest (71.5%), were above the national average (MDS, 2007, p. 10; 2010, p. 5).

As regards the form of water supply, Camargo et al. (2013, p. 168) explains that most of the Bolsa Família households have direct access to the general distribution system (65.6%), and the second most used form is wells or springs (21.9%). This situation is different in the North region, where the use of wells or springs is 40.9%, and the general distribution system covers 45.4% of households, while access to piped water in the South and the Southeast is already higher than 80.0%, surpassing the national average in this indicator (Camargo et al., 2013, p. 168).

The data presented on families' access to electricity and water in their homes reflect the situation of diversity of development in the Brazilian regions. The data show a positive advance of all regions in recent years, even the poorer ones, which now have greater access to energy and water in their homes. This may have an impact as a result of the inclusion of families in the Bolsa Família, contributing to an immediate improvement of living standards and raising the well-being of these families.

Regarding the type of water treatment, in 2009 the most prevalent treatment forms throughout the country were percolation and chlorination (38.2% and 35.5%, respectively) (MDS, 2010, p. 13). It is striking that a high percentage of households did not use any kind of water treatment (21.6%) (MDS, 2010, p. 13). In this respect, the Midwestern and the Southeastern regions were in a better situation in 2009, when it was found that only 13.0% and 15.0% of the households did not have any kind of treated water, respectively. It is also striking that in 2009 36.0% of the program's beneficiaries in the South did not receive treated water, thus holding the last position, while the North, with 26.8% of the households in this situation, occupied the second to last position (MDS, 2010, p. 13). The impact of non-access to treated water is that the health of the population became worse due to the onset of diseases resulting from this situation, which creates a great demand for health programs in order to minimize the consequent water-related illnesses. Ultimately, this situation has a greater impact on the life of the poorer populations, generating more challenges in their living conditions, which are worsened because of their difficulty in accessing clean water and basic health care programs.

In 2006 garbage collection in 65.4% of the households assisted by the Bolsa Família was met by the public collection system, and this figure went up to 68.8% in 2009, 90.6% of the families in urban areas were in this situation (MDS, 2010, p. 13). In this respect, the Southeast, the Midwest and the South stood out because more than 80.0% of the households had access to the public garbage collection system (MDS, 2010, p. 13). At the other extreme the North and the Northeast placed below the national average with 59.6% and 59.7% of the households, respectively, with access to this service (MDS, 2010, p. 13). Again, the states of Maranhão and Piauí showed the lowest percentages of households with garbage collected by the public collection system (39.6% and 43.7%, respectively) (MDS, 2007, p. 11; 2010, p. 13). We consider that garbage collection is an important consideration for the social protection system because the lack of this service has negative consequences on population health.

However, the most precarious situation of the families assisted by the program in Brazil has to do with the sewage system. Only 54.2% of all households had access to a public sewage system or cesspools (an alternative that is also acceptable), and 67.8% of them had access in urban areas (MDS, 2007, p. 10). Again, the Northern region was in the worst situation. There only 34.2% of the households had access to this service (MDS, 2007, p. 10). It was followed by the Northeast with 46.3%, and there Maranhão was the state in the worst situation, as only 29.5% of the households had access to an adequate sewage system (MDS, 2007, p. 10; 2010, p. 13). For Camargo et al. (2013, p. 168), access to sanitary flow is the most precarious item in the profile of the Bolsa Família families, with only 35.7% of them accessing the sewage or storm collector system, and 14.9% do this by means of the septic tank. In the North region only 28.7% of the families have adequate access to this service (Camargo et al., 2013, p. 168).

When satisfactory access to water supply, garbage collection and sewage system is considered, for example the sanitation conditions seen as adequate for the households, the surveys show that in 2009 only 41.8% of the families assisted by the Bolsa Família in Brazil were in that situation, and the figure went up to 54.5% among the households located in urban areas (MDS, 2010, p. 13). This figure shows the inequality of poverty in Brazil when one compares the various regions. While in the Southeast 65.0% of the program's beneficiaries had adequate sanitation, in the Northern region this percentage dropped dramatically to 17.7% and to 32.1% in the Northeast (MDS, 2010, p. 14). In this respect, the Midwest was closer to the national average (41.1%) and the South was above this average, having 53.2% of the households with adequate sanitation conditions (MDS, 2010, p. 14).

Camargo et al. (2013, p. 168) establish a comparison with national percentages, using as reference the 2010 Census, and find that in general the households of the Bolsa Família beneficiaries are in a worse condition regarding all indicators analyzed: in public water supply, the ratio is 82.8% of the general population to 65.6% of the Bolsa Família; in the sewage collecting system or septic tank it is about 66.8% against 50.6% of the Bolsa Família; 87.4% against 64.9% as regards garbage collection and 98.7% against 89.8% of the Bolsa Família as far as electrical lighting is concerned.

In this analysis, one must also consider that simultaneous access to the garbage collection services, sanitary sewerage by public network or septic tank, electrical lighting and public water supply are important conditions for a home infrastructure. From this point of view, only 38.1% of the Bolsa Família families have access to these services at the same time (Camargo et al., 2013, p. 170). Even in the urban area, where these services are more present, this percentage is 48.9% of the beneficiary families, and in the North (14.9%) and Northeast (29.2%) regions the families have smaller proportions of simultaneous access to these services (Camargo et al., 2013, p. 170). In a more precarious situation, only 5.2% of the households in the rural area have simultaneous access to these services, and this situation is extremely serious in the North region, where only 1.5% of the families living in the rural area have simultaneous access to all four services (Camargo et al., 2013, p. 170).

In sum, the data presented above about the beneficiaries of the Bolsa Família and their legal representatives contains relevant indicators that can be regarded as evidence that the program has a significant focus on poor and extremely poor families. This is evident in the predominance of youth among the beneficiaries; the predominance of people of African descent; the concentration of the beneficiary families on the poorest regions, particularly the Northeast; the low level of school education and the predominance of enrollment in public schools. At the same time, it was pointed out as well as precarious, poorly paid and informal jobs or working conditions; precarious simultaneous access to the services of garbage collection, sanitary sewage through a public system or septic tank, electrical lighting and public water supply, which are important conditions for the infrastructure of a household. The lack of social inclusion in major aspects of living conditions more significantly affect the poorest and most vulnerable members of society including racialized groups (black, pardo) and indigenous populations, who continue to exert less power and influence in society. Those groups must receive attention from the social work professional at the community level, offering some education opportunities and facilitating their organization in order to press the state to meet their needs and rights.

Focus and impacts of the Bolsa Família on poverty and inequality

The Bolsa Família's focus is understood in terms of "targeting resources and programs at certain population groups considered vulnerable in society as a whole" (Silva, 2001, p. 13). However, the concept of focus adopted within the sphere of reforms of social programs in Latin America in the 1980s and 1990s, under the influence of neoliberal ideas, reduced focusing to merely compensatory actions. These social programs aimed at mitigating the effects of the structural adjustment on the vulnerable population groups, helping to weaken the struggle for universal social rights and to emphasize, in the agenda of social policies, the option for focusing on targeted social programs to the detriment of universalization.

Several studies on income transfer programs in Brazil highlight their ability to focus on the target public (Soares, Soares, Medeiros, & Osório, 2006; Soares, Osório, Soares, Medeiros, & Zepeda, 2007). Along the same lines, Soares, Ribas and Osório (2007, p. 3), dealing with performance in choosing the beneficiaries of the Bolsa Família, point out that 92% of the non-eligible population did not receive benefits from the program. However, broader studies were conducted by the Instituto Brasileiro de Geografia e Estatística (IBGE – Brazilian Institute of Geography and Statistics) in the context of the PNAD of 2004 and 2006, whose results were published in special supplements – PNAD 2004: Aspectos Complementares de Educação e Acesso a Transferência de Renda de Programas Sociais (Complementary Aspects of Education and Access to Income Transfer from Social Programs); PNAD 2006: Acesso a Transferência de Renda de Programas Sociais (Access to Income Transfer from Social Programs) (IBGE, 2006; 2007).

These studies allow comparing private households that had beneficiaries of money transfer from some government social programs to those without beneficiaries. By comparing the data it was possible to highlight several indicators that allow inferring that the income transfer programs seem to be clearly focused on poor and extremely poor families in Brazil. Among these programs, the Bolsa Família should be underlined because it is a massive program, considering the number of families covered from 2006 onwards and its geographic coverage. Among the indicators inferred on the basis of the two surveys, the concentration of households assisted by money transfer from government social programs in the Northeast, the poorest region of Brazil, should be highlighted. Furthermore, the data showed that the families that received money transfers from government social programs, when compared to those that did not receive this transfer, presented the following characteristics: less monthly mean household income; greater number of residents per household; significantly inferior conditions regarding sanitary sewerage, garbage collection, existence of a telephone and ownership of durable goods; main segment of activity concentrated on agricultural activities; higher rate of informal workers; concentration of coverage in the age range of 0 to 17 years; marked differences as to number of years of schooling and to the illiteracy rates; predominance of blacks and pardos among the people of reference in the households (IBGE, 2007, p. 35).

At the same time as the studies performed by IBGE (2012) showed the good level of focus of income transfer programs on the target population groups, they also presented data evidencing cases where this focus is lacking. This can be seen in the existence of private households with a per capita family income within the inclusion criteria that were not assisted, as well as private households with a per capita family income higher than the eligibility criteria that were included in the aforementioned programs, as shown below.

According to data from PNAD 2004, 1.3% of the private households without a monthly family income per capita and 4.4% with a monthly per capita family income of up to 25% of the minimum wage (R$65.00 [US$18.84]) did not benefit from money transfers from government social programs (IBGE, 2006, p. 21). On the other hand, 11.4% of households with a per capita family income of more than 25% to 50% of the minimum wage (maximum R$130.00 [US$37.68]) also did not receive money transfers from the government (IBGE, 2006, p. 21). If families with an income higher than the eligibility criteria are taken into account, PNAD 2004 recorded that 7.6% of private households with a per capita household income beginning at one minimum wage, and thus above the criterion for inclusion in the Bolsa Família and the Benefício de Prestação Continuada (Continuous Benefit), received a money transfer from government social programs (IBGE, 2006, p. 21).

The reality identified in 2004 is confirmed by the data from PNAD 2006, which revealed that 4.7% of the private households without monthly per capita family income and 10.3% with a monthly per capita family income from 25% to less than 50% of the minimum wage (from R$87.50 [US$25.36] to less than R$175.00 [US$50.72]) did not receive any money transfer from government social programs (IBGE, 2007, p. 118). Further, considering families with incomes higher than those established for inclusion in income transfer programs, PNAD 2006 recorded that 9.4% of the private households with per capita family incomes beginning at one minimum wage and, thus, above the criterion for inclusion in the Bolsa Família and the Benefício de Prestação Continuada received money transfers from government social programs (IBGE, 2007, p. 62).

In previous papers (Silva, 2010a; 2010b; Silva & Lima, 2009), the focusing or targeting of social programs is a difficult mechanism to operate, taking into account the difficulties inherent to applying mechanisms and criteria that could reach all of the target population group of a given program. In other words, the so-called positive discrimination of those who need it most has historically been marked by problems. These problems are aggravated in the case of Brazil by the large territory, by the diversity of economic, social and political realities of the municipalities, which are marked by a so-called patrimonialist culture, or social relations based on favors and misappropriations (Silva, 2010a, 2010b; Silva & Lima, 2009). This situation tends to be more pronounced due to the large number of small municipalities where personal relations tend to be placed above institutional relationships, and often relatives, friends and fellow members of political parties are favored. Social workers in small Brazilian municipalities will confront the reality of personal, clientelistic and patrimonialist relations in their daily practice. The challenging work environment is a result of institutional ties, mostly based on temporary contracts, and a lack of resources and limited training to deal with such situations.

The impacts of the Bolsa Família on the reduction of inequality and poverty in Brazil

Research on the Bolsa Família have assessed the program's impacts on the reduction of inequality and poverty in Brazil, taking into consideration the food and nutritional security of the beneficiaries, possible impacts on the areas of labor, education and health of the assisted families as well as indications of possible impacts on women, who are the main family representatives in the Bolsa Família. In this chapter, I will highlight the program's impact on poverty, and poverty related to inequality (Barros, Carvalho, Franco, & Mendonça, 2007b).

When considering the impacts of the income transfer programs, particularly the Bolsa Família, on the reduction of poverty and inequality in Brazil, many studies point to a continued reduction of poverty and inequality in the country from 2001 onwards. Thus, Barros, Carvalho, Franco and Mendonça (2007a, p. 20) took the Gini Index as one of the most frequently used inequality measurements and found a decrease from 0.594 in 2001 to 0.566 in 2005. This represents a reduction of 4.6% in the period and is regarded as the steepest decline of inequality in the last 30 years (Barros et al., 2007a, p. 7). In another study that covered the same period, Barros et al. (2007b, p. 15) showed that the annual income in Brazil rose by 0.9%, but that the poor benefitted the most from it, whereas the groups that comprised the 10% and 20% wealthiest people had a negative growth (−0.3% and −0.1%, respectively). For the first time in Brazil, poverty decreased mainly due to the reduction of inequality. The PNADs have recorded successive declines in the Gini Index: 0.535 in 2004, 0.532 in 2005, 0.528 in 2006, 0.521 in 2007, 0.513 in 2008, 0.509 in 2009, 0.501 in 2011 and 0.500 in 2012 (IBGE, 2013, p. 59), although income from labor is still very concentrated. Thus, the study by Barros et al. (2007a, p. 8) indicated that 10% of the population with the lowest income levels had only 1% of the country's total income. Conversely, the 10% of the working class with the highest income levels had 44.4% of the total labor income (Barros et al., 2007a, p. 8). This situation places Brazil among the most unequal countries in the world. Brazil will need 20 more years to reach a position similar to the average of the countries with lower inequality levels (Barros et al., 2007b, p. 21). Further, there is a big gap between the two extremes in the distribution of the monthly per capita income among the families that lived in private households. Moreover, this situation is reaffirmed in relation to the family arrangements, since it was found that half of the family arrangements (50.5%) are located in the group that earns up to one minimum wage, whereas only 5.5% of the private households earned more than five minimum wages (IBGE, 2008, p. 58). The situation is confirmed in the distribution by class of the families' per capita average monthly income measured in minimum wages, as 30% earn up to 0.5 minimum wage, 27% between 0.5 and 1, 22% between 1 and 2, 7.1% between 2 and 3, 5.2% between 3 and 5 and 4.1% more than 5 minimum wages (IBGE, 2008, p. 58).

More recent studies show that the decreasing trend of poverty and inequality in Brazil is being maintained. When looking at poverty and wealth in the six largest urban areas of Recife, Salvador, São Paulo, Porto Alegre, Belo Horizonte and Rio de Janeiro in Brazil, it can be seen that the production growth in the country from 2003 to 2007 was accompanied by an improvement in the income of all families and a decrease in the number of poor people. The study also indicated the maintenance of this trend in 2008. Thus, the condition of poverty and indigence was reduced by one-third, decreasing from 35.0% in 2003 to 24.1% in 2007 (Instituto de Pesquisa Econômica Aplicada [IPEA], 2008, p. 7).

The Instituto de Pesquisa Econômica Aplicada (IPEA – Applied Economic Research Institute) conducted another study about inequality and poverty in the same Brazilian metropolitan areas in 2009, during the international financial crisis. It showed that between January (0.514) and June of 2009 (0.493) the Gini Index dropped 4.1% and this was the biggest decrease since 2002 (0.534) (IPEA, 2009, p. 2). In the period from March 2002 to June 2009 the decrease was of 7.6% (IPEA, 2009, p. 2). The same study found that the poverty rate in the metropolitan areas in Brazil dropped 26.8% between March 2002 and June 2009 (IPEA, 2009, p. 3). Thus, it concluded that the social variables were not altered in the context of the severe international crisis that started in the second half of 2008 and that the income transfer from the government to the poor may have contributed to this result (IPEA, 2009, p. 3). This finding demonstrates the importance of social protection in the lives of the poor and in addressing inequality in Brazil, mainly during periods of economic crises.

Subsequently, in 2010 the IPEA (p. 8) carried out another survey on poverty, income inequality and public policies in the world as a whole and in Brazil in recent years. The main sources of data, at the international level, were the United Nations (World Bank and World Income Inequality Database (WILD)) and, at the national level, the PNAD conducted by the IBGE and data from the Ministério do Planejamento, Orçamento e Gestão (SIGPLAN – Ministry of Planning, Budget and Management) and Ministério da Fazenda (SIAFI – Ministry of Finance). As far as Brazil is concerned, this study found that between 1995 and 2008, the annual average decrease in the absolute poverty rate (up to 0.5 minimum wage per capita) was of 0.8% per year (IPEA, 2010, p. 8). In the period between 2003 and 2008, the annual decrease rate was even more significant, it was 3.1%, while the national rate of extreme poverty (up to a quarter of the minimum wage per capita) was of −2.1% per year (Chedieg, 2012, p. 18). The study highlighted that the decline in poverty and indigence has been taking place since the approval of the 1988 Federal Constitution and with the increase in social expenditures in relation to the Gross Domestic Product from 13.3% in 1985 to 21% in 2005 (Chedieg, 2012, p. 18). It also underlined the move toward a decentralization of social policies and toward social participation in the definition, implementation and management of social policies, which contributed to raise the participation of the municipalities from 10.6% to 16.3% in the same period (Chedieg, 2012, p. 18). However, the same study points out that the maintenance of the improvement in the socioeconomic conditions requires sustaining a high rate of economic growth; low inflation rates; direction of the production to goods and services with higher added value and with a high and advanced technological content; alteration of the regressive tax pattern, which places an excessive burden on the basis of the social pyramid; alteration in the policies of use of public funds; improvement of the infrastructure in the whole country and of the effectiveness in the use of public funds (Chedieg, 2012). It emphasized some deficiencies in the coordination, integration and articulation of the whole set of public policies in horizontal terms. It also highlighted, in the case of Brazil, the following causes for the social improvement and consistent decline of poverty and inequality: continuing currency stability; stronger economic expansion; reinforcement of public policies; real increase of the minimum wage; expansion of popular credit programs; reform and extension of the income transfer programs to the lower income groups (Chedieg, 2012).

According to the 2010 Census, 22% of the Brazilian population is poor (about 42 million people) and have a family income of 0.5 minimum wages (IBGE, 2011, p. 100). Of these, 8.5% are indigent (16.2 million), with a monthly income of 0.25 of the minimum wage (IBGE, 2011, p. 100). Further, according to IBGE (2011, p. 100), which is the Brazilian institution responsible for the Censuses and PNADs, from 1998 to 2008 the poor families dropped from 32.4% to 22.6% of the population and, according to IPEA (2010, p. 8), 12.8 million Brazilians rose above the level of poverty between 1998 and 2008.

From a more global and recent perspective, the process of what is called "growth with inclusion" recorded in a report on Indicators of Brazilian Development, based on the compilation of data from different sources and especially from PNAD 2011 (Chedieg, 2012, p. 11) considers that, in the last 10 years, the Brazilian economy was marked by the combination of economic growth and improvement in income distribution, so that the real per capita GDP increased 29%, with a more favorable development of the poorer population's income, and a significant drop in the Gini Index from 0.553 in 2001 to 0.501 in 2011. The same source indicates a growth considered strong and continuous of per capita income per household with a mean rate per year of 4.5% above the inflation since 2004, going from R$687.00 [US$199.13] in 2003 to R$932.00 [US$270.14] in 2011 (Chedieg, 2012, p. 14). More intense growth was recorded in poor regions and for the less favored parcels of the population, which contributes to reducing inequality. Thus, per capita household income, including all sources and transfers, increased throughout the country, with the Northeast being outstanding with a 2.9% increase per year, 65% above the national average. At the same time, the historical inequality had decreased between 2001 and 2011 when the income of the 20% poorest increased at a rate seven times greater than that of the richest (5.1% per year on average above the inflation). This denotes that the monthly median per capita income per household of the 20% poorest went from R$102.00 [US$29.56] in 2001 to R$167.00 [US$48.40] in 2011 (Chedieg, 2012, p. 16). Reflecting this situation, the Gini Index between 2001 and 2011 fell in all the regions, to a level below 0.5 in the South and Southeast regions (Chedieg, 2012, p. 17). However, this level is still high compared to the international situation. For example, in the Northeast and Midwest regions, the distributive situation is worst, and the Gini Index converged to a level of 0.5 (Chedieg, 2012, p. 16).

The most marked improvement was recorded regarding the situation of extreme poverty: between 2001 and 2011 the population with a per capita household income up to US$1.25/day dropped from 14% to 4.2%, a level much lower than the target stipulated by the Millennium Development Goals (12.8%) (Chedieg, 2012, p. 17).

I consider that the quantitative measures of poverty only based on income reduces its multidimensional perspective and renders invisible the structural determination that makes people poor or rich. The consequence is the individualization of situations of poverty, to the detriment of a humanizing and totalizing perspective to deal with it. In this way, the poor people are ultimately blamed for their situation of poverty and considered individually responsible for overcoming this situation. It is up to the state to provide support, including income transfer programs. These programs became prevalent since the 1990s when neoliberalism in Brazil began to guide the country's development and its insertion into the international scenario became hegemonic.

With regard to understanding the causes of diminishing poverty and inequality in recent years, several studies demonstrate that in Brazil the income transfer programs, together with economic growth, monetary stability, reduction of unemployment, increased insertion of workers into social security, the rise in income from work and, especially, the readjustment of the minimum wage above inflation, have contributed to reduced inequality and poverty indexes, especially to the reduction of extreme poverty, diminishing deprivations in the lives of the beneficiary families, but overall are not significant enough to remove them from poverty in most cases (Barros, Carvalho, Franco, & Mendonça, 2006, p. 25; IBGE, 2010, p. 60; IPEA, 2008; 2009; 2010; 2011; Soares et al., 2007, p. 5; Souza & Osório, 2013, p. 39; Souza, Osório, & Soares, 2011). In this context, social work has expanded its professional space, entering the sphere of social policies and social security, with an outstanding participation in the policy of social assistance and in the implementation of income transfer programs, which are considered important in the process of reducing poverty in Brazil.

Conclusion: possibilities and structural limitations of the Bolsa Família

Reflecting on the accomplishments and limitations of the Bolsa Família as a conditional income transfer program focused on the poor and extremely poor families in Brazil requires placing this discussion in the context of Latin America. In this continent, from the 1990s onwards, the adoption of conditional income transfer programs focusing on poverty and extreme poverty has expanded significantly. This form of social protection is situated in the context of the productive restructuring of the world economy under neoliberal ideology. The social policies in Latin America have undergone profound transformations since the 1980s, weakening the social struggle for the universalization of social rights. The movement for their universalization gives place to the implementation of programs focused on poverty and extreme poverty. Poverty on the continent and especially in Brazil is becoming more visible. However, it is seen only as an income deficiency, without taking into account the structural factors that generate structural poverty and social inequality. The main consequence of this view is a diminished debate on structural issues and the reduction of social intervention to a focus on the immediate improvement in the living conditions of the poor. This political choice is limited to maintaining and controlling poverty, while at the same time reinforcing the legitimacy of the state. This system keeps a group of poor people at the threshold of survival, inserted in the circle of marginal consumption. In this process, fundamental structural issues, such as the high concentration of property and extreme social inequality, so markedly and historically present in Brazilian society, become secondary. In this way, such a choice creates the illusion that poverty can be eradicated by social policies through income transfer programs. Although social work interventions and roles have increased since 2000, this reality has an impact on the professional practice of the social workers who continue to be sought above all to implement punctual and compensatory actions whose consequence is the reproduction of poverty, even though it is attenuated.

The universal social protection based on the universal, collective and inalienable social rights of every citizen gives place to the right to a precarious and marginal survival of the people classified as poor and extremely poor solely on the basis of their insufficient income.

This is the context that sustains the prevalence of the income transfer programs focused on poor and extremely poor families in Latin America and in Brazil. Such programs establish moral duties to be fulfilled by the families as conditions in the areas of education and health and, in this way, reaffirm the theory of human capital by viewing people's education and health as conditions that are sufficient to break the vicious cycle of poverty, which is the product of the structural conditions of the way in which capitalist society is organized for economic production and reproduction and social relations. In addition, it must be taken into account that the education and health services offered to the poor and extremely poor are quantitatively insufficient and of poor quality, since the conditions that they must meet are not accompanied by appropriate steps by the state in order to guarantee the expansion, democratization and quality of the services it provides.

To this more general scenario we must add the structural problems of the Bolsa Família mentioned in previous papers (Silva, 2010a, 2010b; Silva & Lima, 2009). In this field we see the adoption of income as the sole criterion for the inclusion of the poor and extremely poor in the program. This criterion is insufficient to account for the structural and multidimensional aspects of poverty. In addition, the program establishes a very low per capita income for the inclusion of the families in it, thus limiting the access of many families that face extreme hardships and difficulties. There is also a discrepancy regarding the focus on the poor and extremely poor families. The financial aid offered by the Bolsa Família is extremely low and varied, thus limiting the possibility of producing a more significant impact on the reduction of the families' poverty. On the other hand, empirical studies have identified the program's fragility in terms of its association with a macroeconomic policy that might guarantee sustainable economic growth and prioritize the redistribution of income. These studies have also shown its fragile association with structuring programs that would give the families access to basic social services and with the development of quality actions in the fields of education, health and work. In this context, the insertion of social work in the sphere of social services offered to the poor may, contradictorily, be an opportunity for these professionals to develop a creative and critical practice, so that they can contribute to the formation of a consciousness of the rights of their public of users.

The reality of the income transfer programs discussed here fosters and disseminates a false moralistic view that underlies these programs, which is reproduced in society by the claim that they create dependence, do not encourage people to work and that families must be educated by meeting conditions. However, this is not meant to deny the relevance of these programs for the families that benefit from them, since they offer concrete possibilities for improving the immediate living conditions for a great part of the Brazilian population.

One cannot deny the ascension of a significant number of Brazilian families that are now above the poverty line and are included in the lower middle class (the so-called C middle class). This ascension is shown, for example, by the fact that these families are consuming more, have more job opportunities and an increased income from work. But pillars of a structural nature such as the concentration of income from work and the concentration of property, as well as the increased income from capital, remain practically unaltered.

However, it is important to highlight that other factors besides the Bolsa Família have contributed to the socioeconomic changes that have been experienced in recent years and very widely disseminated at the national and international level. Some of these factors that should be highlighted are the annual increase of the minimum wage above the inflation rate, the economic growth with the subsequent decrease of unemployment and the increase of regular jobs; the income transfer programs that pay one minimum wage, such as the Benefício de Prestação Continuada (Continuous Benefit) and the Previdência Social Rural (Rural Social Security), as well as the establishment of the minimum wage as the lowest benefit paid by the social security in Brazil since the Federal Constitution of 1988. In addition to these factors there has also been a rise of public expenditures in social programs.

Note

1 The exchange rate between the Brazilian real and the US dollar fluctuates every day, and in this chapter I considered the value of August 5, 2015 (R$3.45).

References

Barros, R.P., Carvalho, M. de, Franco, S., & Mendonça, R. (2006). *Uma análise das principais causas da queda recente na desigualdade de renda Brasileira* [An analysis of the main causes of the recent drop in inequality in Brazilian income]. Rio de Janeiro: IPEA. (Texto para Discussão, n. 1203). Retrieved from www.ipea.gov.br.

Barros, R.P., Carvalho, M. de, Franco, S., & Mendonça, R. (2007a). *A queda recente da desigualdade de renda no Brasil* [The recent drop in income inequality in Brazil]. Rio de Janeiro: IPEA. (Texto para Discussão, n. 1.258). Retrieved from www.ipea.gov.br.

Barros, R.P., Carvalho, M. de, Franco, S., & Mendonça, R. (2007b). *A importância da queda recente da desigualdade na redução da pobreza* [The importance of the recent drop in inequality in reducing poverty]. Rio de Janeiro: IPEA. (Texto para Discussão, n. 1256). Retrieved from www.ipea.gov.br.

Camargo, C.F., Curralero, C.R.B., Licio, E.C., & Mostafa, J. (2013). Perfil socioeconômico dos beneficiários do programa bolsa família: O que o cadastro único revela. [Socioeconomic profile of the Bolsa Família Program beneficiaries: What is revealed by the cadastro unico registry]. In T. Campelo & M.C. Neri (Eds.), *Programa bolsa família: Uma década deinclusão e cidadania* [Bolsa Família Program: A decade of inclusion and citizenship] (pp. 157–178). Brasília: IPEA.

Chedieg, J. (2012). *Relatório indicadores de desenvolvimento Brasileiro* [The importance of the recent drop in inequality in reducing poverty]. Brasília: PNUD Brasil. Retrieved from www.mds.gov.br.

Instituto Brasileiro de Geografia e Estatística. (2006). *Pesquisa nacional por amostra de domicílios PNAD 2004: aspectos complementares de educação e transferência de renda de programas sociais* [National Household Sample Survey – PNAD 2004: Complementary aspects of education and income transfer from social programs]. Rio de Janeiro: Author.

Instituto Brasileiro de Geografia e Estatística. (2007). *Pesquisa nacional por amostra de domicílios – PNAD 2006: Acesso a transferência de renda de programas sociais* [National household sample survey – PNAD 2006: Access to income transfer from social programs]. Vol. 28. Rio de Janeiro: Author.

Instituto Brasileiro de Geografia e Estatística. (2008). *Pesquisa nacional por amostra de domicílios – PNAD 2007* [National household sample survey – PNAD 2007]. Rio de Janeiro: Author.

Instituto Brasileiro de Geografia e Estatística. (2009). *Pesquisa nacional por amostra de domicílios – PNAD 2008* [National household sample survey – PNAD 2008]. Rio de Janeiro: Author.

Instituto Brasileiro de Geografia e Estatística. (2010). *Pesquisa nacional por amostra de domicílios – PNAD 2009* [National Household Sample Survey – PNAD 2009]. Rio de Janeiro: Author.

Instituto Brasileiro de Geografia e Estatística. (2011). *Censo 2010* [2010 Census]. Brasília: Author.

Instituto Brasileiro de Geografia e Estatística. (2013). *Pesquisa nacional por amostra de domicílios – PNAD 2012* [National household sample survey – PNAD 2012]. Rio de Janeiro: Author.

Instituto de Pesquisa Econômica Aplicada. (2008). *Pobreza e riqueza no Brasil metropolitano* [Poverty and wealth in metropolitan Brazil]. Brasília. (Comunicação da Presidência, n. 7). Retrieved from www.ipea.gov.br.

Instituto de Pesquisa Econômica Aplicada. (2009). *Desigualdade e pobreza no Brasil metropolitano durante a crise internacional:primeiros resultados* [Inequality and poverty in metropolitan Brazil during the international crisis: Initial results]. Brasília. (Comunicado do IPEA, n. 25). Retrieved from www.ipea.gov.br.

Instituto de Pesquisa Econômica Aplicada. (2010). *Pobreza, desigualdade e políticas públicas* [Poverty and wealth in metropolitan Brazil]. Brasília. (Comunicado do IPEA, n. 38). Retrieved from www.ipea.gov.br.

Instituto de Pesquisa Econômica Aplicada. (2011). *Mudanças recentes na pobreza brasileira* [Recent changes in Brazilian poverty]. Brasília. (Comunicados do IPEA n. 111). Retrieved from www.ipea.gov.br.

Ministry of Social Development and Fight against Hunger. (2007). *Perfil das famílias beneficiárias do programa bolsa família – 2006* [Profile of the families benefiting from the Bolsa Família Program – 2006]. Brasília: Author.

Ministry of Social Development and Fight against Hunger. (2010). *Perfil das famílias beneficiárias do programa bolsa família – 2009* [Profile of the families benefiting from the Bolsa Família Program – 2009]. Brasília: Author.

Ministry of Social Development and Fight against Hunger. (2015). *Relatório de informações sociais* [Report of social information]. Brasília: Author. Retrieved from http://aplicacoes.mds.gov.br/sagi/RIv3/geral/index.php.

Report from the Transition Government Administration (2002). *Relatório de governo de transição sobre os programas sociais*. Brasília. Mimeo.

Santos, W.G. dos. (1987). *Cidadania e justiça: política social na ordem brasileira* [Citizenship and Justice: Social policy in the Brazilian order] (2nd ed.). Rio de Janeiro: Campus.

Silva, M.O. da S.E. (2001). *O Comunidade solidária: O não enfrentamento da pobreza no Brasil* [Comunidade solidária – Solidarity community: Failure to deal with poverty in Brazil]. São Paulo: Cortez.

Silva, M.O. da S.E. (2010a). *Focalização e impactos do bolsa família na população pobre e extremamente pobre* [Focus and impacts of the Bolsa Família on the poor and extremely poor population]. São Luís. Mimeo.

Silva, M.O. da S.E. (2010b). *Os limites da focalização e a transição para uma renda básica de cidadania: o Bolsa família no Brasil* [The limits of the focus and transition to a basic income for citizenship: The Bolsa Família in Brazil]. International Bien Congress. São Paulo: Basic Income Earth Network.

Silva, M.O. da S.E. (2011). *O Serviço social e o popular: Resgate teórico-metodológico do projeto profissional de ruptura* [Social work and the popular: Theoretical-methodological retrieval of the professional project of rupture] (7th ed.). São Paulo: Cortez.

Silva, M.O. da S.E., & Lima, V.F.S. de A. (2009). *O Bolsa família: a centralidade do debate e da implementação da focalização nas famílias pobres e extremamente pobres no Brasil* [The Bolsa Família: The centrality of the debate and implementation of the focus on poor and extremely poor families in Brazil]. In: Seminário Latinoamericano de Escuelas de Trabajo Social, Quayaquil, Equador: ALAETS. Mimeo.

Silva, M.O. da S.E., Yazbeck, M.C., & Giovanni, G. di (2012). *A política social brasileira no século XXI. A prevalência dos programas de transferência de renda* [Brazilian social policy in the XXI century: The incame transfer programs prevalence] (6th ed.). São Paulo: Cortez.

Soares, F.V., Ribas, R.P., & Osório, R.G. (2007). *Avaliando o impacto do programa bolsa família: uma comparação com programas de transferência condicionada de renda de outros países* [Evaluating the impact of the Bolsa Família program: A comparison with the programs for conditional income transfer in other countries]. IPC evaluation note.

Soares, F.V., Soares, S., Medeiros, M., & Osório, R.G. (2006). *Programas de transferência de renda no Brasil: Impactos sobre a desigualdade e a pobreza* [Programs for conditional income transfer in Brazil, Chile and México: Impact on inequality]. Brasília: IPEA. (Texto para Discussão, n. 1.228). Retrieved from www.ipea.gov.br.

Soares, S., Osório, R.G., Soares, F.V., Medeiros, M., & Zepeda, E. (2007). *Programas de transferência de condicionada de renda no Brasil, Chile e México: Impacto sobre a desigualdade* [Programs for conditional income transfer in Brazil, Chile and México: Impact on inequality]. Brasília: IPEA. (Texto para Discussão, n. 1.293). Retrieved from www.ipea.gov.br.

Souza, P.H.G.F. de, & Osório, R.G. (2013). O Perfil da pobreza no Brasil e as mudanças entre 2003 e 2011 [The profile of poverty in Brazil and the changes between 2003 and 2011]. In T. Campelo & M.C. Neri (Eds.), *Programa Bolsa Família: Uma década de inclusão e cidadania* [Bolsa Família Program: A decade of inclusion and citizenship] (pp. 137–156). Brasília: IPEA.

Souza, P.H.G.F. de, Osório, R.G., & Soares, S.S.D. (2011). *Uma metodologia para simular o programa bolsa família* [A methodology to simulate the Bolsa Família Program]. Brasília. (Texto para Discussão, n. 1654). Retrieved from www.ipea.gov.br.

9 Toward livelihood security through the Mahatma Gandhi National Rural Employment Guarantee Act (MGNREGA)

An initiative of the government of India

Miriam Samuel and Sekar Srinivasan

Introduction

The National Rural Employment Guarantee Act (NREGA) was enacted by the government of India on August 25, 2005, and it came into force as of February 2, 2006. The scheme was subsequently renamed as the Mahatma Gandhi National Rural Employment Guarantee Act (MGNREGA) on October 2, 2009. This is the first ever attempt in India to entrust a legislative capacity to a scheme, and this is important because it empowers the local government with complete decentralization rights from designing to implementation of works. The very salient feature of this Act is that it guarantees a minimum of 100 days of employment to rural households, who are willing to perform unskilled manual labor. The major objectives of this legislation are to combat the ever-growing unemployment problem among the rural population and to mitigate poverty to a large extent. This Act also intends to serve as a multipurpose domain to address various other important social development issues in India such as out-migration of rural population, women's empowerment, economic inclusion of weaker sections of the society, reduce the disparity of wage employment between men and women, infrastructure development in rural areas, uplifting the rural poor, and enhancing the capacity of local governance.

MGNREGA is called the "People's Act" since it was prepared after various levels of consultation with many organizations, and further enshrined an important component of a demand driven by people rather than scheme. This Act empowers the people to demand work. The legislation is empowering the lowest level of the administration to have the highest capacity for development and implementation of the scheme. This Act emphasizes the delegation of authority in all its operations such as planning, allocation, implementation and evaluation of the scheme. It aims to support holistic development in rural India and it establishes legal obligations that no government functionaries could escape from (Mehra, 2009). To ensure transparency, the Act has various components such as provision to conduct concurrent social audits at village level, and to increase the significance of "Gram Sabha." In India the "Gram Sabha" is a body of all persons entered as electors in the electoral of a Gram Panchahyat and is involved in the planning and implementation of the scheme. MGNREGA has attracted the attention of a large number of poor members of scoiety and it has emerged as a ray of hope to address multiple problems. Yet, it is the success of the scheme that should determine whether MGNREGA has served its purpose or not. The following sections in this chapter will provide information to trace its success and challenges since its implementation.

History of the Act

The enactment of MGNREGA has deep roots in the five-year plans of the government of India. India, after its independence, started to accelerate development programs and to address various developmental issues through five-year plans (Chakraborty, 2014). The first five-year plan began in 1952–1957 with a focus on integrated rural development programs (Gupta, 2006) and consecutive five-year plans were designed to address rural development issues in India. India's

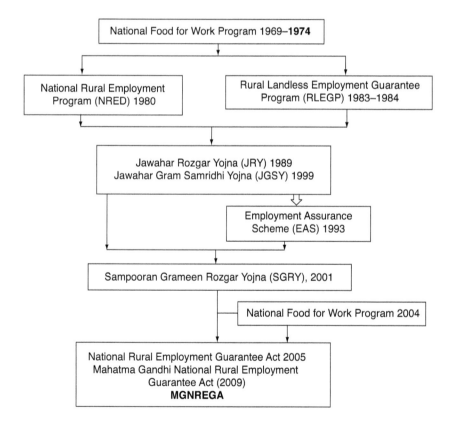

Figure 9.1 Evolution of MGNREGA (Srinivasan, 2008).

development is vastly dependent on the large number of rural villages, and the five-year plans were formulated to ensure inclusion of rural populations in the development process. The first five-year plans gave a conspicuous indication that in order to bring economic development and social development in rural India, the government should create avenues for employment (Varma, 1996). Thus, employment opportunities will cater to the needs of the people and in turn would address poverty, migration, nutrition and health, and foster a strong rural India. These continued efforts of the government have paved the way for the creation of MGNREGA in the year 2005.

Though NREGA/MGNREGA carries the status of legislation as a recent scheme, its origin can be traced back to 1969–1974 with the National Food For Work Program (NFFWP). Since this time, the scheme has undergone many changes and has been consecutively introduced in various names as an employment scheme. Finally, it has evolved as NREGA in the year 2005 and renamed as MGNREGA in the year 2009. Figure 9.1 traces the evolution of NREGA/MGNREGA.

MGNREGA has its origin in several employment schemes introduced in various five-year plans. However, MGNREGA is very distinct and superior to its predecessor schemes because it is a right-based scheme that entrusts all rural eligible households with a minimum of 100 days of employment (Mehra, 2009). All the villages in India were covered in three phases between 2006 and 2008 except Jammu and Kashmir. Jammu and Kashmir have not been included due to political factors and their special status conferred in the Indian Constitution.

Significance of MGNREGA

MGNREGA has been considered as a vibrant scheme that entrusts a legal guarantee to rural households of not less than 100 days of employment to those who are willing to perform unskilled manual work (Mehra, 2009). The scheme is designed to incorporate human rights enshrined in the Constitution of India and the rights listed by United Nations Human Rights Commission. This scheme made its clear commitment to ensure the right to work and food security through its legal guarantee of 100 days of employment (Faizi, 2010). Ravi and Engler (2015) highlighted that wages earned with MGNREGA have reduced the number of meals forgone by the rural households in Andhra Pradesh and contribute to improved nutritional status and food availability. It further emphasized the involvement of disadvantaged groups by way of enhancing participation. Sharma (2010) found that women's participation is well above the statutory minimum of 33% and that 48% of women participated in 2009–2010.

Beyond women's participation, MGNREGA aims to cover a wider array of disadvantaged sections of society such as physically challenged, older people and elders, Scheduled Castes (SC) and Scheduled Tribes (ST). Historically, Indian society has seen social stratification based on the caste system, which is a very unique structure in the Indian culture and such stratification has weakened the SC and ST as the most disadvantaged socio-economic groups in India. In order to protect these most disadvantaged groups MGNREGA encourages their participation. It was found that workforce participation of SC and ST was 49% during the 2009–2010 financial year at the national level (Sharma, 2010). Some of the major objectives are to support the disadvantaged groups and reduce poverty through wage employment. Beyond this, it also aimed at creating economic independence among women and improving the economic condition among the rural poor.

On the other hand, this also ensures parity in the payment of wages for both men and women (Farzana, Mukhopadhyay, & Sahh, 2012) with payments into bank accounts. There are 90 million accounts that have been opened in banks and post offices for the purpose of wage disbursement under this scheme, and it is one of largest financial-inclusion schemes for the rural poor (Sharma, 2010). It has facilitated accessibility to financial institutions and improved saving habits among the beneficiaries. Another important provision is to uphold the 73rd and 74th Amendment in the Constitution by decentralizing authority to the local government. This scheme has empowered the local government by way of giving them complete authority over the decision-making right from selection of work to evaluating the scheme through social auditing. MGNREGA has empowered the "Gram Sabha" or all men and women in the village who are above 18 years of age as well as the village "Panchayat" or local elected government.

Important provisions of MGNREGA

MGNREGA brought a paradigm shift and is unique from previous employment wage schemes of the Indian government (Mann & Pande, 2012), and it has integrated natural resources management and livelihood perspectives. The employment scheme has created wage generation, enhanced livelihood options at the village level, and improved the social security of the rural poor and marginalized groups. The scheme is widely appreciated by different sections of society (National Federation of Indian Women [NFIW], 2008). The scheme aims to reach out to a segment of the population with the clear intention to act as a one-stop solution to address several social issues. The key provisions of the scheme will be discussed in the next section.

Worker entitlements

Any rural household with members 18 years of age and older is eligible to work in the program. Households are entitled to demand work by registration at the local panchayat office (local government office) in person or by writing. The registered households will be provided with a job card within 15 days of registration. Households can seek employment at a panchayat office or at a block development office. A block development office is a cluster level office that oversees and implements rural development schemes. Upon request potential participants are entitled to work within 15 days of their application. If a job is not available the applicant is eligible to receive an unemployment allowance as prescribed by the legislation. It is established that the work site should be within a 5 km radius from the worker's village, and if available employment is beyond this distance, the worker is entitled to a travel allowance of 19% of their salary or paid wages. Workers are entitled to be paid not less than minimum wages prescribed by the Minimum Wages Act and the salary must be paid in 14 days. MGNREGA workers are paid between Rs.100–150 (between US$2–3) per day (Ramsundar & Shubhabrata, 2013). The wages fixed under this scheme are regularly revised by the Ministry of Rural Development with the consent of the parliament.

Work selection

Gram Sabha has the authority to determine the nature and choice of work annually and select the site. The selected work sites are then ratified by the Gram Panchayat. This scheme is viewed as an effective machinery to exercise decentralization of power at the local level (Chakraborty, 2014).

Type of works

The creation of sustainable assets in rural areas is one of the major objectives of MGNREGA (Mann & Pande, 2012). While the types of work to be carried out under this scheme are clearly defined in the clauses of MGNREGA the state government determines the type of work to better meet the needs of their geographical area. MGNREGA provides an opportunity for beneficiaries to choose the type of work and customizes the work based on local needs (Mehra, 2009). The legislation classifies the work into several categories as follows:

Category A: Public Works Relating to Natural Resources Management
This work consists of water conservation and water harvesting; watershed management, irrigation works, afforestation and plantation, and land irrigation.

Category B: Individual Assets for Vulnerable Sections
This includes improving the productivity of lands of vulnerable households, horticulture, sericulture, plantation, farm forestry, development of fallow or waste lands of vulnerable households, creating infrastructure for promotion of poultry and fisheries.

Category C: Common Infrastructure for NRLM (National Rural Livelihood Mission) Self-Help Groups
This work comprises the creation of durable infrastructure for bio-fertilizers and agricultural productivity, creation of common sheds for livelihood activities of self-help groups. Self-help groups are small informal association at the grassroots level organized for mutual help, solidarity, and joint responsibility for economic benefits.

Category D: Rural Infrastructure

This work accommodates rural sanitation related works such as construction of individual latrines, school toilet units, *anganwadi* (courtyard shelters established under Integrated Child Development Services to combat child hunger and malnutrition), toilets and solid and liquid waste management. Rural infrastructure also includes the creation of rural road connectivity, and the construction and maintenance of infrastructure facilities.

(Mahatma Gandhi National Rural Employment Guarantee Act, 2005: Report to the people, 2014)

Transparency and accountability

The MGNREGA is the only scheme implemented with an institutional framework and enacted by legislation (Mehra, 2009). The legislative nature of this scheme entrusts its beneficiaries with a right to approach judicial bodies and to access redressal forums (Sharma, 2010). This scheme incorporated many components to ensure transparency and accountability in all phases and in all levels. For example, the Gram Sabha is authorized to conduct social audits to scrutinize all records and books, and allows the general public to seek information through the right to information about financial disclosure, wage disbursement and any other project related disclosures (Sharma, 2010). It has incorporated the provisions to establish a grievance redressal mechanism to ensure transparency in its implementation (*Mahatma Gandhi National Rural Employment Guarantee Act, 2005: Report to the people*, 2014).

Worksite management

MGNREGA strictly prohibits any type of entry of contractors in performing the work. The scheme further necessitates that work sites should have minimum basic requirements such as safe drinking water, shade for rest, a crèche facility for children, and a first aid box with necessary materials for emergency treatment. The worksite should carry a display mentioning the name of the work, fund allocation details, and the number of employees involved.

The salient features of MGNREGA are unique and comprehensive in order to achieve its objectives. However, the provisions in the scheme are highly appreciable subject to its effective implementation. In the course of the past decade, there have been many appreciations and criticisms of the scheme. Thomas and Bhatia (2012) conducted a study in the state of Gujarat to assess the impact of this scheme on quality of life. It was found that the quality of life changed, especially among the socially disadvantaged groups. According to Chakraborty (2014) there are structural insufficiencies and inefficiencies in the governance of the scheme. He further stated that lapses in wage payment and discriminatory methods of worker selection hampered the effectiveness of this scheme. Despite these criticisms it has been effective in reaching the disadvantaged in rural areas.

MGNREGA implementation structure

The scheme is an initiative of the central Indian government (Union government); however none of the schemes can be implemented effectively without the support of the state government. The scheme is designed in such a way that the power has to be shared equally between the central and state government. The fund allocation for this scheme is shared between governments, and the central government shares 75% of the cost of the work and the state government shares 25% of the cost of the work (*Mahatma Gandhi National Rural Employment Guarantee Act, 2005: Report to the people*, 2014). This scheme is predominantly funded by the central government and administration, and supervision of the scheme is provided by the state and respective local government. MGNREGA is one of the largest schemes initiated by the central government and, moreover, it requires continuous effort by both levels of government for its operation. As already discussed in the provisions, this scheme has vested authority with the local government. It is believed that development will be comprehensive if it is executed through a bottom-up approach (Chakraborty, 2014). On the other hand, delegation of power to local government does not restrict superior authorities from exercising their responsibilities. MGNREGA has a comprehensive chain of command from the top authority to the lowest authority to share the responsibility and to ensure effective implementation. Figure 9.2 provides the implementation structure of MGNREGA.

The comprehensive structure was made to implement the MGNREGA effectively and efficiently. The long chain of command which flows from top to bottom is appreciated by intermediate authorities as a checkpoint to correct any irregularities in an effective manner. The next section of the chapter will discuss MGNREGA in the field.

Current scenario of MGNREGA

MGNREGA is the one of the world's largest employment initiatives and it has generated more employment opportunities in rural areas than any other government scheme or private initiative in post-independence India (Sampth & Rukmini, 2015). At the same time, it has received many critics over its merits and demerits (Chakraborty, 2014; Sampth & Rukmini, 2015). Interestingly and surprisingly, the legislative capacity of the scheme has been sustained under successive governments despite the reality that new governments seek to revise programs in order to claim their success. MGNREGA continues to receive the same level of support with successive governments. The sustainability of the scheme demonstrated its effectiveness and reach with rural populations. MGNREGA continues to receive substantial support and funding in each financial year for the benefit of a large number of participants. It provides employment to around 50 million households every year (*Mahatma Gandhi National Rural Employment Guarantee Act, 2005: Report to the people*, 2014). MGNREGA has been implemented in a phased manner from its inception; it covered 658 districts,

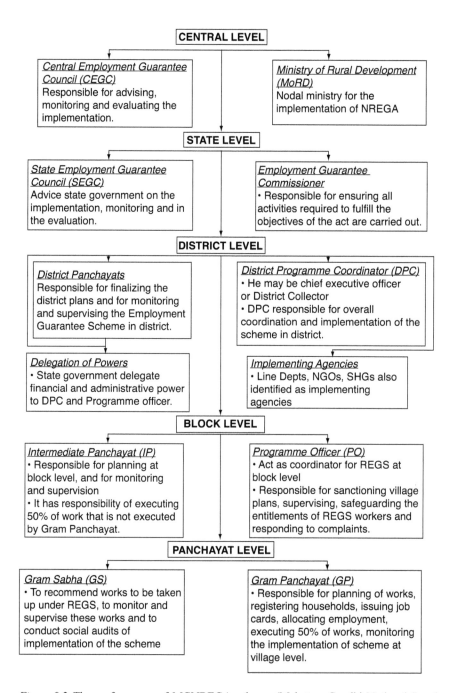

Figure 9.2 The performance of MGNREGA scheme (Mahatma Gandhi National Rural Employment Guarantee Act, 2005: Report to the people, 2014).

6,849 blocks and 250,223 villages across India during the year 2015 (MGNREGA Web page, n.d.).

Table 9.1 indicates the performance of MGNREGA through the total number of households provided with employment, total number of works taken up at the village level, and total number of works that have been completed at the village level. Table 9.1 provides information on the participation of disadvantaged groups; it is found from the table that the participation of SC, ST and women is very significant. The numbers of people participating in this scheme are increasing year to year. Women's participation in this scheme is growing with every year. There were fewer women beneficiaries in 2006–2007, at 40%, yet the number of women continues to increase and is well above the statutory requirement of 33% (National Federation of Indian Women (NFIW), 2008). The figures in the table are huge and it is growing year after year with the hope of bringing effective change in the lives of the poor. It is important to assess the performance of MGNREGA to show its impact, challenges and areas for improvement.

The implementation of MGNREGA is very significant in the improvement of rural livelihood, rural infrastructure, protection of social security, increased participation of disadvantaged groups, reduction of poverty and contributions to the improved socio-economic conditions of the rural poor (Faizi, 2010; Sharma, 2010). During the year 2009–2010, the scheme provided employment to 26.8 million people of which 52.24% of the beneficiaries belonged to SC and ST, and women comprised 50.37% (Faizi, 2010).

MGREGA and social work

The Indian Constitution adopted different mechanisms for meeting the needs of people and communities, and supported programs and policies for poverty reduction, health, welfare of children, women and other marginalized communities such as SC and ST. The earlier sections in this chapter have described the evolution of the scheme leading to its present form. This section will consider the critical role of this scheme as a community development approach in social work. Ife (2002) states that community development is "a process of establishing, or reestablishing structures of human community within which new ways of relating, organizing social life and meeting human needs become possible" (p. 2). In this context, the scheme can be seen as an attempt to facilitate a process of community development and developing structures and processes for meeting human needs, drawing on the resources, expertise and wisdom of the community itself (Ife, 2002, p. 2).

Payne (2005, p. 223), in his book *Modern Social Work Theory*, quotes Henderson and Thomas's (2002) four concepts related to community development. These four concepts are discussed below in relation to the MGNREGA:

- Social capital, which focuses on developing social and community infrastructure as important resources for communities. The MGNREGA strongly focuses on improving the infrastructure and natural resources in

Table 9.1 Implementation structure of MGNREGA (Srinivasan, 2008)

	Year 2006–2007	Year 2007–2008	Year 2008–2009	Year 2009–2010	Year 2010–2011	Year 2011–2012	Year 2012–2013	Year 2013 (December)
Job cards issued (in million)	37.8	64.8	100.1	112.5	119.8	125	127.9	127.2
Employment to households (in million)	21	33.9	45.1	52.6	54.9	50.6	49.8	38.1
Person days (in million)	905	1,435.9	2,163.2	2,835.9	2,571.5	2,187.6	2,298.6	1348
SC	229.5	393.6	633.6	864.5	787.6	484.7	509.6	315.3
	(25%)	(27%)	(29%)	(30%)	(31%)	(22%)	(22%)	(23%)
ST	329.8	420.7	550.2	587.4	536.2	409.2	409.5	210.9
	(36%)	(29%)	(25%)	(21%)	(21%)	(19%)	(18%)	(16%)
Women	364.0	611.5	1,035.7	1,364.0	1,227.4	1,052.7	1,179.3	733.3
	(40%)	(43%)	(48%)	(48%)	(48%)	(48%)	(51%)	(54%)
Others	345.6	621.6	979.5	1,384.0	1,247.8	1,293.8	1,381.4	821.8
	(38%)	(43%)	(45%)	(49%)	(48%)	(59%)	(60%)	(61%)
Total works taken up (in thousands)	835	1,788	2,775	4,617	5,099	8,077	10,651	11,164
Works completed (in thousands)	387	822	1,214	2,259	2,590	2,756	2,560	1,117

the community, such as roads, community buildings, water bodies, land reclamation, afforestation and others.

• Civil society, which involves the formation of informal organizations by ordinary people to work alongside or as an alternative to the government. The functioning and implementation of the scheme has heavily relied on the local governing structure, self-help groups and other informal groups in the villages.

• Capacity-building, which seeks to build up the human resources of communities. Research reports and data presented earlier indicate how the MGNREGA has built the capacity of people and communities by reducing poverty, empowering women and building resources in the community.

• Social inclusion, which ensures that marginalized groups and communities receive assistance to play a stronger role in society. This concept is central to the scheme and mandates that SC, ST and women should benefit from this scheme.

The MGNREGA not only upholds these community development concepts through its mandate, but has within it enshrined the principles practiced in a community development approach in social work. Ife (2002) lists 25 principles of community development that he broadly classifies under ecological principles, social justice principles, valuing the local, process principles and global and local principles. Central to community development is the social justice principle of empowerment, which "means providing people with the resources, opportunities, vocabulary, knowledge and skills to increase their capacity to determine, to participate in and affect the life of their community" (Ife, 2002, p. 208), and the MGNREGA has indirectly, through ensuring security of livelihood for people, increased the "power" of disadvantaged people in the community. The guarantee of work and wages and inclusion of SC, ST and women is a strategy that has influenced the capacity of people.

The MGNREGA is a community development driven approach by and for poorer communities in order to improve economic and social development. There have been many lessons learnt and it is imperative for social workers to critically reflect on MGNREGA as a social protection policy of the Indian government to improve people's lives and communities.

Role of social workers in MGNREGA

The key element of MGNREGA is to ensure transparency and accountability, for which it encourages people to participate in Gram Sabha and social audits in the villages to monitor the effectiveness of the implementation. A social audit is a process by which people work with the government to monitor and evaluate the implementation of this scheme (Burra, 2006). To conduct social audits, many non-governmental organizations (NGOs) and social workers are engaged in training local government institutions and community members to participate in the social audit processes. Burra (2006) found that the Government of Andhra Pradesh (GoAP) actively involved many NGOs, community-based organizations

(CBOs) and volunteers to conduct interviews with beneficiaries, and requested their help in training the beneficiaries on how to conduct social audits. In the process, social workers were actively involved in educating the people on various benefits of this scheme and empowered them in the realization of their right to work. The role of social workers was found to be instrumental in empowering people to access the benefits and enjoy the guaranteed legal entitlements.

MGNREGA and climate change

MGNREGA has contributed to climate change adaptation and mitigation (Singh, Pandey, Gupta, & Ravindranath, 2010). Its contribution can be found in the Category A types of work that prioritizes natural resource management. Major works under MGNREGA were performed on:

1   water conservation and water harvesting;
2   drought proofing including afforestation and tree plantation;
3   irrigation canals including micro and minor irrigation works;
4   provision of irrigation facility, plantation, horticulture and land development;
5   renovation of traditional water bodies; and
6   flood control and protection works.

MGNREGA is not aimed at a single target of reducing poverty but contributes to creating a multitude of benefits (Singh et al., 2010). The impacts of MGNREGA projects have recharged groundwater resources, irrigation canals and water conservation. The renovations of bodies of water have strengthened agricultural productivity (Chakraborty, 2014). It is surprising that 53% of the works supported by MGNREGA were related to soil and water conservation (*Mahatma Gandhi National Rural Employment Guarantee Act, 2005: Report to the people*, 2014). The contribution of MGNREGA to climate change mitigation and adaptation is significant in the rural areas (Singh et al., 2010). For example, activities such as forest restoration, water conservation, rainwater harvesting, land development and afforestation can significantly contribute to climate change mitigation. The impact of MGNREGA works were found to be significant in recharging the groundwater, improving soil fertility and increasing biomass to better improve the ecological systems in rural areas (Singh et al., 2010). MGNREGA projects contribute to sustainable development by enriching and enhancing the natural resources in the rural areas, and reducing poverty.

MGNREGA and migration

One of the important objectives of MGNREGA is to reduce the out-migration from the rural areas to decrease the inflow in urban areas, to reduce slum rates, and to strengthen villages (Jain & Singh, 2013). The recent studies conducted on MGNREGA have indicated that migration from the villages has been substantially reduced (Sharma, 2010). It has reported that post implementation of this scheme, the number of migrating families came down to 45% in 2009–2010 (specifically families which migrate during non-seasons) (*Mahatma Gandhi National Rural Employment Guarantee Act, 2005: Report to the people*, 2014). MGNREGA has emerged as a new source of livelihood option for many rural households. Many rural residents choose to migrate to urban areas due to the non-availability of livelihood options at the village level. Previously villagers had access to agricultural and non-agricultural labor as a main income activity whereas today many unskilled laborers rely on MGNREGA work as a source of income. It has a direct impact on the livelihood of poor rural people and presents as an opportunity to enhance their quality of life (Thomas & Bhatia, 2012). When there is lack of livelihood options, people move out of the villages in search of jobs. MGNREGA has created employment opportunities for the rural poor; it has also reduced out-migration. Mistry and Jaswal (2009) conducted a study in different districts of Gujarat, Maharashtra, Madhya Pradesh and Rajasthan that found 55% of the respondents agreed that this scheme has reduced out-migration in their families. Women's participation in the MGNREGA plays a crucial role in mitigating the migration from rural areas (Jain & Singh, 2013). Verma (2011) found from his studies that out-migration among women and old age people were reduced compared to men. While MGNREGA has played a role in reducing the migration of unemployed rural people from the villages, it has not been able to prevent the migration of men to urban areas in search of higher wage jobs. It provides an avenue for unskilled laborers to get employed; it also creates opportunities for skilled persons to work in block and district level administration (Sharma, 2010).

MGNREGA and women's empowerment

MGNREGA recognizes the necessity to have specific provisions to encourage and enhance women's participation. It aims to contribute to gender equity and women's empowerment by incorporating important provisions in the Act such as equal payment of wages between men and women, ensuring access to work, and decent working conditions for women and their representation in decision-making bodies (Mann & Pande, 2012). MGNREGA statistical reports show that the number of women participating in MGNREGA is steadily increasing year after year. For example, in 2011–2012 women's rate of participation was 48% and in 2012–2013 it increased to 51% (*Mahatma Gandhi National Rural Employment Guarantee Act, 2005: Report to the people*, 2014). It is observed that women are more actively involved MGNREGA than agricultural labor (Ghosh, 2009). On the other hand, parity in wages between men and women is a significant factor that has attracted more women to participate in the scheme (Mann & Pande, 2012). MGNREGA is empowering women by employing them in MGNREGA and contributes to women's economic independence, social security and increased participation in Gram Sabha (Das, 2012).

Women's participation in the scheme has enhanced their economic independence which in turn improves their social status. Traditionally, women were economically dependent on men even for their day-to-day expenses. Post-MGNREGA women are viably economically independent and they have control over their income from MGNREGA (Kelkar, 2011). Women are able to use their income for household needs, health-related expenses and children's education (Jandu, 2008). MGNREGA has empowered women through various other practices such as participating in meetings and social audits. Above all, MGNREGA has created new opportunities for women to better access financial institutions (*Engendering Development through MGNREGS: A Study of Women Workers in the States of Uttar Pradesh, Maharashtra, Karnataka and Andhra Pradesh*, 2011; Ghosh, 2009). All beneficiaries open an account in a bank or post office through which they receive their wage payment. This has further empowered women to access financial institutions independently and exert better control over their income, contributing to economic independence. Srinivasan (2008) conducted a study in Vizhunthamavadi Village Panchayat in Tamil Nadu in South India to understand the impact of MGNREGA in the village. The following case study is an excerpt of the study.

A study on MGNREGA in Nagapattinam District, Tamil Nadu, South India

A quantitative study was conducted in Vizhunthamavadi Village Panchayat, Killayur Block, Nagapattinam District, Tamil Nadu in South India. Vizhunthamavadi village has chosen for the study. Since it has more number of agricultural labours. The goal of the study was to understand the effectiveness of MGNREGA and its influence among 50 beneficiaries. The findings show that among the 50 beneficiaries randomly selected for interviews, 72% of the beneficiaries were women. The beneficiaries of social protection described how the work undertaken improved the rural infrastructure, road connectivity, and water bodies in their villages. There was an increase in the number of water bodies in village such as tanks and wells, and many older water bodies were renovated. The social protection works created more livelihood options for rural landless labourers – with 52% landless agricultural labourers as beneficiaries.

The study identified a number of challenges with implementation. Based on direct observation there were village worksites that lacked adequate facilities that were supposed to be guaranteed by legislation such as safe drinking water, first aid kit, shade for period of rests, crèche facilities for children, and a board displaying the name of the work and other financial details of the works. It was also found that the village clerk is challenged with respect to managing the records and there was a shortage of skilled employees who can take care of these records. The study found that the awareness level of beneficiaries on the features of this scheme was very limited and the rural labourers do not demand work as prescribed in the Act. Most beneficiaries do not know about the unemployment allowance and other benefits related to travel allowance, medical care assistance and compensation for delayed payments. Finally, the study found that women's participation in the scheme was greater compared to men in this village site. There is a need to build awareness of the provisions available in the Act for workers in order to ensure that workers are knowledgeable about their rights.

Source: (S. Srinivasan, 2008)

MGNREGA and marginalized groups

The scheme was designed to incorporate the marginalized sections of the society in the development process in order to foster inclusive growth. MGNREGA aims to reach its objectives by way of providing employment opportunities for marginalized sections of society such as SC and ST. At the national level, the participation of SC and ST in MGNREGA ranges between 40–50% each year (*Mahatma Gandhi National Rural Employment Guarantee Act, 2005: Report to the people*, 2014). This scheme ascertained that marginalized sections of the society should not be excluded from the development processes and they should be given priority in the process so as to keep it inclusive and free from any discrimination. Apart from the employment opportunities, MGNREGA has special provisions in the Act that enforces the renovation of private lands belonging to SC and ST, and increasing their irrigation facilities to improve their livelihood options (Chakraborty, 2014). Along with this, MGNREGA is also empowering the marginalized to participate in the decision-making process by way of participating in the Gram Sabha meetings and taking part in local governance. However, while the scheme aims at bringing every community to come together and work in harmony, there are some people who are not ready to get along with all community members on the same equal platform. For example, the SC families were sent to far-off worksites while upper-caste families were engaged in works at nearby sites (Kumar & Maruthi, 2011). This is a discriminatory and harmful traditional practice based on caste as a form of oppression. The traditional cultural stigma creates many challenges for the local government to ensure that marginalized groups participate in the program in an equitable manner without creating discord in the community. In a recent conversation with a village president in Tamil Nadu, it was found that there are a number of different practices at the village level (Srinivasan, 2014). In order to keep the village free from caste-based violence and discriminatory practices in MGNREGA worksites it is a common practice to group workers together who belong to the same caste/community. MGNREGA strives to foster inclusive growth and bring different caste groups together for work. However, discriminatory caste beliefs prevail and it is a very sensitive issue. If people agree to work in any caste group, they will form a group of their own. But if they resist, groups of the same caste are brought together for work. Another practice is that each caste group will live in different hamlets within the villages. It is a duty of local government to ensure effective implementation of MGNREGA and to maintain communal harmony at the village level.

While MGNREGA has increased the participation of disadvantaged groups the caste-based oppression remains visible at the village level (Kumar & Maruthi, 2011). There is need for structural interventions in order to address this issue and to ensure everyone can work together in an equitable manner. The next section of the chapter will discuss how MGNREGA has impacted agricultural productivity and agricultural sectors.

MGNREGA and agricultural productivity

The agricultural sector is severely affected by the non-availability of water and irrigation facilities in the villages. One of the major contributions made by MGNREGA is that it has increased the number of water bodies and irrigation facilities, and has improved the quality of the soil. The excavated silt from MGNREGA works has improved the soil quality by enhancing the nutrients in the soil (Tiwari et al., 2011). MGNREGA also contributed to enhancing agricultural productivity and cropping patterns. In many places, the existing water bodies were renovated under MGNREGA work to support the agricultural base villages.

MGNREGA is criticized by agricultural farmers for reducing the number and availability of agricultural workers in rural areas and for contributing to an increase in the salary and wage rates of workers (Chakraborty, 2014). The small-scale farmers are largely affected because of these impacts and they are not able to hire a sufficient number of agricultural workers for work in their fields. MGNREGA has been linked with minimum wages in agricultural sectors and fixed wages resulted in new minimum wages in many states (Sharma, 2010). Small-scale farmers claim they are not able to pay the same wage rates as MGNREGA. However, it has been argued that MGNREGA works are carried out during the off-season in order not to affect agricultural activities as a result of the non-availability of workers (Chakraborty, 2014). This is one of the most significant challenges facing the implementing authorities – to ensure that the agricultural sector and MGNREGA go hand in hand. The next section of the chapter will discuss the perspectives of social work and MGNREGA. This section will discuss how community development perspectives have been addressed in the scheme.

Challenges of MGNREGA

MGNREGA is appreciated for its comprehensiveness and multifaceted agenda to reduce poverty and improve rural infrastructure and growth. However, MGNERGA has a number of limitations and inefficiencies. Some of the most frequently encountered challenges across India are structural deficits and cumbersome implementation procedures (Chakraborty, 2014). There is a challenge in the implementation of MGNREGA at the rural level. This results in poor performances of MGNREGA in many villages and stagnation of work schemes in many villages.

MGNREGA has not strengthened the local governance with additional manpower to effectively implement the scheme but entrusted most of the responsibilities to the local government. This affects the way the scheme is implemented. On September 1, 2011, the Ministry of Rural Development released a discussion paper titled "Reforms in MGNREGA Implementation" in order to make the implementation more effective. This paper identified nine major challenges to be addressed:

1   Ensure demand-driven legal entitlements
2   Reduce distress migration from rural areas
3   Reduce delays in wage payments to workers
4   Provide the requisite number of days of work as per demand
5   Improve quality of assets created under MGNREGA and their relevance to the livelihoods of the poor
6   Ensure full payment of wages stipulated under MGNREGA
7   Anchor participatory grassroots planning
8   Sustain regular flow of funds
9   Strengthen grievance redressal mechanisms.

(Source: *Reforms in MGNREGA Implementation* (2011))

The commitment from the Ministry of Rural Development to improve the implementation of MGNREGA is a positive sign that implementing government institutions are aware that there is incompatibility between the provisions enshrined in the legislations and the practice reality. Similarly, the active participation of people is equally compelling for its effective implementation.

Conclusion

MGNREGA is a scheme that has attracted the participation of every section of society, particularly the rural poor. This scheme is one of the largest poverty alleviation initiatives of the government of India. It has encouraged and empowered citizens to feel that they have the right to demand work and to protect themselves with the legal rights enshrined in the legislation. MGNREGA emerged as an effective and vibrant scheme to be implemented in all rural districts; it has reached 658 districts across India. Moreover, it is not just a unidirectional scheme, where government holds all the powers. It is bi-directional where people have equal opportunity for their participation and hold a greater responsibility in decision-making. The processes and stages involved in the scheme created a myriad of opportunities for the local government and people to have better control over the implementation of the scheme. This resulted in the empowerment of local governance and to every member of rural villages.

MGNREGA adopts a community development approach. The Act represents a bottom-up approach rather than a top-down approach. It encouraged people to decide on the type of work, budget allocation for the work selected and it has transferred the accountability to the people rather than government intervening in each step. It has given more freedom to local government to have more power over its implementation than any other authorities. The delegation of responsibility at the village level has empowered the local government and also brought the marginalized sections of the society to become involved in the decision-making process. Moreover, women's empowerment is very visible and evident in most villages (Kelkar, 2011). With respect to women's participation in the scheme, it is very encouraging to see the increase in number every year. For example, during the year 2012–2013, 51.3% of participants were women, the following year there were 52.82% women participants, and in 2014–2015 there were 54.88% women participants (MGNREGA Web page, n.d.). It is a healthy sign for the future of India, to have empowered women who can partake in economically productive activities. Women empowerment is one of the significant contributions of this scheme. It has provided a way for women to have better access to financial institutions, participation in decision-making at home as well as at village level, and provides women with fair treatment in relation to men. MGNREGA's contribution toward reducing poverty and stemming the rural outmigration is a significant result. This scheme enhanced the livelihood opportunities apart from the routine agricultural and non-agricultural labor. The regular revision of wages has influenced salaries in rural areas and contributed to restructured wage payments in other industries. MGNREGA altered the living conditions of the rural poor and contributed to the rural livelihoods. Moreover, it is a community development driven approach, it encourages to create social capital, believes in the capacity building of people and their participation in planning and implementation. It provides opportunities for civil society organizations and social workers' involvement in ensuring transparency and accountability. Thus, MGNREGA incorporates multidisciplinary components with the great vision to establish social protection and social development.

References

Burra, N. (2006). Transparency and accountability in employment programmes: The case of NREGA in Andhra Pradesh. Retrieved from www.levyinstitute.org/pubs/EFFE/Transparency_and_accountability_in_employment_programme_Final_version.pdf.

Chakraborty, B. (2014). MGNREGA policy and application. *International Journal of Sociology and Social Policy, 34*(3/4), 263–300.

Das, D. (2012). Examining India's Mahatma Gandhi national rural employment guarantee act (MGNREGA): Its impact and women's participation. *International Journal of Research in Management, 6*(2), 209–218.

Faizi, A.A.A. (2010). Impact of national rural employment guarantee scheme in strengthening local government institutions in India. *Asia-Pacific Journal of Rural Development, 20*(2), 141–168.

Farzana, A., Mukhopadhyay, A., & Sahh, S. (2012). *Female labour force participation and child education in India: The effect of the national rural employment guarantee scheme*. Discussion Paper No. 6593, Institute for Study of Labour, Bonn.

Ghosh, J. (2009). Equity and inclusion through public expenditure: The potential of the NREGS. International Conference on NREGA. Ministry of Rural Development and ICAR.

Gupta, S. (2006). *Rural development schemes: A study on tribal area in Himachal Pradesh*. New Delhi: Indus Publishing.

Henderson, P., & Thomas, D. (2002). *Skills in neighbourhood work* (3rd ed.). London: Routledge.

Ife, J. (2002). *Community development: Community-based alternatives in an age of globalization* (2nd ed.). Australia: Pearson Education.

Jain, P., & Singh, R.J. (2013). Mahatma Gandhi national rural employment guarantee act (MGNREGA) on the touchstone of social security. *Indian Journal of Applied Research, 3*(2), 227–229.

Jandu, N. (2008). Employment guarantee and women's empowerment in rural India. International Seminar on National Rural Employment Guarantee Scheme in India. New Delhi: Institute for Human Development and Centre de Science Humaines.

Kelkar, G. (2011). MGNREGA: Change and continuity in gender relations. *Journal of Economic and Social Develop, 7*(2), 11–24.

Kumar, P., & Maruthi, I. (2011). *Impact of NREGA on wage rate, food security and rural urban migration in Karnataka.* Bangalore: Institute for Social and Economic Change, Bangalore.

Mahatma Gandhi National Rural Employment Guarantee Act, 2005: Report to the people. (2014). Retrieved from http://nrega.nic.in/Netnrega/Data/English_Annual_report_2010_11.pdf\npapers3://publication/uuid/FEBAB4D2-1FDF-4E15-BF94-AEB-612FA4A32.

Mann, N., & Pande, V. (2012). *MGNREGA Sameeksha: An anthology of research studies on the Mahatma Gandhi National Rural Employment Guarantee Act, 2005 2006–2012.* Orient Blackswan Private Limited.

Mehra, P. (2009, December 27). Village of 2020! Brought to you by NREGA. *Business Today*, pp. 62–66. Retrieved from www.businesstoday.in/magazine/cover-story/village-of-2020!-brought-to-you-by-nrega/story/4965.html.

MGNREGA Web page. (n.d.). Retrieved on September 19, 2015, from http://mnregaweb4.nic.in/netnrega/all_lvl_details_dashboard_new.aspx.

Mistry, P., & Jaswal, A. (2009). Study of the implementation of the National Rural Employment Guarantee Scheme (NREGS).

National Federation of Indian Women. (2008). *A Study by National Federation of Indian Women.* New Delhi: Ministry of Rural Development (MoRD).

Payne, M. (2005). *Modern social work theory* (3rd ed.). Chicago: Lyceum Books.

Ramsundar, B., & Shubhabrata, S. (2013). Case study a critical evaluation of MRNEGA: A study on birbhum district of West Bengal, India. *Management and Administrative Sciences Review, 2*(2), 171–180.

Ravi, S., & Engler, M. (2015). Workfare as an effective way to fight poverty: The case of India's NREGS. *World Development, 67*(C), 57–71.

Reforms in MGNREGA implementation. (2011). New Delhi: Ministry of Rural Development, Government of India.

Sampth, G., & Rukmini, S. (2015, May). Is the MGNREGA being set up for failure? *The Hindu.* Retrieved from www.thehindu.com/sunday-anchor/is-the-mgnrega-being-set-up-for-failure/article7265266.ece.

Sharma, A. (2010). The Mahatma Gandhi National Rural Employment Guarantee Act. *Innovative, 2011*, 271–289.

Singh, V.S., Pandey, D.N., Gupta, A.K., & Ravindranath, N.H. (2010). *Climate change impacts, mitigation and adaptation: Science for generating policy options in Rajasthan, India.* Rajasthan State Pollution Control Board, Jaipur, India.

Srinivasan, S. (2008). A study on implementation of national rural employment guarantee scheme, Vilunthamavadi Village, Nagapatinam, Tamil Nadu, India. Madras Chirstian College affiliated to University of Madras, Chennai.

Srinivasan, S. (2014). Personal communication, August 10, 2014.

Thomas, B., & Bhatia, R. (2012). Impact of NREGA scheme: A study on the overall quality of life of tts beneficiaries (a study undertaken among beneficiaries of 3 districts of Gujarat State). *Asia-Pacific Journal of Social Sciences, 4*(2), 213–227.

Tiwari, R., Somashekhar, H.I., Parama, V.R.R., Murthy, I.K., Kumar, M.S.M., Kumar, B.K.M.,... Ravindranath, N.H. (2011). MGNREGA for environmental service enhancement and vulnerability redution: Rapid appraisal in Chitradurga District, Karnataka. *Economic and Political Weekly*, *46*(20), 39–47.

UN Women – Institute for Human Development. (2011). Engendering development through MGNREGS: A study of women workers in the states of Uttar Pradesh, Maharashtra, Karnataka and Andhra Pradesh. UN Women, South Asia Ofice, New Delhi.

Varma, R.K. (1996). *Policy approach to rural development*. Jaipur: Printwell.

Verma, S. (2011). *MG-NREGA assets and rural water security: Synthesis of field studies in Bihar, Gujarat, Kerala and Rajasthan, Anand*. Gujarat: International Water Management Institute.

10 The South African Child Support Grant and dimensions of social justice

Vivienne Bozalek and Tessa Hochfeld

Introduction

Nancy Fraser (2008; 2009) equates social justice with the social arrangements which make it possible to participate socially on par or equally with each other. This chapter considers the extent to which one such social arrangement, the Child Support Grant in South Africa, provides its recipients with the ability to interact equally with others in relation to three different dimensions. First, with regard to the redistribution of resources, second, with regard to a recognition of work such as caring labor and third, in relation to the representation of people's voices or social inclusion. We have chosen to use Fraser's *trivalent* view of social justice with its economic, cultural and political dimensions to examine a case study about the South African Child Support Grant, for four reasons.

First, we regard the dimensions that she identifies, the economic or distribution of resources, the cultural or recognition of attributes and the political or representation/social inclusion or exclusion, to be useful categories to examine people's life circumstances. Second, Fraser equates social justice with participatory parity, which is a compelling way of comparing people's circumstances and assessing what they are able to be and to do. Third, it is useful because Fraser focuses specifically on the social arrangements which either enable or put barriers up to achieving participatory parity in relation to the three dimensions – the economic, cultural and political. The fourth reason that we find Fraser's conception of justice to be useful for our analysis of forms of social protection such as the South African Child Support Grant, is that it helps us to assess the socially transformative potential of social interventions, as she differentiates between affirmative and transformative outcomes. Thus the analysis from Fraser's perspective allows us to be critically engaged and politically vigilant toward social arrangements such as Child Support Grants and how they can contribute toward social justice. It also makes it possible for a program such as the South African Child Support Grant, which is almost universally considered successful, to be viewed in a more nuanced light.

This chapter is organized in the following way: The first section is an introduction to South Africa's social assistance program, and the second describes the Child Support Grant as a form of social protection. This is followed by an explication of Fraser's social justice framework we use to analyze the data presented in our case study. We then briefly describe the research design, and finally analyze the data using Fraser's dimensions of participatory parity.

Social assistance in South Africa

We begin by describing social assistance in the form of cash transfers in South Africa, one of which is the Child Support Grant. While South Africa is a middle income country with a functional economy and good infrastructure, rates of poverty remain very concerning, at over 50% of the population as a whole (UNICEF, 2010). Unemployment rates for the working age population are high, hovering around 30% depending on the definition used (Woolard et al., 2011, p. 358); the higher percentage includes the "work discouraged" who have given up looking for work. As a result, and due also to poor access to fertile land and water in rural areas significantly reducing the efficacy of subsistence agriculture, almost 26% of the national population face some form of food insecurity (Statistics South Africa [StatsSA], 2014a, p. 57). South Africa has very high income inequalities: in 2007, the Gini co-efficient was 0.63 (UNDP, 2014, p. 170). While the end of apartheid meant significant improvements in services and infrastructure for black people, 14% of all households (mainly residing in urban areas) continue to live in informal housing or slums (StatsSA, 2014a, p. 34) and in some rural parts of the country nearly 20% of households have no potable water (StatsSA, 2014a, p. 40). While access to primary education and primary health care is good, actual outcomes in health and education are deficient due to a variety of factors, resulting in a poor ranking for South Africa on the Human Development Index (UNDP, 2009). Children, women, those living in a rural area, and those of African descent remain the most disadvantaged and the poorest (SAHRC & UNICEF, 2011).

South Africa provides social protection to its population using a number of different instruments, such as a national public works program, a large school feeding scheme, and an extensive social assistance program. Social assistance takes the form of a range of cash transfers, and these have been one of South Africa's most effective mechanisms for redistributing resources in the country. Cash transfers cover over 30% of the population of 51 million and have directly led to improvements in South Africa's national poverty levels (Lund, 2011; Posel & Rogan, 2012; Woolard et al., 2011). The large, well-funded social assistance program is one of the two arms of South Africa's welfare program, the second is a smaller, poorly funded arrangement of social services. Historical, political, leadership and funding challenges have all undermined the effectiveness of social service delivery in South Africa (Patel, 2015). In addition, while democracy has ensured unprecedented access to public services, such as education, these services face massive problems of quality delivery and constantly operate in a state of crisis.

Cash transfers have a long history in South Africa, beginning in 1928 with Old Age Pensions for white citizens, which eventually expanded to include other racial groups. Social grants during the apartheid era were thus well established, publicly funded, and widely accepted, though significantly racially skewed in favor of whites. The current cash transfer program has been hailed as one of the success stories in social protection in the developing world, particularly as it is run and fully funded by the state and not donor organizations. The right to social protection is enshrined in the South African Constitution and formal Acts of Parliament (such as the Social Security Act), and is thus not dependent on the benevolence of the ruling party. It is a large program by the standards of most African countries, reaching more than 16 million poor people monthly (SASSA, 2015, p. 1). By far the transfer with the furthest reach is the Child Support Grant, assisting nearly 70% of the 16 million monthly grant beneficiaries, as illustrated in Table 10.1.

The South African Social Security Agency (SASSA), a national centralized state institution, is the disbursement agency of all grants. Recipients can choose to collect cash at pay points or for the money to be deposited directly into special bank accounts. Funding for all grants is from the state, collected primarily as tax revenue and centrally managed. Further, the system of distribution is largely efficient and free of fraud, therefore almost all of the budget of R120.9 million (approximately US$12 million) in 2014 earmarked for grants actually reached the intended individuals (Patel, 2015). In addition, all the cash transfers are means tested, but because the budget is affordable and there is a legislated right to social security, the means test is set at a relatively generous amount. Therefore, it is not only the completely destitute who benefit from social assistance; the not-so-poor and the working poor are also eligible to access grants.

Because the South African cash transfer system targets individuals in particular vulnerable categories, such as the aged, the disabled and children, adults between the ages of 18 and 60 who are able-bodied have no claim to social assistance. The ideological assumption underlying this design is that able-bodied adults should be engaged in productive activities and therefore ought not need any income support, whereas certain groups of vulnerable people such as the aged are entitled to state care. Even the state acknowledges the falsehood of this notion due to the lack of jobs for working age adults, but does not want to remedy poverty through social assistance measures alone and is rather focused on labor-promoting schemes as its intervention strategy (Barchiesi, 2011; Patel, 2015). The persistent failure of this approach has meant that large numbers of people live in consistently precarious and desperate circumstances.

Although great strides have been made in terms of racial equity in changing social policies which in the past privileged the few, national policies still do not actively recognize that dependency is central for human flourishing and that there is a universal need for care across the phases of human life (Sevenhuijsen, Bozalek, Gouws, & Minnaar-McDonald, 2007). One of the consequences of so many individuals without any direct form of income protection is the phenomenon of income pooling, where a single low value grant might support a whole household as it is the only reliable cash income among the members (Neves, Samson, van Niekerk, Hlatshwayo, & du Toit, 2009).

Table 10.1 Total number of social grants by grant type as of March 31, 2015 (South African Social Security Agency [SASSA], 2015)

Social assistance	Target group	Amount received/month (US$ equivalent)	Number of beneficiaries as at March 2015
Child Support Grant	Paid to the primary caregiver of a child/children up to 18 years old, subject to a means test.	US$25	11,703,165
Old Age Pension	Persons over the age of 60 years old, subject to a means test.	US$106	3,086,851
Disability Grant	Persons medically diagnosed as disabled over the age of 18 years old, subject to a means test.	US$106	1,112,663
Smaller grants (consolidated)	Foster Care Grant; Care Dependency Grant; Grant-in-Aid; War Veterans' Grant	Ranges from US$23 – US$100	739,964
Total number			16,642,643

The Child Support Grant

In this section of the chapter, we describe the Child Support Grant and make reference to its considerable achievements in working toward socially just conditions. We also examine the complexities of this form of state intervention for its contribution to social justice outcomes.

The Child Support Grant (CSG) was created in 1998 by the first democratic government in order to reach poor children who were largely uncovered by social assistance measures at the time, with the specific intention of improving nutrition for young children. It is a cash transfer program that reaches 11.7 million poor children every month (SASSA, 2015, p. 1) which is over 60% of the total population of children in South Africa (StatsSA, 2014b, p. 9). It is distributed via the primary caregiver of the child. Caregivers are predominantly women, and are often the biological mothers or grandmothers of the child (Vorster & de Waal, 2008), although they do not need to be biologically related. The design of the grant, born as it was in the heady early days of the new democratic South Africa, is unusually progressive. The "follow the child" principle means that the CSG goes to the child's primary caregiver, whomever that may be. This design was due to expansive kinship structures and high levels of economic migration in South Africa, resulting in children being frequently cared for by adults other than their biological parents. While, however, the gender-neutral language means CSGs can go to male or female caregivers, biologically related or not, the gendered nature of care means very few men (approximately 4%) claim the grant for children in their care (Vorster & de Waal, 2008).

The CSG is disbursed on the condition that children attend school, but since there was almost universal primary school enrollment prior to the institution of this regulation, to all intents and purposes this functions as an unconditional grant (Lund, 2011). The amount disbursed per grant is small (R320, approximately US$25, per month as at mid 2015). Research indicates the CSG is spent primarily on food, but also covers school related costs, health costs, and other household expenses (Delany, Ismail, Graham, & Ramkisson, 2008; Neves et al., 2009; Patel, Hochfeld, Moodley, & Mutwali, 2012).

Despite the low monetary value of the CSG, research on its impact has indicated substantial positive effects as a cash transfer (SAHRC & UNICEF, 2014), an extraordinary achievement. The CSG has led to improved food security for the children getting the grant as well as the households in which they live (Agüero, Carter, & Woolard 2006; Delany et al., 2008; Department of Social Development, South African Social Security Agency, & UNICEF, 2012; Woolard et al., 2011), and improved health outcomes for children (Department of Social Development et al., 2012). It has contributed to more regular school attendance and is helping to keep children in school longer via the purchase of uniforms, books and school transport (Delany et al., 2008; Department of Social Development et al., 2012; Neves et al., 2009). The grant has been shown to have had a positive effect on children's care in the household, as recipient caregivers are spending more time than caregivers *not* getting a CSG in activities such as doing homework with children, playing and reading to them, watching television together, and walking them to school (Patel et al., 2012). The grant is important as a labor-promoting tool for unemployed caregivers, who use it to start small businesses and to pay for transport to look for work (Woolard et al., 2011). Finally, research has shown that the CSG is supporting women's empowerment in relation to the control over resources and decision-making in the household (Adato & Bassett, 2008; Patel & Hochfeld, 2011; Patel et al., 2012). As so many of the social impacts accrue in the first instance to the caregiver recipient, this chapter engages with the benefits and challenges of the CSG in relation to these women caregivers.

In the following section of the chapter we outline Nancy Fraser's trivalent conception of social justice, which we use as a lens to examine the case study regarding the CSG in this chapter.

Fraser's trivalent conception of social justice

Nancy Fraser, an eminent US political scientist, views social justice as the ability to socially interact as peers or on an equal footing, which she refers to as participatory parity. Participatory parity refers to social interaction in the public and private spheres, in institutions such as schools and universities, in the workplace, in community organizations and in formal and informal political organizations (Fraser & Honneth, 2003). In order to achieve participatory parity in society, social arrangements would have to be put in place which would make it possible for individuals to interact on a par with each other.

Originally, Fraser regarded participatory parity as involving two dimensions – an economic or class-based dimension which would require *redistribution* and a cultural dimension which would require *recognition* for participatory parity to be possible (Fraser, 2000; Fraser & Honneth, 2003). In later years, Fraser (2008, 2009, 2012) added another dimension, making it a trivalent view of social justice, incorporating economic, cultural and political dimensions. The addition of the political arose because Fraser argues that in the current era issues which transcend national boundaries should receive our attention due to the profound impact of globalization. She calls this a post-Westphalian theory of social justice, where the importance of national boundaries can no longer be assumed in the impact on people's abilities to participate as equals. For example, the International Monetary Fund conditions of financial support have severe consequences on resource-constrained environments which are forced to enter into negotiations to obtain funding, and the digital divide is impacting on access to knowledge and other goods across national boundaries.

Fraser (2008; 2009) sees all three dimensions of social justice as being intertwined and influencing each other reciprocally, but each as analytically separate and not reducible to the other. Fraser's (2008, p. 282) slogan "No redistribution or recognition without representation" is indicative of her insistence that for social justice to be possible each dimension must be considered.

Each of the three dimensions of social justice can be viewed either from an affirmative or transformative perspective according to Fraser. From an affirmative perspective, social justice can be redressed by attending to the inequitable outcomes of social arrangements in ways which make ameliorative changes. Transformative approaches to social justice, on the other hand, address the root causes of the three dimensions through restructuring the generative framework which has given rise to impairment of participatory parity. In the section that follows, each dimension – the economic, cultural and political – will be briefly discussed.

Redistribution and maldistribution

With regard to social justice, people can be prevented from participating as equals by economic constraints through obstacles in structures which deprive them of access to material resources through poorly paid or exploitative work or lack of access to income-generating work and disparities in work, leisure time and responsibilities. This dimension pertains to economic or class-based issues which are related to the means of production and includes access to resources such as education, knowledge, housing, food, water, electricity, health care, and for our particular focus in this chapter, on social protection or the South African CSG. In terms of affirmative and transformative approaches to the economic dimension, affirmative approaches would incorporate liberal welfare state initiatives where income is redistributed through income-generating projects or social security such as the CSG, which reallocate existing goods to other groups of people who do not have access to them. Transformative approaches to the economic dimension would require changes to the division of labor, the setting of responsibilities – who gets to do what work and how this is valued (e.g., the paid and unpaid caring work in society) (Tronto, 2013), challenging property ownership, or universalizing benefits so that certain groups are not devalued in receiving these benefits.

Recognition and misrecognition

Another way in which people can be prevented from interacting with each other on a par socially is the ways in which their attributes or the activities or practices they are engaged with are valued or devalued. Fraser is interested in the institutionalized hierarchies of cultural value or the status positions rather than the psychological effects of being devalued (Fraser & Honneth, 2003). In this dimension, status inequality or misrecognition would occur when some categories of people and the attributes associated with them are depreciated or devalued.

Forms of status inequality or misrecognition would include cultural domination, where members of particular groups are "inferiorized" or "othered" through institutional practices perpetuated through processes like colonialism by settler groups, or where the values and attributes of certain groups are backgrounded and rendered invisible through mass media and other interpretative practices. Attributes of marginalized groups may also be actively maligned, for example the ways in which the attributes of refugees and migrants have been disparaged in the South African context.

Injustices regarding misrecognition would pertain to those groups who were accorded less respect and esteem than others in terms of cultural categories such as race, gender, sexuality, ability, nationality, etc. Examples of institutional practices which would affect misrecognition would be institutional policies and practices which assume a normative social actor, such as white, male, middle class, heterosexual, and where the attributes of other groups are implicitly regarded as deficient or inferior. Other examples include welfare policies which stigmatize certain groups of people such as single mothers, or language policies in higher education institutions which value certain groups of people, as well as normative categories such as male-headed households, nuclear families and so on.

In order to address misrecognition, Fraser is clear that she is not interested in psychic reparation on an individual level but rather in overcoming subordination claims for recognition in status by deinstitutionalizing patterns of cultural value which impede participatory parity on a social level of particular groups of people. In terms of affirmative and transformative approaches to misrecognition, affirmative approaches would concentrate on revaluing disrespected identities or devalued traits of maligned groups, while transformative approaches go further in deconstructing the binary categories themselves, thus destabilizing symbolic oppositions in institutionalized patterns of cultural value.

Affirmative strategies may have the effect of reifying groups of people such as black people, or women, along a single axis, in this way simplifying complexity and multiplicity of situations of misrecognition or encouraging identifications with particular categories. An example of the use of an affirmative approach to misrecognition would be gay identity politics in revaluing gay sexuality, and a transformative approach would be queer politics which questions and deconstructs the binaries between homo- and heterosexuality, thus destabilizing sexualities and going beyond identity politics.

Representation, misrepresentation and misframing

Representation, misrepresentation and misframing constitutes the third, political, dimension which has recently been added by Fraser to the dimensions of distribution and recognition, and pertains to who counts as a member of a community – who is included and belongs socially and, conversely, who is excluded.

Fraser distinguishes between two forms of misrepresentation – the ordinary political one which has the national territorial state as its frame, where particular groups of people on the basis of social markers such as gender, race and ability are prevented from participation in their national political processes. The second form of misrepresentation is more serious, and concerns how political boundaries are set and who can be a member or not. In this way, people can be excluded from participating altogether, and those who are poor or devalued have no way of making any claims about their positions – this she refers to as *misframing*. Misframing is the most serious form of injustice as it can be regarded as a political death – such as Jews in Nazi Germany, Palestinians in Israel, and refugees in many countries. Those who are included within the set political boundaries belong socially and are the ones who can air their claims regarding social justice. However, those who are excluded are regarded as non-persons and do not even get to petition their position as rights-claimants, and are thus denied any possibility of interacting on an equal footing with others.

Fraser sees misframing as the defining form of injustice currently, as the global poor are powerless in challenging their positions. The injustices they experience are misframed as it is not acknowledged that it is the international corporations such as the International Monetary Fund (IMF), or situations like being excluded from the knowledge economy by the digital divide, and so on, which are responsible for the lack of participatory parity, rather than only being disadvantaged in their own nation state. In the political dimension, affirmative approaches would still accept that the territorial state is the most appropriate context in which to contest issues of injustice as members of a political community, and would see injustices of representation and belonging as arising from and being resolved within the context of the territorial state itself, rather than outside its boundaries. From a transformative perspective, while it would be recognized that while the state-territorial perspective would remain salient in some instances of injustice, it would not be regarded as relevant in all cases. For example, structural injustices pertaining to international or global issues such as climate and other environmental issues, the digital divide and differential access to knowledge production and consumption, global market policies, disease, drugs, weapons, etc. all impact groups of people across national territories.

Fraser's "all affected" principle addresses how these common issues affect the life chances and ability to participate as equals of those affected by these across geopolitical contexts. In this case, the most effective way of addressing these issues would be through international social movements such as the basic income grant movement, which would give affected groups of people a collective voice to express their concerns about being affected by these forms of injustices.

We now turn to a discussion of how the CSG is experienced by a female caregiver who receives the grant on behalf of children in her care. This micro-view is useful in order to understand the real lives behind the statistics that describe the effects of the CSG nationally. From this vantage point it is possible to ask the question: How is it experienced by individuals for whom this is a critical livelihood?

Research design

The data used in this chapter is drawn from a study that investigated the social impacts of the CSG in a Johannesburg setting. Tessa Hochfeld conducted this research using a narrative inquiry framework. Between 2011 and 2013 she generated data with six women receiving CSGs for their children via multiple interviews, observations and participatory research methods. This chapter uses data from one of the women's stories as a case study to illustrate Fraser's notion of participatory parity and how it can be applied to an individual life.

The woman we have chosen to focus on, Jane,[1] is an articulate, confident, educated woman who has fallen on hard times. She lives with her boyfriend, Nathi, and with five of her six children, plus takes care of two young relatives. The family lives in a small three-bedroom apartment in run-down accommodation in the city of Johannesburg. Jane, a qualified teacher with the Department of Basic Education, was dismissed from her job while in hospital with severe depression, a result of extreme trauma from the abduction and murder of her late husband. Her boyfriend gets varying and unpredictable income from work as a freelance plumber. Their only other income is three CSGs.

Redistribution

Grant recipients point to the critical role the CSG plays in their survival and in keeping them from destitution (Department of Social Development, South African Social Security Agency, & UNICEF, 2011; Hochfeld & Plagerson, 2011; SAHRC & UNICEF, 2014), and this is supported by the research on the positive impact the grant has on food security (Department of Social Development et al., 2012; SAHRC & UNICEF, 2014). These material effects are also clear in Jane's case. She describes the importance of the grant for her children's food security as follows:

JANE: I am really trying [to manage], I can say thank you [for the grant] because I can buy food for the kids … it is very hard when they are crying for bread. [When I get the grant] I feel very great, like a good mother, because, I know with kids its not like you can … well, you [an adult] can go hungry but not the kids. But [with the grant] I manage to buy them food. I don't buy groceries like I used to do when I was working. I just buy those important things that they need, then I must make sure that we've got the money that is left to buy bread as bread is needed every day. But the grant doesn't last the whole month, yes, it doesn't last us even half a month.

Jane's three CSGs and her boyfriends' patchy and irregular income supports a family of nine, thus it is not surprising that she comments that the grants do not last out the month.

An example of the multiple positive material effects of the CSG is how it can assist with needs beyond food security. Jane experienced the grant as key to achieving good health. At the time of our interviews, Jane was struggling with serious depression, but she was no longer taking medication as her private medical insurance was suspended when she was dismissed and unable to pay premiums, and the waiting list to see a specialist at the public hospital was months long. This depression prevented her from looking for casual work, intermittently interfered with her ability to care for her children, and caused suicidal thoughts. Her previous private psychiatrist offered to see her for free, but Jane said to me:

JANE: Even though that is so kind of her, I could not make an appointment. It is because I don't have money to go there. You see it's right in town so I need two taxis[2] [to get there] and then again two when I come home. So when I get the grant next month then I can go, only when I will be having that money.

The grant offers material resources that have a small but significant positive effect on people's lives. This example also illustrates the value of *choice* which comes from the disbursement of cash rather than other forms of income protection (such as vouchers): needs and priorities shift over time and cash offers users control over identifying essential needs (Holmes & Jones, 2013).

It can therefore be regarded as highly effective in redistributing income to caregivers who are struggling to survive, offering poor women recipients one of the three of Fraser's dimensions of participatory parity, despite the low monetary value of the grant. It would be regarded as an affirmative rather than transformative approach to redistribution in that the benefits are not universalized for everyone, it is a small amount of money in relation to the need, and it does nothing to change the macro socio-economic circumstances that render finding and keeping a stable income a precarious and difficult process. In addition, the major burden of the caring work continues to fall on Jane as the primary female caregiver, so the CSG does not change entrenched gender roles and norms in relation to responsibility for caring activities.

Recognition

Recognition is how people are valued socially, which allows them to be able to participate equally in social life. This spans different spheres, from the micro, such as intra-household practices, to the practices common in broader social and public life.

Recipients of the CSG in South Africa are regularly regarded with suspicion by members of the public, as the mass media tends to deplore the notion of "dependency." The public assumption is that receiving a grant makes people lazy, and amounts to fleecing "good citizens" of public funds. These views are even expressed by senior public officials who do not want people to rely on "hand-outs" (Hassim, 2006). This negative perception of welfare recipients is echoed worldwide in conservative circles (Fraser, 2013). The centrality of dependence in human existence, and the necessity to generate alternative income in addition to the CSG due to its low monetary value, is unacknowledged.

The demonization of dependence in public discourse and the fact that the grant is not universal immediately makes the recipients see themselves as pathologized (Fraser, 2013), set apart from others in society in relation to having their needs met, and makes recipients strongly wish to survive on their own without the sense that they are relying on the state (Hochfeld & Plagerson, 2011). Jane's boyfriend, Nathi, expressed this as follows:

NATHI: I don't like that I must raise my kids with grant money. If I had a good job I would … not allow my kids to get a grant from the state. I would really like raise my kids with my own money because I don't want that in the future my kids say that they were raised by grant money. I must raise my kids from my own money. I want my kids to say that daddy did everything for me.

By getting a grant, recipients are acknowledging their need for help in meeting the dependency needs of their family members due to socio-economic structural conditions over which they have no control. They are often harshly judged for needing support, and in turn judge themselves harshly, perceiving this as a kind of personal failure. This is exacerbated by gendered normative expectations of men who are perceived to be the primary breadwinners (Fraser, 2013). Thus social needs that have been individualized and pathologized powerfully misrecognizes grant recipients.

In addition, while notions of the deserving/undeserving poor have not explicitly driven policy and legislation, they do pervade discourses of ordinary people. Behaviors that are common in South Africa across socio-economic divides, but which are frowned upon if the person is a grant recipient, such as high indebtedness, high alcohol consumption, and motherhood at a young age, are strongly disapproved of if the individual is a grant recipient (Department of Social Development et al., 2011; Makiwane, 2010). So pervasive are these "undeserving" discourses that recipients themselves hold these views, believing that they are among the very few who receive grants and use the money in "acceptable" ways (Hochfeld & Plagerson, 2011). The humiliation that comes with being categorized as "deserving" or "undeserving" is a strong form of misrecognition.

Other forms of misrecognition can strongly influence, and often undermine, the impact of the grant. For instance, Jane could previously have been regarded as "functional and self-sufficient" through access to income-generating employment; having a professional job gave her the means to care for her large family successfully. She was thus not a candidate for state support. But the multiple effects of the murder of her husband and the dismissal from her job drastically changed her position and ability to care for her dependent children. Being dismissed during a bout of severe illness is not just in contravention of the law, but is a powerful way of communicating "erasure" of Jane's status as an employed and economically independent member of society, in other words, she was subjected to a severe form of misrecognition. Her experience of the dismissal is expressed in the following narrative:

JANE: [Rebecca] was here as a social worker from the Department of Basic Education to witness [the dismissal]. So she called me one day, she says I was worried when we brought you the [dismissal letter that day]. Do you know, do you remember what happened? I told her I don't know what you are talking about, then she said, I did see that, you didn't see what was happening, it was wrong for us to give you the letter of a dismissal on that condition you were. You looked very sick and you looked confused.

INTERVIEWER: So she could see for herself?

JANE: Ja, she said it was wrong because you cannot fire someone who has got a severe depression and more especially the way, the looks of it, she did see that something was not right … I was here at home. 'Cause they gave me [strong medication]. I couldn't remember anything 'cause even when I was coming from hospital, I didn't even know my kids, that I have got kids that I have got to attend to. According to [eldest daughter], she said that the doctor also said they must tell me who is this, who they are and they must remind me that I have got kids, this happened to me so, because I didn't know anybody. Even my colleagues they say they came here, I know them, then I was asking who are they, what do they want? Why are so many people coming in this house?… [Rebecca] even tried to talk to the hospital social workers then they said, it was wrong [what they did to me], there was no one [before in their experience] who was having a severe depression who was dismissed so that thing is wrong.

Jane was further misrecognized due to the dominant discourse which pathologies dependency and under-values unpaid caregiving activities (Fraser, 2013). This would intensify the lack of participatory parity in terms of the status shift that Jane experienced in the loss of her formal paid employment.

The state as a monolithic and lumbering instrument can also, inadvertently, result in profound misrecognition. Jane twice had the strange experience of being accused of grant fraud: routine state check-ups on the employment status of recipients led to the immediate cancellation of her grants as the Department of Basic Education still had her recorded as employed as the unfair dismissal case was still pending. Just when she needed help the most, she was accused of fraudulently getting grants for personal enrichment, rendering her very real struggle for survival and for caring for her family invisible. The experience is captured in the following conversation:

JANE: I am, my heart [can't take the stress]. So now I have got a case whereby, they said I have done … fraud and corruption, yes, [they say] I am getting the grants illegally and they have [cancelled] them, oh…. Anything I fix, the other one breaks. [If I was working] I would not even go to the Social Services to ask for the grant, why would I, and even if they can check, I applied for the grant last year [2010] and I was dismissed in 2009. So with this now we didn't get the grant last month…. Now we are suffering. I don't even have … the money to buy soap and to buy them bread tomorrow. There is nothing in the kitchen. [Jane begins to sob].

These examples of multiple misrecognition have great relevance for social work as a profession. The humiliation, disrespect and disappointments created by the experiences recorded above are not intentionally produced by the design or implementation processes of the CSG, but rather from the interaction of the CSG as a social protection mechanism and the current social, economic and political context in South Africa. Thus while they are unintended consequences of a largely successful and well-designed cash transfer, they are real and harmful for the individuals involved. Social workers therefore have a responsibility to respond not just therapeutically and supportively, but politically and as a social advocate for those whose experiences are patently unjust.

Representation

With regard to representation and framing, the number of children receiving the grant has been continually expanding due to extensive lobbying to extend the age limit of children over the years since its implementation. This has been very successful as a civil society campaign as the age criteria of 0–7 years was incrementally increased to 0–18 years. However, the amount of the grant is still limited and its means-tested nature still tends to demonize a particular group of people, which may be avoided if it was universalized and extended to all caregivers of dependents.

Another area of misrepresentation can have an impact on the participatory parity in relation to CSGs. Jane's Mozambiquan boyfriend, Nathi, was powerless to prevent the destruction of his travel and identity documents giving him permission to live and work in South Africa. She describes this experience as follows:

JANE: Things are very very tough. Because you see Nathi, he doesn't have a job. He doesn't have an ID that is why. The problem is he doesn't have papers, he is from Mozambique. You see he had papers, all the right ones, but they [the police] destroyed them. Even if he wants to go home he is stuck.
INTERVIEWER: How can the police do that?
JANE: They always do. I have seen them.... Even when the papers are all perfect, they say they can make your life a misery and they just tear them [right there like with Nathi] and they don't care, they just go away. There are very cruel people out there.

Nathi is in a position of being socially and economically excluded from South African society because he is a migrant from another African country. This according to Fraser is the most severe form of injustice in that he is prevented from being a rights claimant in South Africa. This has a profound knock-on effect on the other dimensions – economic exclusion and gross misrecognition or even abuse. The CSG may then be even less adequate in meeting the needs of everyone in the household under these circumstances. In addition, Nathi's illegal position makes him politically and socially invisible, and makes it impossible to earn a living to support his children independently, increasing the family's dependence on state support.

A final consideration of misrepresentation is revealed when we return to Jane's experience of being accused of fraud. This not only resulted in misrecognition, but also misrepresentation, as it cancelled her political rights to social assistance. In addition, to get the grant reinstated was not just a case of presenting the right documents, but also a fight for political voice and entitlements.

Redistribution, recognition and representation

We have already alluded to the multiple ways in which participatory parity is affected by a combination of redistribution, recognition and representation in terms of one instrument of social protection, the CSG. This leads us to a consideration of the complex ways these dimensions are intertwined, although they can be regarded as analytically separate.

Circumstances that result in maldistribution, misrecognition and misrepresentation in relation to the CSG occur, for example, when the failures of other services erode the benefits of the grant. While this has been identified as an economic, and thus distributive, concern, such as when grant money is used to pay for health care or educational costs that should be free (Patel & Hochfeld, 2011), it can be also be as a result of misrecognition and misrepresentation. Receiving the grant should entitle the caregiver to a range of poverty alleviation mechanisms as a "package" of "care" for those who need it. Instead, benefits often have to be fought for, and sometimes lost, individually. In addition to this, some categories of people, such as those who are homeless or do not have the correct documentation, are excluded from receiving the CSG. This was Jane's experience when trying to access benefits to which she is entitled: Jane looks after her sister's seven-year-old daughter, Thenjiwe, for whom she receives a CSG. Jane's sister is a drug addict and lives on the streets. I asked if she was receiving a school fee waiver (called a fee exemption), to which she should be entitled, and she replied thus:

JANE: So when I apply for an exemption, they tell me that I must have the full custody of the child from court. And I cannot, my sister is alive. I am just helping because I cannot just ignore the child. They said I must go to court for it and I can't do that. And then they make me walk around the streets to look for my sister to sign the forms, I found her in Joubert Park but she would not come with me so I made her sign there on the street. But the school, they said every year she had to come every time if she doesn't make her life better so it's up to her and then they won't give the child the exemption.

Here it can be seen that Jane's sister's child, Thenjiwe, is affected by her mother's misrecognized status and that she is excluded from access to free schooling. This means that the redistributive value of Thenjiwe's CSG is devalued as Jane has to use it to pay for school fees. The punitive system toward those whose status is devalued and who are excluded from the system thus has a knock-on effect on the redistributive power of the CSG.

Conclusions

The dismantling of apartheid has led to greater participatory parity and access to the CSG is one instance of this. The CSG is widely regarded as a successful and efficient mechanism of social protection (Department of Social Development et al., 2012; SAHRC & UNICEF 2014; Woolard et al., 2011). The purpose of this analysis is not to contradict this view, but rather to illustrate, using Fraser's work, that attaining social justice is a complex political journey that cannot rely on a single social protection instrument. Therefore, while income support such as the CSG is critical for vast numbers of people in South Africa, their needs extend beyond cash, and delivery falls short in a number of areas of broader social security and social investment.

Service failures in areas such as housing, health, education, welfare service support, urban bias and job creation are not experienced by individuals in isolation from one another. The erosion of the value of the CSG due to the breakdowns and non-delivery of public services has been noted as a major weakness in the social protection of South Africa (Patel, Hochfeld, & Moodley, 2013). If services which claim to be free (such as education and primary health care) were really free of all costs, then the CSG would be assisting to a greater extent to achieve participatory parity from an economic perspective.

Therefore, while the CSG can be seen to contribute to redistribution of resources, recognition of dependency work and social inclusion, more is needed to counter the still existing severe inequalities in South African society. Since 1994 South Africa has established progressive policies. However, it often remains difficult to operationalize them, with poor implementation and weak accountability (SAHRC & UNICEF, 2014).

A further advantage of Fraser's approach is the refusal to psychologize and individualize social inequalities such as viewing struggling families as "dysfunctional," unemployed adults as "lazy" and claimants as "untrustworthy" or "undeserving"; rather it allows us to see structural determinants of social problems as critical points of departure.

This chapter has shown that Nancy Fraser's conception of social justice, which is *participatory parity*, is a useful way of evaluating social protection. It provides a number of dimensions for assessing the extent to which social arrangements such as the CSG can contribute toward achieving participatory parity. Social protection can be evaluated as a contribution to social justice against each dimension separately, as well as in combination. The value of this trivalent approach to evaluating social protection is in the levels of nuance that are exposed. The approach offers us the opportunity to see how policy instruments have different layers of impact, some of which have affirmative effects, some transformative effects, and some even have unintended effects of preventing participatory parity through, for example, the misrecognition of beneficiaries.

While the CSG is an example of a functional social protection mechanism which should be used and embraced by social work practitioners, this analysis demonstrates how social workers are always required to be a critical voice in relation to the real-life consequences of policy programs. The existence of effective social protection mechanisms does not absolve social workers from remaining vigilant about a wide spectrum of injustices that people continue to experience in both public and private domains. Social protection is not the end in itself; it is merely one tool we use as a means to travel toward social justice.

Notes

1 Names and some identifying details have been changed.
2 Privately run mini-bus taxis are the primary form of transport for the majority of South Africa's population.

References

Adato, M., & Bassett, L. (2008). *What is the potential of cash transfers to strengthen families affected by HIV and AIDS? A review of the evidence on impacts and key policy debates*. Boston: Joint Learning Initiative on Children and AIDS.

Agüero, J.M., Carter, M.R., & Woolard, I. (2006). *The impact of unconditional cash transfers on nutrition: The South African child support grant*. SALDRU Working Papers 8, Southern Africa Labour and Development Research Unit, University of Cape Town.

Barchiesi, F. (2011). *Precarious liberation: Workers, the state, and contested social citizenship in postapartheid South Africa*. Durban: University of KwaZulu Natal Press.

Delany, A., Ismail, Z., Graham, L., & Ramkisson, Y. (2008). *Review of the child support grant: Uses, implementation and obstacles*. Johannesburg: Department of Social Development, CASE, SASSA and UNICEF.

Department of Social Development, South African Social Security Agency, & UNICEF. (2011). *Child support grant evaluation 2010: Qualitative research report*. Pretoria: UNICEF South Africa.

Department of Social Development, South African Social Security Agency, & UNICEF. (2012). *The South African child support grant impact assessment: Evidence from a survey of children, adolescents and their households*. Pretoria: UNICEF South Africa.

Fraser, N. (2000). Rethinking recognition. *New Left Review*, *3*, 107–120.

Fraser, N. (2008). Reframing justice in a globalizing world. *New Left Review*, *36*, 69–88.

Fraser, N. (2009). *Scales of justice: Reimagining political space in a globalizing world*. New York: Columbia University Press.

Fraser, N. (2012). Feminism, capitalism, and the cunning of history: An introduction. *FMSH-WP-2012-17*. Retrieved on December 25, 2015, from www.ssnpstudents.com/wp/wp-content/uploads/2015/03/Feminism-Capitalism.pdf.

Fraser, N. (2013). *Fortunes of feminism: From state-managed capitalism to neoliberal crisis*. London: Verso.

Fraser, N., & Honneth, A. (2003). *Redistribution or recognition? A political-philosophical exchange*. London: Verso.

Hassim, S. (2006). Gender equality and developmental social welfare in South Africa. In S. Razavi & S. Hassim (Eds.), *Gender and social policy in a global context: Uncovering the gendered structure of the "social"* (pp. 109–129). Basingstoke: Palgrave.

Hochfeld, T., & Plagerson, S. (2011). Dignity and stigma among South African female cash transfer recipients. *IDS Bulletin*, *42*, 53–59.

Holmes, R., & Jones, N. (2013). *Gender and social protection in the developing world: Beyond mothers and safety nets*. London: Zed Books.

Lund, F. (2011). A step in the wrong direction: Linking the South African child support grant to school attendance. *Journal of Poverty and Social Justice, 19*, 5–14.

Makiwane, M. (2010). The child support grant and teenage childbearing in South Africa. *Development Southern Africa, 27*, 193–204.

Neves, D., Samson, M., van Niekerk, I., Hlatshwayo, S., & du Toit, A. (2009). *The use and effectiveness of social grants in South Africa.* Cape Town: FinMark Trust, Institute for Poverty, Land and Agrarian Studies, and Economic Policy Research Institute.

Patel, L. (2015). *Social welfare and social development in South Africa* (2nd ed.). Cape Town: Oxford University Press.

Patel, L., & Hochfeld, T. (2011). It buys food but does it change gender relations? Child support grants in Soweto, South Africa. *Gender and Development, 19*, 229–240.

Patel, L., Hochfeld, T., & Moodley, J. (2013). Gender and child sensitive social protection in South Africa. *Development Southern Africa, 30*, 69–83.

Patel, L., Hochfeld, T., Moodley, J., & Mutwali, R. (2012). *The gender dynamics and impact of the child support grant in Doornkop, Soweto.* Johannesburg: University of Johannesburg.

Posel, D., & Rogan, M. (2012). Gendered trends in poverty in the post-apartheid period, 1997–2006. *Development Southern Africa, 29*, 97–113.

SAHRC & UNICEF. (2011). South African Human Rights Commission (SAHRC) and UNICEF bring together experts from government, civil society and academia to focus the spotlight on children's rights. Retrieved on December 25, 2015, from www.unicef. org/media/media_58031.html.

SAHRC & UNICEF. (2014). *Poverty traps and social exclusion among children in South Africa.* Pretoria: SAHRC.

Sevenhuijsen, S., Bozalek, V., Gouws, A., & Minnaar-McDonald, M. (2007) South African social welfare policy: An analysis using the ethic of care. *Critical Social Policy, 23*(3), 299–321.

South African Social Security Agency (SASSA). (2015). *Fact sheet: Issue no 3 of 2015: A statistical summary of social grants in South Africa.* Pretoria: SASSA. Retrieved from www.sassa.gov.za/index.php/knowledge-centre/statistical-reports.

Statistics South Africa (StatsSA). (2014a). *General household survey, 2014, statistical release P0318.* Pretoria: StatsSA.

Statistics South Africa (StatsSA). (2014b). *Mid-year population estimates, 2014, statistical release P0302.* Pretoria: StatsSA.

Tronto, J.C. (2013). *Caring democracy markets, equality, and justice.* New York: New York University Press.

UNDP (United Nations Development Programme). (2009). *Human development report 2009. Overcoming barriers: Human mobility and development.* New York: UNDP. Retrieved from: http://hdr.undp.org/en/reports/global/hdr2009/.

UNDP (United Nations Development Programme). (2014). *Human development report. Sustaining human progress: Reducing vulnerabilities and building resilience.* New York: United Nations.

UNICEF (United Nations Children's Fund). (2010). *Inequities in the fulfillment of children's rights in South Africa: A statistical review.* Background Document for UNICEF's Strategic Moment of Reflection: October 2010. Pretoria: UNICEF South Africa.

Vorster, J., & de Waal, L. (2008). Beneficiaries of the child support grant: Findings from a national survey. *The Social Work Practitioner-Researcher, 20*, 233–248.

Woolard, I., Harttgen, K., & Klasen, S. (2011). The history and impact of social security in South Africa: Experiences and lessons. *Canadian Journal of Development Studies, 32*, 357–380.

11 Social protection in Ghana

Old challenges and new initiatives

Ziblim Abukari and Linda Kreitzer

Introduction

Social protection is now widely considered an important development strategy to reduce poverty and vulnerabilities of poor and marginalized populations and strengthen their coping capacities. In lower income countries where few state-established social safety net programs exist, social protection initiatives play a crucial role in reducing vulnerabilities and enhancing capabilities to weather shocks such as hunger, drought, floods, and diseases. Hurrell, Mertens, and Pellerano (2011) describe social protection as programs that are designed to increase coping capabilities and reduce social exclusion in poor countries. In their opinion, social protection can be effective in supporting specific social groups such as reducing gender inequality and inter-generational transmission of poverty. According to the Ghana National Social Protection Strategy (NSPS) office, social protection "consists of a set of formal and informal mechanisms directed towards the provision of social assistance and capacity enhancements to the vulnerable and excluded in society" (Government of Ghana, 2007, p. 8). The NSPS identifies impoverished individuals, households, and communities that lack access to basic social services as target beneficiaries of the government social protection programs. As if in acknowledgment of the failure of its developmental philosophy and neoliberal policy in Africa, the World Bank policy framework in 2002 advised African governments to consider social protection as an *investment* rather than *charity* (emphasis added) (Heitzmann, Canagarajah, & Siegel, 2002).

Ghana, like many lower income countries, has experienced profound economic, political, and social changes since the end of colonial rule in 1957. The most notable among these changes in the past two decades are market and political liberalization, privatization of government-owned enterprises, devolution of central authority and planning to district assemblies, and globalization, all of which were part of the International Financial Institutions' Structural Adjustment Programs. As Heitzmann et al. (2002) rightly point out, such changes brought significant stress on social arrangements that have traditionally served as informal safety nets. Similarly, the economic restructuring instigated by the World Bank and the International Monetary Fund (IMF) mandated cutbacks on government expenditure that directly affected formal social safety net programs including health care, education, and agriculture, thereby elevating the risks of many poor households' inability to cope with these changes.

This chapter will review social protection programs in Ghana within the context of the Livelihood Empowerment Against Poverty (LEAP) and its complimentary programs including the National Health Insurance Scheme and the Education Capitation Grant. We examine the prospects as well as challenges of these programs within the framework of the government's national social protection strategy.

Background of social protection in Ghana

With a relatively steady economic growth and political stability in the past two decades, Ghana is considered a development success story for Africa. Results of the latest Ghana Living Standards Survey (GLSS6, 2014) and other reports show that the country has met the UN Millennium Development Goal (MDG1) of cutting poverty by half by 2015 ahead of the deadline (Ghana Statistical Service, 2014; IMF, 2012; Okudzejo, Mariki, Lal, & Senu, 2015; UNDP, 2012). Despite these improvements, 24.2% of Ghanaians still live in poverty and 8.4% of those people live in extreme poverty and are unable to meet the basic necessities of life such as adequate nutrition, shelter, safe drinking water, and health care (Ghana Statistical Service, 2014). Recognizing that microeconomic growth and stability may not necessarily translate into real social development (Midgley, 1995), or pull people out of poverty and protect vulnerable people from shocks such as diseases, natural disasters, and food crisis, the government of Ghana developed a National Social Protection Strategy (NSPS) to provide more targeted interventions to the impoverished or chronic poor through new safety net programs that reduce vulnerability and marginalization. Before we delve into the new safety net programs we are quick to add that social protection is not a new phenomenon in Ghana. In fact, long before the arrival of Europeans and the creation of the modern states, traditional African societies and, for that matter, Ghanaian society, already had in place institutional arrangements for major contingencies through collective security and mutual help to one another.

Informal social protection

Before colonialism, Africa was a continent with a rich history of micro-nations (Maathai, 2009) whose people created informal networks that sustained and cared for people in these nations. "People carried their cultural practices, stories and sense of the world around them in their oral traditions, which were rich and meaningful. They lived in harmony with the other species and the natural environment and they protected that world" (Maathai, 2009, pp. 161–162). It was a vibrant continent with a long and complex history in which diverse ethnic groups lived and created infrastructure that met the economic, social, and political needs of the group (Apt & Blavo, 1997). The region, now known as West Africa, was divided into tribal kingdoms, notable among them, the Asante Kingdom, and life was mainly rural with the main social system being that of the kinship institution (Ray, 1986), and solidarity as the embodiment of Ghanaian traditional culture (UNICEF, 2009). Kinship efficiently met the needs of the family and was based on the notion of large families. These institutions protected family members from poverty and isolation. For example, the extended family was a revered institution that provided social and economic support to its members during times of need, and to aging members who were threatened by economic deprivation, disability, and social isolation (Kumado & Gockel, 2003). According to Ghanaian legend, "traditional extended family practices transcended socio-economic protection to offering psychological stability and moral upliftment" (Kumado & Gockel, 2003, p. 1). The extended family, neighbors, and clan members had a duty to make sure a child was treated well. Fostering a child was a common practice among relatives (Nukunya, 1992). Older people were respected and given high honor, and children were expected to look after them.

The invasion of the British of the region and subsequent colonization deeply affected this social protection system of the past. Colonial rule was based on the needs of the colonizer and this intrusion weakened the kings (Ray, 1986) and the clans by drawing borders that were unnatural and which caused additional conflicts (Nukunya, 1992). It weakened the kinship system (Nukunya, 1992) and weakened family ties and responsibilities to child-raising through exploitation, formal education, labor opportunities in other regions, and Western values of individualism. Kings were manipulated by the British as pawns for furthering the colonial agenda and families were divided.

Formal social protection

From the 1940s onwards various social protection strategies were implemented in Ghana. Table 11.1 summarizes the major social protection services implemented over the next few decades. Among the first were the trade union movement, beginning as early as the 1920s, and the youth movement in the 1930s. The services listed in Table 11.1 have been beneficial for some Ghanaians, primarily public sector workers. However, for those who work in the informal sector, these benefits did not help them escape poverty. These include subsistence farmers, fishermen, domestic service workers, workers in small establishments, and street vendors. Asamoah and Nortey (1987) conclude that "Social security schemes can never hope to carry the full burden of achieving social equality or raising the general standard of living. At present, the system favors urban moderate and high income earners" (p. 60). These schemes needed to be constantly evaluated for their effectiveness to the changing Ghanaian society. However, the political and economic situation that Ghana found itself in after independence affected the efficiency of these systems.

Table 11.1 Chronology of social protection programs in Ghana prior to 2000 (Asamoah & Norty, 1987; Kumado & Gockel, 2003)

Agency or program	Description
The National Pension Scheme – CAP 30 1946	Name derived from Chapter 30 of the Pension Ordinance of 1946; provided pension to civil servants and members of the Ghana Armed Forces prior to 1972.
Department of Social Welfare and Housing 1946	Regulated operations of orphanages; training of disabled and mentally ill.
Department of Social welfare and Community Development 1952	Responsible for juvenile crime non-formal education.
Education Act of 1961	Guaranteed free primary education for all Ghanaians up to six years.
Voluntary organizations and personal social services	1930–1960s – run by missionaries, church groups, international organizations, and tribal organizations.
Social Security Act of 1965, 1972, 1991	Set up the Social Security and National Insurance Trust (SSNIT). Provident Fund Scheme; old age, invalidity, and survivors' benefits, pension scheme.
State Insurance Corporation 1955	Provide non-life insurance needs including fire and motor accidents.
Interstate Succession Law 1984	Protects inheritance rights of widows and children.

Economic reforms

Once the colonizer had left in 1957, Ghana was looking forward to a better future for the country. Pan-Africanism was strong and the continent as a whole was ready to take control of its own destiny. The early days of Kwame Nkrumah (first president of Ghana, 1957–1966) were marked by progress in education, health and development. However, by the end of his presidency, the country was deep in debt and political unrest was dominating the country with several military coups attempted. From 1981 to 1992, a military government led by J.J. Rawlings led the country through economic, political and social reforms, called the Economic Recovery Program (ERP), through the lending programs of the IMF and the World Bank. At first, the lending was generous with medium-term loans. However, the unexpected oil crisis and world economic recession in the 1980s caused the lower income countries' debts to triple and plunged countries like Ghana into a debt crisis from which they have never fully recovered (Lewis, 2005; Sachs, 2005; Sewpaul, 2006; UNICEF, 1989; Yunus, 2007). Cutbacks in social investments, the privatization of social programs, the abandonment of social planning and similar policy developments had a negative impact on health, education and welfare in many lower income countries (Midgley, 1995) including Ghana. Children were most affected negatively by these programs (UNICEF,

2001). To alleviate the suffering, Ghana introduced the Program of Action to Mitigate the Social Costs of Adjustment (PAMSCAD), which was basically money spent on financing small community development projects (Ninsin, 1991). Critics claim that this program was a band aid solution to an economic adjustment and was not effective (Overseas Development Institute [ODI], 1996; UNICEF, 1989) with poor administration whereby funding was diverted and used for political purposes (Herbst, 1993; Hutchful, 1997). In retrospect, these structural adjustment programs were devastating to Ghana's social development (Konadu-Agyemang, 2000).

With the breakdown of the extended family, the shift to semi-formal institutionalized social security systems and the mixed results of the economic programs of the 1980s and 1990s (Kumado & Gockel, 2003) there was a growing need to develop a National Social Protection Scheme that would benefit the majority of Ghanaians, in particular the poorer section of society. This change has been influenced by a steady growth in GDP since 2000 and the discovery of oil in 2010 in the Western Region (Okudzejo et al., 2015; Sultan & Schrofer, 2008). Recent data show that revenue from oil is becoming a major contributory factor to Ghana's GDP, rising from a modest 24.5 million barrels a year in 2011 to 40 million barrels annually in 2014, contributing 6.3% to GDP in 2014 (Okudzejo et al., 2015, p. 4).

Current social protection strategies

Since independence from colonial rule in 1957, Ghana has implemented several social protection schemes with limited coverage and success as discussed earlier. The major problem always appears to be the challenge of including workers in the informal sector, who constitute the majority of the population (Osei-Boateng & Ampratwum, 2011). There is also a problem of how to integrate women, children, older persons, and people with disabilities into social protection schemes since they have been historically excluded from major government policy strategies (Gbedemah, Jones, & Pereznieto, 2010). These excluded groups are more likely to experience chronic poverty. With a recognition that microeconomic growth and mainstream development strategies have failed to reduce extreme poverty particularly among vulnerable groups, the government launched two programs to ameliorate the situation of vulnerable groups that will also protect them against economic disasters and shocks. These were the NSPS and Ghana Poverty Reduction Strategy (GPRS I & II). The primary goal of these programs was to reduce poverty and vulnerability through the Livelihood Empowerment Against Poverty (LEAP), cash transfer program, and other complementary programs – the National Health Insurance Scheme (NHIS), and the Education Capitation Grant, which are examined in this chapter.

An overview of cash transfer programs

Cash transfer programs have emerged as a quintessential component of poverty reduction strategies in many low income countries in recent years. Since the development of social protection programs in Ghana is so closely affected by social protection programs in other parts of the world, particularly Latin America, a brief review of some existing social protection programs in those regions is necessary. Started in South America in the 1990s in Brazil and Mexico, cash transfer as a form of assistance to the poorest members of the population consists of two types: conditional and unconditional cash transfers.

Conditional cash transfers

Conditional cash transfers (CCTs) represent a new generation of development initiatives "that seek to foster human capital accumulation among the young as a means to breaking the inter-generational cycle of poverty" (Rawlings & Rubio, 2003, p. 3). As the name implies, CCT programs provide cash to poor families and households with a condition to fulfill certain requirements including continuous enrollment of young children in school, clinic attendance for growth monitoring of young children, and regular pre- and postnatal clinic attendance for pregnant and lactating mothers (Johannsen, Tejerina, & Glassman 2009; Sewall, 2008). Among the best known conditional cash transfer initiatives in lower income countries are the Bolsa Família in Brazil and Opportunidades in Mexico, which have inspired similar programs in the region as well as Asia and sub-Saharan Africa. For example, the LEAP program in Ghana (more on this later) provides cash benefits to eligible beneficiaries on a regular basis who meet the conditions outlined above including school enrollment and attendance, clinic visits and immunization, and caregivers of orphans and vulnerable children (Government of Ghana, 2007).

Unconditional cash transfers

Other forms of social cash transfers have been widely discussed in a few African countries as well. For example, the Kenyan government designed an unconditional cash transfer program for orphans and vulnerable children (OVC) that face poverty and despair to provide cash transfers directly to the poorest households containing OVC (International Policy Center, 2012).

Similar pilot unconditional cash transfer programs in Zambia, Malawi, and South Africa reveal challenges in institutionalizing social cash transfer within the countries' mainstream social policies. According to Wietler (2007), Zambia's pilot cash transfer program has enabled many destitute people to engage in productive activities that generate employment for other members of their communities. However, Wietler observes that the transfers are inadequate to cover all the needs of beneficiaries or all eligible members due to institutional constraints.

One may ask if either of these cash transfers is more effective in Africa. In one experimental study, Baird, McIntosh, and Ozler (2011) compared educational outcomes and risky behaviors among young people in Malawi who were enrolled in a conditional cash transfer (CCT) program to a control group enrolled in an unconditional cash transfer (UCT) program. The authors reveal that while there was only a marginal decline in the dropout rate in the UCT group, the dropout rate fell by 43% in the CCT group (Baird et al., 2011, p. 4). Students in the CCT also outperformed their counterparts in a test of reading comprehension. But Baird et al. (2011) discovered that even with the marginal outcomes, the UCT program had some notable latent effects on the participants. For example, the authors observe that rates of teenage pregnancy and early marriages were substantially lower in UCT among girls who dropped out of school, a further proof of the power of cash transfers in reducing vulnerabilities of at-risk populations regardless of the type. Keeping this in mind, the next section discusses social protection programs in Ghana today.

Livelihood Empowerment Against Poverty (LEAP)

Livelihood Empowerment Against Poverty (LEAP) is a cash transfer program that was established in 2008 as a pilot program in 74 out of 178 districts to provide social grants to the poorest segments of society to help them "leap" out of poverty (Government of Ghana, 2007). Starting with 26,000 households in 2009, LEAP reached 68,000 households by the end of 2012 and is projected to reach 165,000 households by 2015 (Daily Graphic, 2012, as cited in Dako-Gyeke & Oduro, 2013, p. 241; Gbedemah et al., 2010). LEAP is being implemented by Ghana's Ministry of Gender, Children and Social Protection, to reduce poverty by providing direct financial support to orphan and vulnerable children (OVC), people with severe disabilities, and persons aged 65 years and older (Government of Ghana, 2007). LEAP implementation is based on a combination of conditional and unconditional cash transfers and eligibility is based on poverty and having a household containing an OVC, elderly poor, or a person with extreme disability who is unable to work (Government of Ghana, 2007).

Program framework

Like other cash transfer programs, the LEAP cash transfer imposes a time limit of three years for beneficiaries to "graduate" from the program (Government of Ghana, 2007). The question of whether beneficiaries become self-sufficient afterwards should be an inquiry for further studies. Nonetheless, it is expected by the NSPS (Government of Ghana, 2007) that LEAP will have resulted in the following outcomes after the implementation:

- A substantial reduction in poverty, hunger, and starvation among elderly poor and people with disabilities who are unable to work.
- Better access to health and education services by extremely poor orphans and vulnerable children younger than 15 years and those living with HIV/AIDS.
- Better and enhanced livelihood for women and children during pregnancy and a reduction in mother-to-child transmission of HIV/AIDS among beneficiaries (pp. 36–37).

LEAP social grants, as they are called, are divided into four main categories:

1   social grants for subsistence crop farmers and fishermen;
2   social grants for extremely poor elderly persons aged 65 years and older;
3   a grant for caregivers of orphans and vulnerable children, particularly children living with HIV/AIDS and with severe disabilities; and
4   social grants for pregnant women and breastfeeding mothers (Government of Ghana, 2007).

Beneficiary individuals and households receive a monthly cash transfer of between $6 and $12 depending on the number of eligible individuals in a household (e.g., for every additional eligible household member the amount will be increased by $2 until the maximum limit of four per household is reached and the amount capped at $12) (Akyeampong, 2011; Government of Ghana, 2007).

The cash transfers are distributed through Ghana Postal Company and payments are made every two months. Unlike the UCT component that is paid to people who are unable to work, CCTs aim to build human capital and reduce vulnerabilities and are guided by the following conditions:

1   enroll all school-age children in school;
2   children are not engaged in child labor;
3   enrollment of all family members on the National Health Insurance Scheme (NHIS);
4   birth and death registration of all children;
5   attend required pre/post-natal clinics and complete required immunization; and
6   not to allow children to be trafficked or engage in any activities considered as the worst form of child labor (Government of Ghana, 2007).

Impact of LEAP on reducing economic and social vulnerabilities

The existing knowledge base regarding the impact of this program remains limited and mixed at best. A nationwide evaluation of the impact of the program reveals that while progress has been generally positive, performance has been mixed across indicators and beneficiary groups. For example, significant progress has been reported in some key LEAP programs such as increasing school enrollment and access to health (Handa, Park, Darko, Osei-Akoto, Davis, & Diadone, 2013), but the overall pace of progress, based on current trends, is marginal. According to Handa and colleagues, LEAP has had a greater impact on older children's schooling; that is, the enrollment of 13–17-year-olds increased significantly, particularly among boys, and there was continuous attendance and fewer grade repetitions among girls. A significant number of LEAP beneficiaries have also enrolled in the NHIS (Handa et al., 2013). However, the report notes that LEAP assistance has not improved food consumption and the number of beneficiaries is still too small to make an impact on the community. This is consistent with the findings of Dako-Gyeke and Oduro (2013), who reveal the marginal impact of LEAP cash transfers on beneficiaries' nutrition, health, and educational needs and outcomes. Focusing on the effect of household size on CCT utilization, Dako-Gyeke and Oduro found that cash transfers were used for all members of the household, including non-LEAP eligible children, a practice that negatively affected LEAP-eligible children's school attendance, access to health care, and nutritional needs. This has revealed a larger socio-cultural issue that will make it difficult for LEAP to make a big impact – the unique challenge of defining an African family due to a large network of extended family members. Presently, the total number of eligible household members is capped at four, the average national household size in 2013. However, this number is below the average family size of poor families in many parts of the country including the three savannah regions where average household size is 5.5 in some places (Ghana Statistical Service, 2014).

Other studies have reported similar mixed impacts of the program on beneficiary households in the northern region. While beneficiaries reported being relatively happier as a result of LEAP, they lament the inadequacy of the grants for sustainable livelihood (Gbedemah et al., 2010). Without providing statistics for school enrollment and attendance, the authors also report that children were happy to go to school and not worry about food or school uniforms and supplies that hitherto had been the major reasons for not attending school. Regarding gender vulnerabilities, Amuzu, Jones, and Pereznieto (2010) observe that while the program is helping households meet a range of practical needs such as food, health care, and school supplies, the amount is inadequate for women to start small businesses.

Notwithstanding the mixed achievements of the LEAP program, Ghana has achieved the MDG1 of reducing the proportion of people living in extreme poverty by half before the 2015 deadline even though spatial inequalities exist (Ghana Statistical Service, 2014). The direct consequence of this is that LEAP, together with the school feeding program, has resulted in a slow but steady decline in hunger, childhood malnutrition, and children born with low birth weight (World Food Program, 2007), which some studies on childhood development in general, and cash transfer programs, suggest have a direct effect on children's cognitive development and learning outcomes (Del Rosso, 1999; Hutchison, 2013; World Bank, 2011).

National Health Insurance Scheme (NHIS)

At independence in 1957, Ghana implemented a universal health care system which provided health care services at virtually no cost to its citizens and financed solely by government through taxes. In the newly independent country that had no physical infrastructure, less skilled labor, and a weak institutional framework to implement, monitor, and assess these programs coupled with weak economic growth, the health care system eventually collapsed in the early 1980s. This led to the introduction of the now infamous "cash-and-carry" system, a fee for service system mandated by structural adjustment policies, thereby reducing access to health care for many Ghanaians particularly the poor and the vulnerable. To address this issue, the NHIS was established by the National Health Insurance Act 650 in 2003 to provide equitable health insurance for all Ghanaians (UNICEF, 2009). The NHIS replaced the "cash and carry" system and is being funded by Ghanaian taxpayers through payroll deductions and sales tax, and presently covers 68% of the population of Ghana (Ghana Statistical Service, 2014). Furthermore, two-thirds of those enrolled in the NHIS are under the exempt category and do not pay the required insurance premium, including retired public servants, persons aged 70 years and older, pregnant women, children under 18 years, and the extremely poor (Ministry of Health, 2015). Although still below the projected coverage, the popularity of the scheme is attributed to a large extent to the emergence of community mutual health organizations (HMOs), which were mandated by the NHIS law (Sulzbach, Garshong, & Owusu-Banahene, 2005). This is a departure from the structural adjustment era healthcare reform where hospitals and physicians demanded payment before treatment. Except people in the exempt category listed above, people who pay the minimum membership fee or premium are entitled to government supported medical services relating to many health issues. Also, LEAP beneficiaries are required to enroll in the NHIS.

A recent review of specific national health indicators shows a slow but steady improvement in many areas over the years. According to the Ministry of Health (2015), national under-five mortality rate (per 1,000 live births) in 2014 was 60, down from 155 per 1,000 in 1988. However, spatial differences are prevalent, suggesting an uneven coverage of the scheme. For example, in the more urbanized and prosperous regions of Greater Accra and Ashanti, the under-five mortality rate dropped from 103.8 and 142.2 respectively in 1988 to 50.0 and 80.0 respectively in 2008 (Ghana Health Service, 2010, p. 10). During the same period under-five mortality rates in the Northern and Upper West Regions, two of the most deprived in the country, saw a decline of 221.8 each in 1988 to 137.0 and 142.0 respectively in 2008 (p. 10). Although the percentage drop in the northern regions is larger it is evident that under-five mortality rate is still almost twice the national average (p. 10). These data suggest that health care coverage is still low among the poor in the poorest regions of the country.

Reducing vulnerabilities among children

Along with the LEAP and NHIS are two other social protection programs targeting the education of children in Ghana. These are related directly to the United Nations Millennium Development Goals (United Nations, 2010) 2 and 3: universal primary education for school age children everywhere, and elimination of gender disparity in primary and secondary education. In Ghana, although there has been an increase in school attendance, this goal was far from being achieved, as shown by UNICEF (2009) that in 2006 the primary school net attendance ratio was 75.3%. As a response to this increasing concern that children are in need of social protection the Education Capitation Grant (ECG) and the Ghana

School Feeding Program (GSFP) were introduced. Each will be explained briefly here.

The Education Capitation Grant

Ghana introduced the first free compulsory basic education policy immediately after independence from colonial rule under the Education Act of 1961 (Foster, 1965). This policy guaranteed free primary education nationwide but the benefits were expanded to cover secondary education in northern Ghana and covered textbooks, uniforms, and school supplies (Foster, 1965; McWilliam & Kwamena-Poh, 1975). Under the 1987 education reforms, a new policy known as Free Compulsory Universal Basic Education (FCUBE) was introduced. This policy restructured the entire pre-university education system and reduced the number of years of pre-tertiary education from 17 to 12. Under FCUBE basic education was free but students were still required to pay a number of user-fees including uniforms, textbooks, and PTA dues, which constituted a burden for many poor children (Osei, Owusu, Asem, & Afutu-Kotey, 2009). Thus, under the Poverty Reduction Strategies set out by the government of Ghana, the Capitation Grant was adopted "as a school fees abolition policy" (Ampratwum & Armah-attoh, 2010, p. 2) to help meet those goals for all Ghanaian children. The grant gives each public primary school around US$3.00 per pupil enrolled each year and is supposed to include direct and indirect costs including "tuition fees, costs of textbooks, supplies and uniforms, PTA contributions, costs related to sports and other school activities, cost related to transportation, contributions to teachers' salaries, etc." (Osei et al., 2009, p. 5).

The effectiveness of the capitation scheme in Ghana

Research findings of the Capitation Grant show both positive gains and challenges to this system. In their study of the program, Ampratwum and Armah-attoh (2010) found that the transference of money was inconsistent partly due to delays and poor record keeping. They also found that the money was not adequate for all it was intended for, and schools were still charging levies/fees for some items like examination fees. Some schools were spending their money on unapproved procurements. Finally, only a few people felt that this grant reduced the financial burden of most parents. On a more positive note, there was an increased attendance of children after the grant was introduced (UNICEF, 2009) and there was overall satisfaction with the grant from school authorities, teachers, and parents.

In another study, Osei et al. (2009) came up with similar results as the above study. Enrollment increased by 10%, "bringing total primary enrollment of 92.4 per cent nationwide" (p. 5). Girls' enrollment increased slightly above that of boys. Some of the challenges to the grant scheme were the decrease in pupil/ teacher ratio, demand for more space, teaching materials and teachers, the smooth and timely release of funds through the districts, and lack of transparency at the school level. Their research found that in 2005–2007 the Capitation Grant amount due was never fully released to any of the districts. One important finding is that the research does not measure the quality of education now given, particularly when teacher to pupil ratio has decreased. The program is now in all public schools in the country and "its value was increased by 50% in the 2009 budget" (UNICEF, 2009, p. 44). Proponents of school fee abolition praise the Capitation Grant as a success and point to high school enrollment numbers and a near parity in enrollments of boys and girls in Ghana and other African countries who have implemented similar school fee abolishing regimes such as Uganda, Tanzania, Zambia, and Malawi (Osei et al., 2009). With the positive outcomes and challenges, "the capitation grant alone cannot deliver on important education outcomes as enshrined in the Millennium Development Goals (MDGs)" (Osei et al., 2009, p. 22). With this in mind another crucial social protection scheme was introduced in 2004 to augment the Education Capitation Grant – the Ghana School Feeding Program.

Ghana School Feeding Program

The School Feeding Program began in 2005 with the primary goal of "increasing school enrollment and retention by providing at least one daily meal to children in deprived districts" (UNICEF, 2009, p. 44). According to Del Rosso (1999), "weak health and poor nutrition among school-age children diminish their cognitive development either through physiological changes or by reducing their ability to participate in learning experiences-or both" (p. 5). Other countries in the world, who have started a feeding program, have found increased enrollment, improved attendance, and improvement in learning (Del Rosso, 1999). In Ghana, the primary concept of the program is to "provide children in public primary schools and kindergartens in the poorest areas of the country with one hot, nutritious meal per day, using locally-grown foodstuffs" (Afoakwa, 2010, p. 1). The immediate objectives are "(i) reducing hunger and malnutrition, (ii) increasing school enrollment, attendance and retention and (iii) boosting domestic food production" (p. 1). What is unique about this particular model is that it emphasizes improving rural farmers' income by using a ready-made market where farmers can sell their produce in their community, and that improves food security taken away by structural adjustment programs of the past. The home-grown school feeding model also has the potential of not only reducing hunger and malnutrition in the rural communities but also breaking the inter-generational cycle of poverty as more children receive formal education.

The effectiveness of the program

This program has been successful in that more children are attending school across the country. In 2005, 69,000 pupils were being fed daily and this number jumped to 656,624 in 2009 (Afoakwa, 2010). According to a news release on December 8, 2014 by the Ministry for Local Government and Rural Development, at the end of

2014 the program fed 1,728,682 children in beneficiary schools and it is projected to reach 2.5 million children by the end of 2015 (Afoakwa, 2010, p. 1). Another positive impact of the School Feeding Program is that it provides school children with healthy and nutritious food that is important for their learning and development. Evidence suggests that health factors are important determinants of when a child is enrolled in school (Akyeampong, Djangmah, Oduro, Seidu, & Hunt, 2007), and that health status has important implications for attendance, retention, and dropout, with hunger, malaria, headache, and poor vision noted as major causes of absenteeism and dropping out of school in Ghana (Fentiman, Hall, & Bundy, 2001). The Ministry for Local Government and Rural Development further revealed in a December 8, 2014 Communiqué that the School Feeding Program, which now covers all the 216 districts in the 10 regions of the country, has resulted in an overall increase in school enrollment by 18% in beneficiary schools nationwide between 2005 and 2011 (p. 1). In the same news release the ministry further notes that dropout rates in the beneficiary schools fell to an all-time low of 1.4% in 2012 (p. 1). These notwithstanding, some challenges remain. For example, a study by Akyeampong (2011) on the impact of the Capitation Grant and the School Feeding Program in two districts in Ghana – one each from the southern and northern regions of the country, revealed mixed outcomes, with more nuances on gender and locality. For example, while his research revealed an observable increase in enrollment, a high dropout rate persists for both districts with a higher dropout rate for girls, particularly in the Savelugu-Nanton district in the Northern Region. This may be attributed to negative socio-cultural practices that tend to discourage female education in favor of early marriage as well as practical challenges such as lack of sanitary kits and latrines, factors that have been identified as barriers to female education in Ghana as girls reach puberty (Dunne, 2007; Dunne, Leach, Chilisa, Maundeni, Tabulawa, & Kutor, 2005). Another challenge is that the increased attendance rate is putting a huge strain on school structures, equipment, and textbooks. Increased funding is therefore needed for the expansion of schools to meet the growing enrollment of children.

In sum, the Education Capitation Grant and the School Feeding Program are playing vitally important roles that have propelled Ghana to achieve gross enrollment target and moving closer to achieving net enrollment for all children. These two programs, coupled with LEAP, are helping more and more Ghanaians with social assistance that will hopefully improve their lives and their children's lives. Recent data released by government of Ghana show that the country has achieved gross primary school enrollment targets as at 2013 but will miss the net enrollment targets, which is attributed to government's renewed push in education in the Capitation Grant, School Feeding Program, and free school uniforms (Ghana Statistical Service, 2014). The report further shows that the net enrollment rate for boys and girls in the urban coastal regions were 88% and 81% respectively in 2013 compared to 63% each for both sexes in rural savannah regions during the same period. While gender parity in enrollment at both primary and junior high levels has stagnated in the past five years, these data show that the target of ensuring gender parity has significantly narrowed. Nonetheless, the Capitation Grant and School Feeding Program have had a profound impact on educational outcomes, suggesting that a political will supported by goal-directed planning can produce real results and positive school outcomes.

Challenges for implementation of social protection programs in Ghana

It is apparent from our analysis that a number of important vulnerabilities have been identified and the Ghana government has developed a number of programs to address them. It has also emerged that formal social protection programs in Ghana suffer from a number of challenges including poor targeting, ineffective coordination, and weak institutional capacity.

Poor targeting

Despite the popularity of cash transfer programs, their impacts are currently limited by high levels of poverty in Ghana. Under such circumstances, cash transfer programs are "targeted" to "deserving poor" households and communities, thereby excluding a significant proportion of the population. This approach is in contrast to the concept of social development, which Midgley (1995) defined as "a process of planned social change designed to promote the well-being of the population as a whole in conjunction with the dynamic process of economic development" (p. 25). However, the targeting of the "deserving poor" under the Ghana social protection program needs to be put in context giving the present rate of poverty in the country. Hurrell et al. (2011) point out two challenges in cash transfer programs in Kenya that resonate with most sub-Saharan African countries including Ghana. Focusing on targeting, the authors observe that high poverty rates in many countries complicate the process of establishing eligibility of beneficiaries since targeting everyone below the poverty line could mean more than half the population, which is not financially feasible. The second challenge, according to Hurrell et al. (2011), is institutional and human resource capacity. As is commonly known, African social welfare ministries are traditionally weak due to resource constraints. As a result, the human and technical capacity may not exist in these institutions responsible for the implementation of cash transfer programs.

The preceding example suggests that targeting is not straightforward and, in poorer countries like Ghana, may be influenced by politics. According to UNICEF (2009), given the high level of poverty in Ghana targeting specific groups of people has political implications as such programs may be used for political propaganda. Moreover, it appears that Ghana's quest to become a middle income country has made targeting the "deserving poor" a prominent theme in the debate around social protection (UNICEF, 2009). For example, in the GSPS (Government of Ghana, 2007), a number of vulnerable target groups were identified, as discussed under the LEAP. However, the recognition that such vulnerable groups should be supported in order to reduce poverty and vulnerability risks is time-bound (three years), a time span too short to lift extremely poor people out of poverty. It has also been observed that although spatial poverty targeting (using poverty maps) is specifically mentioned as the criteria for regional, district, and community selection, the LEAP design in particular involves several criteria without any clear weights, making the selection process less transparent (UNICEF, 2009).

Inadequate cash and delay transfers

Another major challenge adversely affecting the successful implementation of LEAP is the inadequacy of the cash amount, as noted earlier, and delays in transfers coupled with the ambiguity of the eligibility criteria. An official of LEAP reported a delay in the payment of LEAP grants for 10 months to 53,000 beneficiary households in 83 districts nationwide in 2011, which was attributed to bureaucratic procedures at the Bank of Ghana and late submission of grant requests from the districts (Abebrese, 2011). Sadly, the delays persist in the release of LEAP grants even today. On July 25, 2013 the Ghana News Agency reported that LEAP grant payments had been in arrears for 10 months in some districts in Ashanti and other regions of the country.

Lack of credible eligibility criteria

We have already discussed the ambiguity of the eligibility criteria of LEAP and noted that a lack of baseline data and a reliable database makes the selection of beneficiaries less transparent. Coupled with these, observers have noted that the criteria set out by government in the NSPS are not being enforced, making it difficult to determine how the funds are being used and what their impacts are (Abebrese, 2011; Sultan & Schrofer, 2008). Furthermore, because noncompliance does not result in disqualification or immediate loss of benefits, some analysts (Amuzu et al., 2010; UNICEF, 2009) have characterized LEAP conditions as "quasi-conditional," noting that although beneficiaries must meet the eligibility criteria discussed earlier, these conditions are seen as public education measures rather than sanctions to be obeyed.

Regarding the Capitation Grant and the School Feeding Program, gross enrollment rates have surpassed 100% in urban areas with near parity between the sexes (Ghana Statistical Service, 2013, p. 18) as discussed in previous sections. But it has been observed that a large number of children, particularly in rural areas, still experience inadequate access to education, poor quality teaching and learning due to weak management at all levels (Ampratwum & Armah-attoh, 2010; Ghana Statistical Service, 2014). The Capitation Grant and School Feeding Program are implemented through the district assemblies, and school implementation committees at the local level that work collaboratively with school management committees (SMCs) and parent–teacher associations (PTAs) (Afoakwa, 2010). In their review of the Capitation Grant, Ampratwum and Armah-attoh (2010) discovered that schools with functioning PTAs and SMCs managed the capitation grant funding better, and that improper record-keeping is pervasive in all schools. According to the Ghana Education Service (2010), despite the good intentions and contributions of these programs, many children of school-going age in rural areas either fail to enroll or drop out of school for reasons of parental poverty and lack of teachers.

Beyond the statistics these sentiments underscore the practical realities in the country particularly in poor rural districts. For example, fee-free education and a daily hot meal would be meaningless to a rural child who sees a teacher once a week or, in some cases, once a month or not all, coupled with inadequate school supplies. In a more recent report the Ghana News Agency (2012) reported that an alarming 113 primary schools and 83 kindergartens in West Mamprusi District in the Northern Region did not have teachers. Even more worrisome, the Ghana News Agency (2012) report added that the pupil to teacher ratio in the district is 101:1 and 90:1 respectively for kindergarten and primary schools, suggesting that while the cash transfer grants may be raising enrollment rates, ensuring that children receive a quality education remains a mirage for some children (p. 1). These challenges were further underscored by a recent Education for All Global Monitoring Report 2012 by UNESCO which raised concerns about the quality of education and achievement in Ghana, and noted that girls' school enrollment is still lower nationally with 53% of girls in the three Northern Regions having never attended school.

Exacerbating these problems at the primary level is the problem of corruption and political manipulation. For example, the School Feeding Program was supposed to reach 1.5 million students by the end of the first phase from 2005 to 2010 but reached only 713,631 students (Abebrese, 2011). While financing problems were partly blamed for the low coverage, other problems were due to targeting problems. Abebrese (2011) reports that ineffective targeting and political decisions resulted in selecting schools that were not eligible and needy schools were left out. Efforts to re-target the eligible schools based on poverty and food security maps resulted in delays and hence lowering the coverage.

Poor inter-agency coordination

Another major problem facing the implementation of social protection programs is poor coordination among government agencies (UNICEF, 2009). While support for the social protection program is strong, the government has acknowledged that "uncoordinated delivery and targeting of most of the existing interventions has resulted in limited coverage and impact" (Government of Ghana, 2007, p. 10). The Department of Community Development and the Ministry of Gender, Children, and Social Protection, as the implementing agencies, lack the resources and technical expertise to implement these programs. The NSPS assigns the overall coordinating role for social protection to the Ministry of Gender, Children, and Social Protection but given the present relatively weak status of the ministry, effective change is unlikely without building technical and financial support, as well as buy-in from other agencies involved in the process.

Moreover, the inefficient inter-agency linkages discussed above are exacerbated by a poor data management system to make evidence-based policy decisions with no centralized database, a rigorous baseline or an effective monitoring and evaluation system.

Institutional constraints and political interference

Compared with its neighbors, Ghana is considered a model for multiparty democracy. The relative peace and stability, consolidated by two decades of constitutional rule, has made Ghana a suitable place for implementation of social protection programs. Despite this, some analysts still characterize the country as "a neo-patrimonial state, wherein patronage politics, rather than explicit development objectives and legal rules, dominate the decision making process" (UNICEF, 2009, p. 51). This characterization is reinforced by the haphazard manner in which some of the social protection programs are run without recourse to regional and district poverty profiles.

Implications for social work

One of the fundamental values of social work is a commitment to social justice issues globally, including concern about the growing gap between the rich and the poor in the world that may result in marginalization and vulnerability. In this regard, social workers have always worked with the more vulnerable in society including the poorest peoples. Within the context of Ghana's LEAP program the focus on marginalized and vulnerable populations is palpable, ensuring that these groups have access to services that reduce their vulnerability. Prevention is also at the forefront of the program by mandating immunization, school attendance, clinic attendance for pre- and postnatal care, among others for health and wellness, in addition to breaking the inter-generational cycle of poverty. Through these programs social workers in Ghana deliver critical services to the poorest of the poor to meet basic needs of food, clothing, health, education, water, sanitation, and shelter. Moreover, social work's values and ethics are upheld and the respect for the inherent worth and dignity of all people is realized.

In addition, given that economic and social vulnerability are multidimensional, social workers can play a pivotal role in program design, case assessment, and evaluation using a bio-psychosocial perspective. At the policy level, inter-agency collaboration is necessary for the attainment of the goals of the government social protection agenda. In this light, the government should harness the opportunity for synchronizing data collection, monitoring, and evaluation to form the foundation for informed policy decision-making.

Conclusion

Ghana has experienced many different forms of social protection, from relying on indigenous social protection systems, to post-colonial Western systems and finally to ones that are targeting the most vulnerable today. Cash transfer programs are increasingly emerging as an important strand of social protection with a great potential to reduce economic and social vulnerabilities. Less than a decade since the new social protection initiatives were launched the country has made important strides toward reducing poverty and social exclusion by developing a national strategic framework for social protection that has a strong focus on vulnerable populations. Although still at their rudimentary stages, these programs have made useful contributions to tackle the myriad of economic and social vulnerabilities. Notwithstanding these achievements, the programs have not kept pace with demand, exacerbated by delays in processing payments coupled with poor monitoring of the use of funds or enforcing programs' eligibility sanctions.

References

Abebrese, J. (2011). *Social protection in Ghana: An overview of existing programs and their prospects and challenges.* Accra: Friedrich Ebert Stiftung.

Afoakwa, E.O. (2010). *Homegrown school feeding program: The Ghanaian model as icon for Africa.* A paper presented at a forum on child nutrition organized by the Global Child Nutrition Foundation.

Akyeampong, K. (2011). *(Re)Assessing the impact of school capitation grants on educational access in Ghana.* Research Monograph No. 71. Sussex: CREATE, University of Sussex Centre for International Education.

Akyeampong, K., Djangmah, J., Oduro, A., Seidu, A., & Hunt, F. (2007). *Access to basic education in Ghana: The evidence and the issues.* Brighton: CREATE, University of Sussex. Retrieved from www.sussex.ac.uk/education.

Ampratwum, E., & Armah-attoh, D. (2010). Tracking capitation grant in public primary schools in Ghana. *Ghana Centre for Democratic Development, 10*, 1–8.

Amuzu, C., Jones, N., & Pereznieto, P. (2010). *Gendered risks, poverty and vulnerability in Ghana: To what extent is the LEAP cash transfer program making a difference?* London: Overseas Development Institute (ODI).

Apt, A.A., & Blavo, E.Q. (1997). Ghana. In N.S. Mayadas, T.D. Watts, & D. Elliott (Eds.), *International handbook on social work theory* (pp. 320–343). Westport: Greenwood Press.

Asamoah, Y.W., & Nortey, D.N.A. (1987). Ghana. In J. Dixon (Ed.), *Social welfare in Africa* (pp. 22–68). Beckenham: Croom Helm.

Baird, S., McIntosh, C., & Ozler, B. (2011). Cash or condition? Evidence from a cash transfer experiment. *The Quarterly Journal of Economics, 126*, 1709–1753.

Dako-Gyeke, M., & Oduro, R. (2013). Effects of household size on cash transfer utilization for orphans and vulnerable children in rural Ghana. *Academic Journal of Interdisciplinary Studies, 2*, 239–251.

Del Rosso, M. (1999). *School feeding programs: Improving effectiveness and increasing the benefits to education. A guide for program managers.* Oxford: Partnership for Child Development.

Dunne, M. (2007). Gender, sexuality, and schooling: Everyday life in junior secondary schools in Botswana and Ghana. *International Journal of Educational Development, 27*, 499–511.

Dunne, M., Leach, F., Chilisa, B., Maundeni, T., Tabulawa, R., & Kutor, N. (2005). *Gendered school experiences: The impact on retention and achievement in Botswana and Ghana. Educational papers.* London: Department for International Development.

Fentiman, A., Hall, A., & Bundy, D. (2001). Health and cultural factors associated with enrollment in basic education: A study in rural Ghana. *Social Science and Medicine, 52,* 429–439.

Foster, P. (1965). *Education and social change in Ghana.* Chicago: University of Chicago Press.

Gbedemah, C., Jones, N., & Pereznieto, P. (2010). *Gendered risks, poverty and vulnerability in Ghana: Is the LEAP cash transfer program making a difference?* Project Briefing No. 52. London: Overseas Development Institute (ODI).

Ghana Education Service. (2010). *Education sector performance report.* Accra: Ghana Education Service.

Ghana Health Service. (2010). *The health sector in Ghana: Facts and figures.* Accra: Ghana Health Service.

Ghana News Agency. (2012). *About 113 classrooms in West Mamprusi without teachers.* Retrieved from www.ghananewsagency.org/education/about-113-classrooms-in-west-mamprusi-without-teachers-54429.

Ghana News Agency. (2013). *LEAP grants in arrears for 10 months.* Retrieved from www.ghananewsagency.org/economics/leap-grant-in-10-months-arrears-62605.

Ghana Statistical Service. (2013). *2010 population and housing census report: Millennium development goals in Ghana.* Accra: Ghana Statistical Service and UNDP.

Ghana Statistical Service. (2014). *Ghana living standards survey: Report of the 5th round.* Accra: Government of Ghana.

Government of Ghana. (2007). *The national social protection strategy: Investing in people.* Accra: Ministry of Manpower, Youth and Employment.

Handa, S., Park, M., Darko, R.O., Osei-Akoto, I., David, B., & Diadone, S. (2013). *Livelihood empowerment against poverty program impact evaluation.* Chapel Hill: Carolina Population Center, University of North Carolina.

Heitzmann, K., Canagarajah, R.S., & Siegel, P.B. (2002). *Guidelines for assessing the sources of risk and vulnerability.* Social Protection Discussion Paper #0218. Washington, DC: World Bank.

Herbst, J. (1993). *The politics of reform in Ghana, 1982–1991.* Berkeley: University of California Press.

Hurrell, A., Mertens, F., & Pellerano, L. (2011). *Effective targeting of cash transfer programs in an African context: Lessons learned from the on-going evaluation of two cash transfer programs in Kenya.* A paper presented at the Special IARIW-SSA Conference on Measuring National Income, Wealth, Poverty, and Inequality in African Countries in Cape Town, South Africa, September 28–October 1, 2011.

Hutchful, E. (1997). *The institutional and political framework or macro-economic management in Ghana.* Geneva: United Nations Research Institute for Social Development.

Hutchison, E.D. (2013). *Essentials of human behavior: Integrating person, environment, and the life course.* Los Angeles: Sage Publications.

IMF. (2012). *Ghana poverty reduction strategy paper: Medium-term national development policy framework.* IMF Country Report No. 12/203. Washington, DC: Author.

International Policy Center. (2012). *Does the unconditional Kenya's cash transfer for orphans and vulnerable children have impacts on schooling?* One Pager No. 147. Brazil: UNDP.

Johannsen, J., Tejerina, L., & Glassman, A. (2009). *Conditional cash transfers in Latin*

America: Problems and opportunities. Washington, DC: IDB Social Protection and Health Division SCL/SPH.

Konadu-Agyemang, K. (2000). The best of times and the worst of times: Structural adjustment programs and uneven development in Africa: The case of Ghana. *The Canadian Geographer, 52*, 469–483.

Kumado, K., & Gockel, A.F. (2003). *A study on social security in Ghana*. Accra: Friedrich Ebert Stiftung.

Lewis, S. (2005). *Race against time*. Toronto: Anansi.

Maathai, W. (2009). *The challenge for Africa*. New York: Pantheon.

McWilliam, H.O.A., & Kwamena-Poh, M.A. (1975). *The development of education in Ghana*. London: Longman.

Midgley, J. (1995). *Social development: The development perspective in social welfare*. London: Sage Publications.

Ministry of Health (2015). *Holistic assessment of the health sector program of work 2014*. Accra: Government of Ghana.

Ministry for Local Government and Rural Development. (2014). *Building on the success stories and addressing challenges to sustain the Ghana school feeding program*. Accra: Government of Ghana. Retrieved from www.schoolfeeding.gov.gh/.

Ninsin, K.A. (1991). The PNDC and the problem of legitimacy. In D. Rothchild (Ed.), *Ghana: The political economy of recovery* (pp. 49–68). Boulder: Lynne Rienner.

Nukunya, G.K. (1992). *Tradition and change in Ghana: An introduction to sociology*. Accra: Ghana Universities Press.

Okudzejo, E., Mariki, W.A., Lal, R., & Senu, S.S. (2015). *Ghana country report: African economic outlook*. Accra: African Development Bank, UNDP. Retrieved from www.africaneconomicoutlook.org/en/country-notes/west-africa/ghana/.

Osei, R.D., Owusu, G.A., Asem, F.E., & Afutu-Kotey, R.L. (2009). *Effects of capitation grant on education outcomes in Ghana*. Accra: Institute of Statistical Social and Economic Research.

Osei-Boateng, C., & Ampratwum, E. (2011). *The informal sector in Ghana*. Accra: Friedrich Ebert Stiftung.

Overseas Development Institute. (1996). *Adjustment, poverty and PAMSCAD*. ODI Briefing Paper 2/96. London: Overseas Development Institute.

Rawlings, L.B., & Rubio, G.M. (2003). *Evaluating the impact of conditional cash transfer programs: Lessons from Latin America*. Policy Research Working Paper No. 3119. Washington, DC: The World Bank.

Ray, D.I. (1986). *Ghana: Politics, economics and society*. Boulder: Lynne Rienner.

Sachs, J. (2005). *The end of poverty: How we can make it happen in our lifetime*. London: Penguin.

Sewall, R.G. (2008). Conditional cash transfer programs in Latin America. *SAIS Review, 28*, 175–187.

Sewpaul, V. (2006). The global-local dialectic: Challenges for African scholarship and social work in a post-colonial world. *British Journal of Social Work, 36*, 419–434.

Sultan, S.M., & Schrofer, T.T. (2008). Building support to have targeted social protection interventions for the poorest: The case of Ghana. In *Social protection for the poorest in Africa*. Compendium of papers presented during the International Conference on Social Protection, September 9–10, Kampala, Uganda.

Sulzbach, S., Garshong, B., & Owusu-Banahene, G. (2005). *Evaluating the effects of the national health insurance act in Ghana: Baseline report*. Bethesda: The Partners for Health Reform *plus* Project, Abt Associates Inc.

UNDP. (2012). *2010 Ghana millennium development goals report.* Accra: UNDP and Government of Ghana.

UNESCO. (2012). *EFA global monitoring report 2012: Youth and skills: Putting education to work.* Paris: UNESCO.

UNICEF. (1989). *The state of the world's children.* Oxford: Oxford University Press.

UNICEF. (2001). *The state of the world's children.* Oxford: Oxford University Press.

UNICEF. (2009). *Social protection and children: Opportunities and challenges in Ghana.* Accra: Ministry of Employment and Social Welfare and UNICEF Ghana.

United Nations. (2010). *United Nations Millennium Development Goals (UNMDG).* Retrieved from www.un.org/millenniumgoals.

Wietler, K. (2007). *The impact of social cash transfer on informal safety nets in Kalomo District, Zambia: A qualitative study.* Berlin: German Technical Cooperation (GTZ).

World Bank. (2011). *Republic of Ghana: Improving the targeting of social programs.* Report No. 55578-GH. Washington, DC: World Bank.

World Food Program (2007). *Home-grown school feeding field case study, Ghana.* Rome: WFP.

Yunus, M. (2007). *Creating a world without poverty: Social business and the future of capitalism.* New York: Public Affairs.

12 Child-sensitive social protection initiatives in Nigeria

A role for indigenous social care

Augusta Y. Olaore, Vickie Ogunlade, and Chidimma Aham-Chiabuotu

Introduction

Social protection has been recognized internationally as a means to foster social development and to address the impacts of social vulnerability and exclusion driven by poverty (UNICEF, 2015). According to Devereux and Sabates-Wheeler (2004), transformative social protection is a term that describes:

> public and private initiatives that provide income or consumption transfers to the poor, protect the vulnerable against livelihood risks, and enhance the social status and rights of the marginalized; with the overall objective of reducing the economic and social vulnerability of poor, vulnerable and marginalized groups.
>
> (p. iii)

The Asian Development Bank's (2003) discussion of social protection strategy made a note of five primary areas of contemporary systems within society for the purpose of protection. These systems were identified as:

> Labor markets policies and programs designed to promote employment and protect workers; social insurance programs; social assistance and welfare services programs; micro- and area-based schemes to address vulnerability at the community level such as micro insurance and social funds: child-protection programs to ensure the healthy and productive development of children.
>
> (ADB, 2003, p. iii)

These five areas of social protection are aligned with the United Nations' Millennium Development Goals (MDGs), and the new Sustainable Development Goals that aim to address the critical needs of developing and industrialized countries affected by poverty and hostile economic policies (UN, 2008; 2015). As the most populous African county with the largest economy, Nigeria has continued its struggle to develop, implement, and strengthen social protection policies for its citizens in need. Despite efforts, there are significant gaps in the nation's development of social protection initiatives. This lag in progress continues to impact the most vulnerable within Nigeria's society. As Nigeria seeks to create, advance, and improve social protection initiatives, it is important to take notice of the important contributions of indigenous knowledge, beliefs, and social care practices, which strengthen and promote the well-being of children and families. These informal systems and practices have sustained social well-being in traditional and community settings. In the following section a number of traditional practices will be discussed.

Traditional practices and social protection

Social protection is an inherited custom within the African culture, with traditional practices aimed to meet the needs and provide protection for the poor, the vulnerable, and those at risk. Although not viewed as a structured organizational scheme, social protection has existed in African communities as a norm. In Nigeria, social protections have been implemented by heads of households and traditional rulers who have accepted leadership roles in the community. These community leaders have routinely accepted the responsibility of providing collective protection for the vulnerable; ensuring that community members at-risk are provided for and protected from increased risks. The extended family system has also supported this process, fulfilling the critical role of cushioning the impact of poverty, in the context of widowhood and for children deprived of parents (e.g., orphans).

Indigenous social care practices persisted as a prominent means of social protection within the Nigerian community setting until groups such as the Salvation Army and the Green Triangle emerged as pioneers of modern social work in Nigeria (Kazeem, 2011). The primary foci of these non-governmental organizations were delinquency problems among youth. Efforts resulted in the establishment of industrial schools, and the organization of boys' and girls' clubs (Atolagbe, 1989; Kazeem, 2011). During the late 1940s, the colonial government exhibited an interest in organized social work, with the appointment of Mr. Donald Faulkner as the first social welfare officer (Kazeem, 2011).

In addition to the presence of social work as an emerging profession within the community, socio-economic instabilities impacted the provision of indigenous social care practices. The impetuses for such instabilities were numerous changes, which erupted on a macro level. These changes emerged as the result of population growth, urbanization, globalization, climate change, socio-political unrest, wars and their aftermath. With the growing need and desire for evidence-based social protection programs, technological advancements manifested as a challenge to traditional social protective measures, overwhelming and disorganizing facilitators of indigenous social care practices.

Human rights and social justice: the needs of Nigerian children

Social justice is a first order ethical principal: It speaks to "the right to live in an egalitarian society where economic and social differences between social classes and groups are markedly reduced" (Jansson, 2001, p. 24). The profession of social work is an outgrowth of social justice efforts in support of the marginalized, and a commitment to the development of social welfare policies and social protection initiatives to ameliorate social inequalities (Jansson, 2001). Historically, the professional activities have centered on the "helping of individuals, groups, communities [to] enhance or restore their capacity for social functioning and creating social conditions favorable to this goal" (NASW, 1973, pp. 4–5). Children and the issue of human rights is a critical component of social work activity. Due to developmental stages and various states of dependency, children are reliant upon others for their survival needs and protection. Jansson (2001) expressed that children fall within an unusual status, as members of a "dependent out-group … dependent upon the goodwill of adults for requisite services, housing and resources" (p. 23). Without political clout, parental protection, and the commitment of advocates to ameliorate inequalities such as the lack of food, shelter, clothing, education, health care, and protection, children become victims. As victims, children face the risk of suffering a disproportionate share of social maladies, emerging as economic out-group members, residing at the lower echelons of the populace (Jansson, 2001).

Contemporary social protection in Nigeria

Despite the presence of social work practice and its commitment to social care, the effective development and implementation of social protection initiatives have persisted as a challenge for Nigeria. For example, Sanubi (2011) assessed that for the ordinary Nigerian, social protection is not only a strange concept, it is also not recognized as a right to be obtained from the government, as a result of citizenship. Poverty, economic vulnerability, and inequality are frequently viewed as a result of destiny rather than the result of economic policies or hostile conditions. Simultaneously, in lieu of social programs provided by the government, citizens of developing countries, such as Nigeria, believe that it is their moral obligation to give alms to the poor, be it Christianity, Islam, or African Traditional religion (Ogunkan, 2011; Uche & Ogugua, 2013). This perspective has impacted public actions driven by government policies. Those who develop policies and programs view "social protection initiatives more as an altruistic move of government than a furtherance of a well-deserved social contract in a democracy" (Sanubi, 2011, p. 1). Subsequently, in a seemingly democratic polity as Nigeria, social protection programs (and especially social assistance and welfare services) have been particularly inadequate as a greater proportion of the population remain trapped, suffering as a result of economic and social vulnerabilities (Sanubi, 2011).

Contemporary social protection initiatives

This section will provide an overview of two forms of contemporary social protection initiatives, *In Care of the People Cash Transfer Program (COPE CCT)* and the *Family Nutritional Support Program (FNSP)*. Currently implemented in Nigeria, these programs were initiated to address the needs of various groups within Nigeria who have been recognized as vulnerable and economically dependent. These groups include families impacted by extreme poverty, orphaned and vulnerable children (OVC) and those suffering with HIV/AIDS. Discussion of these programs will highlight their service packages, eligibility criteria and major challenges.

In Care of the People Cash Transfer Program (COPE CCT)

The "In Care of the People" (COPE CCT) is a conditional cash transfer program that focuses on eradicating inter-generational poverty in Nigeria. Initiated in 2008, the COPE Program was originally entitled the Care of the POOR CCT Program. COPE CCT Program was the outcome of Nigeria's negotiation regarding a debt relief agreement with the Paris Club and the World Bank in 2005. Nigeria was mandated to direct debt relief funds toward the alleviation of extreme poverty and actualization of the MDGs (United Nations, 2015). In 2008, the social protection program, COPE CCT, was launched under the administration of the National Poverty Eradication Program (World Bank, 2011). In the pilot phase, two states each from the six geo-political zones of the country were selected, due to a very low Human Capacity Development Index (HCDI) (Akinola, 2014).

Identified as a transformative social protection program, COPE's primary foci were the reduction in the vulnerability of the poorest within society, and the enhancement of recipients' capacities to contribute productively to the nation (Holmes, Samson, Magoronga, Akinrimisi, & Morgan, 2012). Programing goals included the identification of 3,000 eligible households located in 12 pilot states by the end of 2009. Eligible households were located in communities targeted with proxy means testing, to determine the poorest communities (Kidd & Wylde, 2011). Further eligibility guidelines were as follows:

*   female-headed households;
*   aged-parent headed households;
*   physically challenged people headed households (e.g., leprosy patients);
*   the transient-poor headed households (e.g., seasonal farmers);
*   Vesicovaginal Fistula (VVF) patients;
*   HIV affected households (Fiszbein & Schady, 2009).

Other eligibility guidelines were specified as attendance in available community based training programs in basic health, sanitation, life and vocational skills, as well as the participation of qualified children less than five years of age in all government free basic health programs. Such health programs included Vitamin A supplementation and National Polio Immunization (Akinola, 2014). Further specifications were indicated as documentation for antenatal care by pregnant women within benefiting households, and the 80% monthly school attendance rate of enrolled school age children, up to the basic education level (i.e., from the primary to junior secondary educational level). Selection processes of participants have relied heavily on a strong community involvement, participation and ownership of the program's requirements for monthly savings. Birth registration and non-involvement in harmful forms of child labor were additional conditions for receipt of COPE CCT (Akinola, 2014).

The amount of funds received via the COPE cash transfer program is dependent upon the number of children. Eligible households receive a Basic Income Guarantee (BIG) of approximately US$10 per child on a monthly basis, with the maximum amount of US$33 for four or more children per month, for a period of one year. The family is expected to graduate from the program at the end of the year, at which time they receive a lump-sum of US$560 – the Poverty Reduction Accelerator Investment (PRAI), for the establishment of viable micro-enterprises (Fiszbein & Schady, 2009).

The extent to which the COPE CCT Program has impacted the participants in terms of poverty alleviation and human capital development is debatable, as there is limited data on impact assessment of the program. COPE's limited success has been recognized as the assistance of participants in the purchasing of basic household items during a short-term period, the support of obtaining daily consumption needs of the recipients, as well as some improvements in the beneficiaries' access to education and health care (Akinola, 2014; Holmes et al., 2012).

However, discussion of the program's outcomes has also drawn attention to COPE's current difficulty in meeting the long-term goals of reducing vulnerabilities and inter-generational poverty, resulting in a very minimal impact on the empowerment of women via sustainable poverty alleviation. Driven by outcomes from community fieldwork executed by Olabanji Akinola (2014) within Ibadan, Oyo state, Southwest Nigeria, between May and October 2013, several limitations were identified for this transformative social protection program. Specific limitations were associated with the designated one year of program involvement, which limits the long-term development of the human capital – with a focus on children. The one-year duration does not respect the challenges families face due to the infrastructural challenges associated with the health and educational systems (Akinola, 2014). Also, the coverage of COPE has been very low, covering only about 22,000 households, which was estimated to be less than 0.001% of poor households (Hagen-Zanker & Holmes, 2012, p. vi). Such limited scope of households deemed as eligible for this cash transfer program has persisted despite an increase in economic suffering due to global and subsequent community vulnerabilities related to income, food, and fuel crises. Concurrently, the marginal income and assets transfers to be utilized by graduating program participants for sustainability have proven to be too low to successfully develop and operate an income-generating trade within Nigeria. It has been further assessed that due to the high cost of production and the challenging macroeconomic environment within Nigeria, various households who have received income via this social protection program remain exposed to the same, similar, or even worse susceptibilities, despite their involvement in COPE (Akinola, 2014).

The Family Nutritional Support Program (FNSP)

The Family Nutritional Support Program (FNSP) was initiated in 2008, as a component of a project in Nigeria, Maximizing Agricultural Revenues for Key Enterprises in Targeted Sites (MARKETS). Funded by the United States President's Emergency Plan for AIDS Relief (PEPFAR)/United States Agency for International Development (USAID), the program commenced in five states (Bauchi, Kano, Lagos, Benue, and Cross River) with the goal to improve the socio-economic status of OVC households affected by HIV/AIDS. The first component addressed the immediate nutritional needs of OVC and their families through food fortification. The second component targeted the long-term nutritional and economic needs of the identified 7,500 households with OVC through a program that promotes home gardening (Samuels, Blake, & Akinrimisi, 2012, p. 42). The package provided OVC with fortified and nutritional food supplements. Simultaneously, OVC caregivers were identified to receive training and income-generating activity (IGA) to support their long-term economic and nutritional status. The target was to improve the socio-economic status of 7,500 OVC households affected by HIV/AIDS in five states (Bauchi, Kano, Lagos, Benue, and Cross River) (Devex Impact, 2015, p. 1). In order to ensure the success of the program, partnerships were formed with two Nigerian agro-processing firms, Grand Cereals and Oil Mills Limited (GCOML) and Dala Foods. These partnerships enabled the production of nutritional supplements, to address the immediate nutritional needs of more than 25,000 OVCs, at a minimal profit margin (Devex Impact, 2015, p. 1).

At present, the overall impact of the FNSP is still unknown, as no comprehensive assessment of the program has been documented. However, though this program was implemented in only five out of 36 states, it has yet to address the nutritional needs of the entire vulnerable group, which has met the eligibility requirements. Also, while the focus on the OVC population was expedient, there remain other families, not affected or infected by HIV/AIDS, but who are as equally poor and vulnerable in need of such services.

It can be concluded from the above discussions that as social protection initiatives, COPE CCT and FNSP have not been able to address the needs and vulnerabilities of the Nigerian population. Nigeria is Africa's most populous country, with an estimated population of about 178.5 million people in 2014 (World Population Review, 2015, p. 1). Though Nigeria was identified as Africa's largest economy, with a 2014 GDP estimated at US \$479 billion, the "economic diversification and strong growth have not translated into a significant decline in poverty levels" (CIA, 2013–2014, Section 5). The Central Intelligence Agency (CIA) (2013–2014) World Factbook data revealed that within Nigeria, over 62% of the nation's population lives in extreme poverty, with nearly 73 (72.7) deaths recorded per 1,000 live births, with a life expectancy (at birth) identified as 53.02 years. For children under the age of five years, it has been estimated that 31% are documented as underweight (CIA, 2013–2014, Section 3). Hagen-Zanker and Holmes (2012) also observed stunting and wasting as a significant phenomenon for children under the age of five. Regarding the impact of HIV/AIDS, data outcomes revealed that 3,228,600 individuals were estimated as infected with this disease. By the following year (2014), it was assessed that 174,300 individuals would have died from this disease, the highest number internationally, during a calendar year (CIA, 2013–2014, Section 3).

The presence of extreme poverty, high infant mortality rates, underweight conditions for children under five, projected shorter life spans, and the high rate of HIV/AIDs and related deaths, point to the need for a systematic and comprehensive social protection system. An additional indicator of the need for social protection programs is dependency ratios. The Central Intelligence Agency (2013–2014) World Factbook discussion indicated that Nigerian dependency ratios (a measure of the age structure) revealed the total number of individuals likely to be economically "dependent" on others' support as 87.7%. The total dependency ratio in Nigeria reflected the ratio of combined youth population (ages 0–14: 82.6%) and elderly population (ages 65+: 5.1%) per 100 people of working age (15–64 years) (CIA, 2013–2014, Section 5). This dependency ratio also projected a greater burden for the working-age population, as well as the overall economy, in the support and provision of social protection programs for those who are often economically dependent, such as children, the youth, and the elderly (CIA, 2013–2014).

The following discussion presents the various vulnerabilities experienced by Nigerian children in the face of an inadequate social protection.

Vulnerabilities experienced by children

Vulnerabilities suffered by Nigerian children include discriminatory socio-cultural attitudes and practices, environmental shocks; bio-psychosocial effects of domestic violence and family fragmentation, societal violence and conflict social exclusion, educational deprivation, in addition to health disparities (Jones, Presler-Marshall, Cooke, & Akinrimisi, 2012). The presence of extreme poverty, high infant mortality rates, underweight conditions for children under age five, and projected shorter life spans point to the shocks children experience within the Nigerian society. Despite being ranked as the 12th largest producer of oil internationally, and the largest oil producer in Africa (Oxford Business Group, 2013, p. 117), Nigeria's ranking on the United Nations Development Program (UNDP) Human Development Index (HDI) points to its lack of progress in meeting the needs of the population that faces life-cycle or structural vulnerabilities. "Nigeria's HDI value for 2013 is 0.504 – which is in the low human development category-positioning the country at 152 out of 187 countries and territories" (UNDP, 2014, p. 2). Nigeria'multi-layered struggles in its efforts to address overwhelming bio-socio-economic issues have continued to devastate children and youth (Avert, 2012; Dioka, 2014; NACA, 2012). The HIV/AIDS epidemic is an example of how family systems are crippled in their efforts to function as the primary support of their children – who are dependent for the provision of survival needs, education and health care, as well protection from emotional and physical harm.

> Children are affected by HIV/AIDS through mother-to-child transmission infection or through the loss of one or both parents from AIDS. The 2008 National Situation Assessment and Analysis (SAA) on orphaned and vulnerable children (OVC) showed that not only has HIV and AIDS been a major cause of death of parents, especially in households where both parents have died, but also before the loss of a parent, social and economic vulnerability is exacerbated by serious illness of a parent or other adult member of the household. When parents fall chronically ill from AIDS, children migrate between households. Many of the households taking on these children find it difficult to afford their support. Of 17.5 million vulnerable children, an estimated 7.3 million have lost one or both parents due to various causes. Of these, 2.23 million were orphaned by HIV/AIDS, while about 260,000 children are living with HIV/AIDS. About 20.3% OVC are not regular school attendant, and 18% have been victims of sexual abuse.
>
> (NACA, 2012, p. 23)

Impact of poverty

Poverty is a driver of the HIV/AIDS epidemic, with devastating outcomes for families and children. Trafficking, abuse, and forced labor are also socio-economic traumas, propelled by poverty and devastating to children. The 2015 1st Quarter Report of the National Agency for the Prohibition of Trafficking in Persons revealed the following outcomes. By the end of the first quarter of 2015, within Nigeria a total of 130 cases of human trafficking and other related matters were reported by NAPTIP (2015, p. 1). The majority of the cases were associated with child labor (24.6%) and external trafficking for sexual exploitation (23.4%). Other cases reported were child abuse (16.9%), kidnapping from guardianship (8.5%), and sexual abuse/rape (3.8%). Cases of baby sales, illegal adoption, Almajiri – children experiencing years of begging (Ifeadikanwa, 2013), as well as missing and abandoned children were grouped together to make up 14.6% of the total reported cases. Meanwhile, out of a total of 107 suspected child trafficking perpetrators, only four were prosecuted and convicted (NAPTIP, 2015, p. 1). The next section will briefly discuss the presence of trafficking, abuse, and labor demands of children and youth – forms of victimization exercised as a means to economic survival within Nigerian communities.

Child trafficking

Nigeria has been identified as major factor in the supply and consumption of human trafficking, as well as a major transit route for those victimized (NAPTIP,

2007). This form of victimization is perpetrated by varied entities including individuals, families, communities, institutions, and organizations. Out of the 1.2 million children who are trafficked globally, 32% of them are from Africa (UNICEF, 2007a, p. 1). The National Agency for the Prohibition of Traffic of Persons review of crimes report indicated that on average, 10 children are trafficked across the Nigerian borders on a daily basis (Lladan, 2011, p. 5). Children trafficked are transported out of the country either by road, air, or sea to neighboring African countries such as the Republic of Benin, Niger, Chad, Ghana. While, within Nigeria, almost every state has a variant of this form of victimization, with child trafficking occurring from rural to urban areas or from one urban area to another (Huntley, 2013).

Outcomes for children who are victimized by trafficking are varied. Children are found to be abducted, coerced, or hired for exploitative labor as domestic servants, beggars, prostitutes, car wash and factory workers, or agents in armed conflicts. They are also coerced to be involved in entertainment and pornography or used for ritual purposes or sources of body parts (Agbu, 2008; NAPTIP, 2007; 2015). Olagbegi (2006) surmised that the glamour of urban areas lures children and their families to seek out traffickers in order to access opportunities available in cosmopolitan cities. Informal relative foster care encourages more affluent relatives to take on the care of less privileged children, moving them away from their parents offering the hope of better education. Unfortunately there are children who exploited, while their educational and developmental needs are not met. A new trend of child trafficking in Nigeria has been the establishment of baby factories, where adolescent girls are confined and non-pregnant victims are forcefully impregnated. Upon delivery, the girls are forced to deliver and the babies are subsequently sold for illegal adoption, ritual purposes, or child labor (Eseadi, Achagh, Ikechukwu-Ilomuanya, & Ogbuabor, 2015; Huntley, 2013).

Child labor

A child working beside their parents as part of their social development is a culturally acceptable occurrence in Nigeria. However, making a distinction between labor that is age-appropriate and labor that is exploitative and harmful has proven difficult (UNICEF Nigeria, 2006). Traditionally, children acquire skills for adulthood by working alongside their parents, which also assists the family, in its effort to survive economically (Amao & Akinlade, 2014). The transition to a cash economy has maneuvered children into earning wages to help the family, as well as exposed them to adverse situations (Jones et al., 2012). Subsequently, for the purpose of this discussion a working definition of child labor would be the utilization of children to earn wages primarily for financial benefits to the family; labor that is age-inappropriate and harmful for their overall growth and development. Therefore, age, hours, and type of work performed and specific conditions under which a child works are factors that must be taken into consideration in a discussion of child labor (Okpukpara & Odurukwe, 2006). In Nigeria, it is a common occurrence for children to be forced into long hours or dangerous situations that are developmentally inappropriate. Such labor requirements commonly observed encompass females engulfed in the role of domestics from an early; boys working as ticket conductors on rolling buses; children functioning as hired farm hands, hawking goods, or begging for alms on behalf of handicapped parents.

Poverty presents as a key factor in the victimization of children, as laborers within inappropriate settings and for extensive timeframes. Children who are members of an impoverished family system find themselves unable to pay school fees, forced to combine school with work. Outcomes of such realities include poor academic performance, coupled with exposure dangers to hazardous environments, including busy highways, crime, violence, and clandestine activities. The missing of school due to street hawking leads to missed school classes or entire days. In addition, Nigerian children between five and nine years of age average nearly 18 hours per week in unpaid domestic chores (Okpukpara & Odurukwe, 2006).

Child abuse

Child abuse continues to exist, constituting a serious threat to the health, welfare, and overall development of Nigerian children (Jones et al., 2012). Battering, along with child labor, stigmatization, discrimination, and all forms child sexual exploitation (including rape) appear to be common occurrences within Nigeria. There are minimal to no enforcements of legal standards, as stipulated in the Child Rights Act. Consequently, there are inadequate structure and resources for the protection and support of victims and their families.

The vulnerability of children to different forms of abuse has been exacerbated by the increased number of orphans and vulnerable children as a result of the HIV/AIDS pandemic (Samuels et al., 2012). Disabilities of any kind have also increased children's vulnerability to all forms of abuse, discrimination, and neglect. Early marriage, a common practice in rural areas and Islamic northern states, is also a significant contributor in the perpetuation of child abuse and its consequences (Jones et al., 2012).

The vulnerabilities of Nigerian children are further compounded by their dependence on adults who themselves are exposed to risks, such as gender inequalities, and spatial location (Jones et al., 2012). Since children, particularly during early childhood, are dependent for care, support, and protection, the caregivers' risks and vulnerabilities compromise their abilities to provide adequate care and support. Such deficits compound the individual vulnerabilities of children. Therefore, from a family systems perspective, there is a need for the conceptualization and implementation of social protection, which are child sensitive, with a focus on intervention goals committed to meeting the needs of parents and caregivers (DFID et al., 2009). The following section will discuss the integrated framework of child-sensitive social protection and current initiatives, which address the vulnerabilities of Nigerian children.

Child-sensitive social protection

Child-sensitive social protection helps to build a protective environment by reducing socio-economic barriers through initiatives that contribute to economic security, ensure access to basic social services, and contribute to the prevention of violence and exploitation (Jones et al., 2012). Social protection programs, which are expected to accommodate child protection, include preventing and responding to violence, exploitation, and abuse, and unnecessary separation from family (UNICEF Nigeria, 2006). Thus, child-sensitive social protection has been described as an evidence-based approach, with an aim to maximize opportunities and developmental outcomes, with a consideration of the different dimensions of a child's well-being (DFID et al., 2009). It has been recommended as an essential framework for addressing the vulnerabilities of children (even in Nigeria) whether they are the primary targets of the social protection programs or not (DFID et al., 2009; Holmes et al., 2012). In the Joint Statement for Advancing Child-Sensitive Social Protection, it was recognized that this approach addresses the immediate vulnerabilities of children, while adopting proactive strategies to address vulnerabilities that a child maybe born into, as well future susceptibilities as of a result of external bio-socio-economic traumas (DFID et al., 2009, p. 2). Following is a summary of the principles for planning, implementing, and evaluating effective comprehensive child-sensitive social protection programs as recommended by the Department for International Development (DFID et al., 2009).

- Avoid adverse impacts on children, and reduce or mitigate social and economic risks that directly affect children's lives.
- Intervene as early as possible where children are at risk, in order to prevent irreversible impairment or harm.
- Consider the age- and gender-specific risks and vulnerabilities of children throughout the life-cycle.
- Mitigate the effects of shocks, exclusion and poverty on families, recognizing that families raising children need support to ensure equal opportunity.
- Make special provision to reach children who are particularly vulnerable and excluded, including children without parental care, and those who are marginalized within their families or communities due to their gender, disability, ethnicity, HIV and AIDS or other factors.
- Consider the mechanisms and intra-household dynamics that may affect how children are reached, with particular attention paid to the balance of power between men and women within the household and broader community.
- Include the voices and opinions of children, their caregivers and youth in the understanding and design of social protection systems and programs (DFID et al., 2009, p. 3)

The development, implementation, and evaluation of child-sensitive social protection initiatives are imperative processes for comprehensive, effective programs designated for the most dependent and vulnerable of those in need. As the primary means of support of children, who are dependent for their survival needs, education, and health care, as well protection from emotional and physical harm, the distress and oftentimes devastation of family systems point to the critical need for a systematic and comprehensive social protection system. Effective child-sensitive social protection initiatives have the potential for benefiting not only children, but will also support family systems, communities, and national development and sustainability (Holmes et al., 2012).

Legislation and policy responses to children's vulnerabilities

As a nation, Nigeria continues the struggle to hash out legislation, develop policies, and implement programs to address the harsh realities of child protection deficits. Nigeria has moved forward in its efforts to protect the children within its society, with the hope of negating the indifference of the general population. The following discussion highlights various legislation and policies put forth to address the human rights issue faced by children – trafficking, exploitative labor, and abuse, as well as needs experienced due to living with HIV/AIDS.

Current child and person living with HIV (PLHIV) initiatives

While the National Policy on AIDS is still in place in Nigeria (NACA, 2010), Nigeria has continued to fall short in meeting HIV goals, lagging behind in terms of laws and policies that protect vulnerable sub-populations, and Persons Living With HIV (PLHIV) against discrimination. There are challenges in terms of obtaining traction regarding the systematic application of social protection measures for HIV and AIDS. The gaps are more visible when moving from national- to state- and then to local government levels for policy implementation (Jones et al., 2012). This may be due to lack of resources, funding, or capacity, or simply poor political will to address the HIV epidemic and its impact on individuals, families, and communities (Amanyeiwe et al., 2008)

Child's Rights Act

Protection of children in Nigeria is undergirded by the Child's Rights Act, which was initiated in 2003. This act was legislated as the country's attempt to domesticate the Convention on the Rights of a Child by the United Nations General Assembly in 1989 (*The Bill*, 2003; UN, 1989; UNICEF, 2007b). The Child's Rights Act addresses child abuse, labor, and trafficking, with children defined as persons under the age of 18 years. The legislation includes sanctions and penalties for violations, which range from monetary fines to imprisonment. Sections 21–23 prohibit the marriage of a child under the age of 18 years, along with fines and sanctions of imprisonment.

Child labor in Nigeria is also specified in the Child's Rights Act (*The Bill*, 2003). Sections 28 and 29 stipulate sanctions against exploitative labor. These sections also reinforce relevant sections of the Labor Act. Children under the age of 14 are to be paid on a daily wage basis and must return to their residence at night. Sections 21, 31, and 32 prohibits the placement of tattoos and marks on the skin of a child, as well as engaging in sexual intercourse with a child. Sanctions range from a fine of approximately US$25.00 (N5,000) to life imprisonment.

It has been observed that although the passage of the Child's Rights Act is a major milestone for Nigerian children, implementation and enforcement has been weak, as a result of cultural norms and beliefs that parents have ultimate responsibility and rights regarding the care of their children. Subsequently, it is typical to see children "hawking" in major cities, without parents' apprehension of law enforcement, as stipulated in the Child's Rights Act. Also, in various states, it is known that marriages with minors are openly contracted, without parental concern of legal enforcement of the law.

Trafficking in Persons (Prohibition) Law Enforcement and Administration Act

The Trafficking in Persons (Prohibition) Law Enforcement and Administration Act was passed in 2003, along with the Child's Rights Act. This legislation has also informed the establishment of the national agency (NAPTIP, 2007, 2015), which enforces and prosecutes violators of this legislation.

National Program on the Elimination of Child Labor

In 2002, Nigeria signed a memorandum of understanding with the International Labor Organization (ILO) to eradicate adverse forms of child labor, and part-nered with the ILO to establish the National Program on the Elimination of Child Labor (NPECL) (ILO, 2005). The labor act stipulates a minimum age of 12 years for employment and apprenticeships, not including light agricultural or domestic work performed for the family. It prohibits children under the age of 12 years from carrying any load that could inhibit physical development, and those under the age of 15 years from industrial work and maritime employment. Minors younger than 16 years are prohibited from working at night, underground, hand-ling machines, working no more than four consecutive hours or more than eight hours a day. This effort to eliminate adverse forms of labor also points to a further need for social protection initiatives to ensure the human rights of chil-dren (ILO, 2005).

While government agencies have been historically involved and responsible for ensuring social protection for their citizens, a reality common to current social protection policies and programs is a lack of awareness by the general population. Barrientos's (2007) examination of lessons learned from social pro-tection initiatives implemented by low income countries is grounded by the fol-lowing observations:

It is taken for granted that the challenges of establishing and developing social protection are that much harder in low-income countries. There are several dimensions to this issue. The demand for formal social protection instruments is weaker in economies that are predominantly rural. Informal support systems and social norms are commonly in place to ensure a measure of protection. Economic development and urbanization strengthen the demand for more extensive social protection institutions. Present day low-income countries generally have weaker, and perhaps fragmented, political systems and labor organizations, with the implication that wider social contracts and solidarity are very limited in scope. In most cases, low-income countries have large deficiencies in state capacity to collect taxes and to design, as well as support and deliver, social protection. The list of dimensions could be usefully extended, but these factors – underdevelopment, politics, finance and administration – are key constraints in establishing effective social protection instruments in low-income countries.

(pp. 1–2)

Enforcement of legislations is weak and awareness-raising campaigns are inconsistent and barely funded. There is inadequate coordination, programming fragmentation, inconsistent planning, and data limitations, in addition to inadequate and vulnerable budgets. Subsequently, the inclusion of grassroots community practices in active collaborative social protection initiatives may undergird, enhance, and lean to the sustainability of governmental social protection initiatives (Vaughan, 1995).

Indigenous Social Care and social protection

As a an element of grassroots community initiatives, Indigenous Social Care (ISC) practices are presented as one system that celebrates community based care systems, which are deeply rooted in native experiences and knowledge. ISC includes a system of indigenous knowledge and beliefs. Spirituality and connectedness with the land as identified by Ife (2001) drives indigenous social care practices. The experiences of the individual community member impacts the collective; and group actions influence the life events of the individual (Belgrave & Allison, 2006). Embedded in the fabric of the community, ISC practices promote the well-being of children and families. Such practices include kinship care for children and the elderly, mutual financial aids, festivals and ceremonies that promote unity and self-esteem. Presently, in Nigeria, there is increasing interest in learning how traditional and indigenous practices, such as the extended family, clan obligations, and mutual aid societies, can build capacities to meet human needs (Olaore & Drolet, submitted).

Social care practices include the provision of social support, social work, personal care, and protection of children in need or at risk, and to strengthening of their families and caregivers. Child-sensitive social protection is to be cognizant of ensuring that provisions reach children who are vulnerable and excluded, including children without parental care, and those who are marginalized within their families or communities due to their gender, disability, ethnicity, HIV and

AIDS, or other factors. Jones et al. (2012) also discussed the importance of considering the mechanisms and intra-household dynamics that may affect how children are reached, with particular attention paid to the balance of power between men and women within the household and broader community. It is vital that the voices and opinions of children, their caregivers, and youth are to be included in the understanding and design of social protection systems and programs. Children are born into communities of extended family and village involvement in Nigeria, and biological parents have an expectation of support in the birthing of an infant. Extended family members are available as caregivers when parents need respite. This extensive community network also serves to monitor and ensure that children are not subjected to harm or maltreatment.

ISC practices: complementary measures of child-sensitive social protection

Jones et al. (2012) posit that "maximizing the effectiveness of social protection requires complementary measures, which may not be considered a core component of social protection, but are necessary to ensure an effective enabling environment to achieve social protection objectives" (p. 3). It was also recommended that transformative approaches require that governmental agencies establish linkages with "complementary" non-governmental structures. This section discusses in specific terms how ISC practices and beliefs may be explored to address some of the social protection gaps for children and PLHIV in Nigeria.

Historically, social protection and social security were the sole responsibility of the family and community systems. Urbanization and modernization has weakened the traditional systems in Nigeria, which has resulted in a social crisis that is only partially met by the government. The primary focus of the government has been the provision of basic education and health care for the influx of rural immigrants to the cities. The need for support of working families with young children in the cities has been untouched by governmental policies and programs. Ensuing is a review of ISC practices, which may be employed as complementary social protection measures within the Nigerian community.

Indigenous financial support

Poverty is a major driver of child protection deficits in Nigeria. A transformative approach to social protection encourages the strengthening of financial capacities of households. Kay (2011) highlights a preference for collective forms of production, the value of labor and an imperative to work the land, as well as the importance of networks of kin, neighbors, and friends in militating poverty, by pooling and exchanging material, resources, and labor as practiced in rural Nigeria. Specific forms of indigenous financial support practices are cash transfer practices; the inclusion of community based non-governmental organizations, traditional celebratory gatherings of community members, and shared farming.

Indigenous cash transfer practices

Informed by the need for economic stability, indigenous cash transfer practices such as the *Ajo/Esusu/Adashe/Alajeseku* have the potential to be recognized and supported by the government as a viable poverty alleviation ISC practice. *Ajo/Esusu/Adashe/Alajeseku* involves the coming together of a group of people who agree to contribute a certain amount of money to a mutual pot. Each month every member of the group gives their monies to a designated member of the group. The individual who receives the lump sum may use the funds to invest in sustaining actions, such as investing in a business, real estate, their children's education, obtaining household equipment, or the financing of a family project. This mode of contribution is rotated to each group member until everyone has the opportunity to receive the designated lump sum, thus completing the cycle. Due to the mutual contribution and expectations, everyone is held accountable: This safeguards against defaulting. *Ajo/Esusu/Adashe/Alajeseku* also encourages the discipline of saving a portion of the income, no matter how little. Such savings make large sums of money available for big projects without the burden of a loan. Planning ahead is also encouraged. An individual who may have a major financial need may utilize the option to request their collection of funds during a future period, when the financial need is to occur.

Esusu (akawo) or ajo: A modified form of the *esusu* (*akawo*) or *ajo* is practiced amongst market women, traders, and artisans in indigenous communities in Nigeria. There is usually an appointed person, who collects a specified amount of money at the end of the day, week, or month from members of the group. The collector is given a percentage of the contribution as compensation for the work of going from person to person or business to business, maintaining accurate records and disbursing the monies to the beneficiaries at any given time.

The inclusion of social protection stakeholders such as governmental agencies, NGOs, and religious organizations may serve in monitoring and mediatory roles to ensure that monies collected by families are utilized for children's education or investment in lucrative businesses, which would have a positive impact on household income levels. Child labor and trafficking has been linked to the inability of caregivers to pay for educational expenses or provide for the basic needs of the families. Subsequently, children are pulled out of school to sell goods on the streets by hawking or to be used as farm hands to increase farm produce for sale or sustenance. Promoting *Ajo/Esusu/Adashe/Alajeseku* has the potential to increase the availability of funds available for households, thus reducing the need to engage children in child labor or trafficking.

Traditional events and gatherings such as naming ceremonies may be utilized for awareness campaigns. Advocated for by social workers, the sharing of information during communal gatherings may reduce barriers, allowing community members to embrace social protection initiatives as valid resources they could possibly apply for and benefit from, as Nigerian citizens. Such advocacy actions could allow for the sharing of information and requirements of critical services, such as cash transfer programs (COPE CCT and FNSP).

Communal farming is a significant resource in indigenous communities. The option of communal farming increases the productivity of individual households. When neighbors come around to assist each other with farm work, it increases the acreage of farmland, thus boosting the potential harvest and income for the family. In addition, monies from the sale of community farm produce may be channeled into supporting the government by funding cash transfer programs such as COPE CCT and FNSP.

Implications for social protection and social work

Having established that the Nigerian people have continued to value their indigenous social care practices, it becomes expedient to consider developing partnerships with grassroots social protection programs. Such partnerships will not only enhance community understanding of the concept of evidence-based social protection programs, but will also increase the likelihood of community ownership of programs and increased commitment. The following discussions present examples of such partnerships, as well as other indigenous practices that can be harnessed for future collaborations.

Community partnerships for care of OVC in Sagamu, Ogun State – Nigeria

Sagamu Community Centre is an NGO in Sagamu local government. A unique feature of this NGO is a collaborative model in which the organization is managed by the local community, Olabisi Onabanjo Teaching Hospital, and the local government. One recent program, funded by HOPE World Wide, is for the care of OVC through the provision of quality education and enhancement of household income. The program package includes a loan of approximately US$10.00 (N2,000): Funds are paid over a period of 22 weeks, in weekly installments. Funds are for the payment of school fees, uniforms, and books for the OVC within the households. Families that receive the loans are trained to engage in small-scale businesses, which will support the provision of their daily needs and enable the payment of the loans.

During the initial phase of the program, community members had an active role in the identification of households with OVC. Also, after a period of about one year, individuals and community groups, including the local chiefs, businessmen, and civil society organizations, were invited to partner with the NGO to ensure sustainability of the program. At present, this program continues to function, with over 50 families benefiting from this social protection initiative (Uko, 2015).

Youth vigilante groups: grassroots partners against child labor, trafficking and abuse and for HIV awareness campaigns

Youth groups provide support for tackling the menace of child trafficking, abuse, and labor, as well as HIV awareness. Jones et al. (2012) reported that currently in Nigeria, the governmental response to child trafficking has been legislative – in the form of anti-trafficking laws. These laws resulted in the creation of the National Agency for the Prohibition of Traffic in Persons (NAPTIP). The NAPTIP approach has included a collaborative relationship with the police force and border/immigration patrol, for the purpose of policing, investigating, and prosecuting perpetrators. This reactionary approach has yielded limited results: Reports revealed that only 12 traffickers have been persecuted between 2003 and 2011 (Jones et al., 2012). Age grade groupings called *Egbe* (Yoruba)/*otu ebiri* (Igbo) are possible resources for combating child labor, trafficking, and abuse.

Rural youth groups currently perform disciplinary functions among their peers.

It was noted that current child labor laws do not apply to children who are hired for domestic services, thus many children are exploited as child laborers with no legal protection. Also, it has been observed that community groups are privy to information or have native knowledge that otherwise may be unknown to official bodies. Such information may be utilized in locating and identifying human traffickers.

Partnering with the community-based youth groups could be a valid model by both governmental and non-governmental agencies. Providing incentives to community members empowers them to develop, implement, and monitor preventive and responsive interventions. Collaborative efforts could also be enhanced via empowerment by incentives to act as a neighborhood watch against child labor and trafficking. Youth groups could collaborate with government and other agencies to address the issue of inappropriate engagement of children in labor, tracking down child traffickers, and reporting or arresting families that are engaged in child labor. Organizations or agencies involved with combating child trafficking, such as the NGO Women Trafficking and Child Labor Eradication Foundation (WOTCLEF), the governmental agency, NAPTIP, or other civil society agencies could donate vehicles, which would aid rapid response and effective monitoring.

A primary goal of the National Policy on AIDS is to increase the awareness of HIV/AIDS among the youth. *Egbe* (Yoruba)/*otu ebiri* (Igbo), could prove invaluable in the context of ISC. The youth group leaders could be utilized as outreach resources, to engage young people, serving as facilitators, mobilizers, and organizers of HIV rallies or walks. Youthfulness and creativity would support the development of engaging dances and drama as public health messages, to promote safe sex practices and non-stigmatization of PLHIV.

Kinship and community care: increased capacity for social protection

The traditional Nigerian culture accepts that child abuse and child protection is the responsibility of the entire community. The provision of kinship care by extended family members is important for caring for one another. Such a belief system can be encouraged and supported through a caregiver subsidy from the government. However, the exploitation of children living with relatives as domestic servants is sometimes due to financial constraints on the part of the caregiver. Remunerating relative caregivers in the Nigerian system may serve as a good incentive to provide adequate care and alleviate the hardship of caring for non-biological children. Relative caregivers may be recipients of COPE, FNSP, and other cash transfer programs. The financial support provided would entitle the government to monitor the care of the children – guarding against child abuse and neglect, which may come as a result of informal foster care (Jones et al., 2012).

Discussion

Indigenous Social Care (ISC), a direct product of strong indigenous Nigerian communities, is a set of practices committed to the creation and enhancement of a caring living environment: A community may be recognized by its physical location, substance, and practices within the setting, as well as a consortium of undertakings throughout the various communal areas or within varied sub-groups. The pattern of norms, beliefs, and values, which guide activities, defines the setting as a community (McDowell, 2006). In the context of Nigeria, this includes villages and townships – communities located in primarily rural settings.

The strategies of building strong families are intrinsically embedded in traditional practices in native communities in Nigeria. The most prominent example of how traditional practices enhance social capital is the Nigerian extended family system. People do not live in isolation in Nigeria. Community contributory cash transfer schemes such as *esusu* in South East Nigeria or *egbe alajesheku* or *ajo* in the South West will not only improve individual and family income but also build social capital. Everyone looks out for everyone, while age-grade youth vigilante groups and traditional leadership enforce discipline, safety, and foster a mindset.

The extended family and expected community responsibility demonstrated in ceremonies, care of widows, and other practices that celebrate the child, give a sense of identity and self-esteem, and prevent child abuse and neglect. Being a good neighbor is the norm in native Nigerian communities and is a preventive and protective factor against child maltreatment. The US Advisory Board on Child Abuse and Neglect (1993) discussed the role of possible neighbor involvement in the monitoring of child maltreatment. Different forms of child maltreatment can be abated when neighbors are alert, supportive, and responsive to harmful behaviors that compromise the safety and protection of children in their environment (US Advisory Board on Child Abuse and Neglect, 1993). Campaigns created via community-based collaborations with coordinated social workers have the potential of increasing prevention initiatives directed toward the issue of child cruelty.

Indigenous beliefs and shared values in native communities also promote cohesiveness. Pebley and Sastry (2003) posited that when communities are cohesive, they are more likely to share attitudes, beliefs, and values about childrearing, safety, and related matters. As a result, community norms are more apparent, enforcing children's adherence to behavioral expectations. Parents' enforcement of behavioral norms for their children is viewed as acceptable and customary, due to the knowledge that neighbors share their beliefs and values (McDonnell & Melton, 2008).

Child maltreatment, such as child labor, trafficking, and abuse, as identified in this chapter, is grounded in relationships, and requires community and family based intervention processes that cannot be effectively addressed in narrow policies and programs. The vision of the Strong Communities initiative is for building systems of support for families of young children beyond social welfare offices, police stations, and courtrooms. This makes child protection part of everyday life. This included the involvement of societal and neighborhood institutions apart from governmental efforts (McDonnell & Melton, 2008).

Biological parents are not regarded as the sole owners of the child. Every child belongs to the entire community: It is believed that the success and prosperity of that child is the prosperity of the community. For example, in some parts of South Eastern Nigeria among the Ibos, it is a taboo for a parent to beat a child who ran into the neighbor's house for shelter. Regardless of the gravity of the offense, once a child escapes to another person's house, the beating must stop. The neighbor assumes the responsibility for investigation and intervening in the matter. Where the child is at fault, the neighbor will correct the child in an age-appropriate manner. It is expected that the child will not repeat that offence, because he/she is motivated to be in favor with the neighbor who was the savior. Sometimes, the child may spend a day or two in the neighbor's house while the neighbor monitors the mood of the parent, just to ensure that the anger has dissipated before the child is taken home. The process ensures that the child will be protected.

The presence of grandparents in homes is another protective factor for children in Nigeria, for grandparents are protective of their grandchildren. Sometimes the protection is so pronounced that parents avoid sending their children to the grandparents because they believe they will be significantly spoilt or indulged. For most Nigerian children, it is a privilege to have grandparents in the home. The grandparents tend to protect the children from both physical and psychological abuse. It is unacceptable to maltreat a child in the presence of the grandparent, to express a negative word, or yell at a child when the grandparents are close by. The grandparents affirm the child by calling them legendary names as practiced in the Oriki, a practice of the Yoruba culture.

Traditional power structures

Traditional power structures are critical in child labor interventions where communities mobilized by local leaders are more likely to engage in reducing child labor and to see positive outcomes. In the Nigerian setting, traditional rulers are referred to as *Obas/Eze/Sultans/Obongs*. There is also an advisory council, which is usually composed of chiefs, heads of kindred and age group heads. Women are also represented in the Yoruba culture by the *Iyalode* (head of all the women) or *Iya loja* (head of all the market women). These leaders are the voices of women, representing their needs and feminine perspectives, thus promoting gender balance.

Traditional rulers are believed to be representative of deities on earth and are highly revered by the people. They serve as gatekeepers for the communities. Social services professionals may collaborate with these local power structures in promoting positive social care systems and preventing practices that jeopardize the social well-being of the citizens. Social workers may also collaborate with traditional rulers by utilizing their palace facilities to disseminate information or conduct community outreaches such as health screening, HIV counseling, award ceremonies for youth groups who have contributed to the battle against human trafficking or child labor.

Village meetings and festivals for education and awareness

Festive sacred cultural gatherings, such as the Igbo New Yam Festival (Ikejiani, 2015), are rallying points, when people come together to celebrate as a part of village life. Masquerades are believed to be gods coming to visit the earth. Subsequently, even members of the community who reside in the cities return to the villages to participate in such festivities to partake of the blessings from the gods. A social worker who collaborates with the indigenous facilitators of village meetings and festivals to stimulate community awareness would be linkages and brokers of information – critical factors in effective public social protection processes.

Many Nigerians either do not know or refuse to accept that trafficking is a crime. Effective governmental monitoring can occur if the population at large understands child labor laws and are willing to report violations. The use of statutory village meetings and festivals can support the processes of educating and creating awareness of the need and realities of child protection deficits in Nigeria. Subsequently, social workers may collaborate with elders and leaders for the inclusion of public education presentations within village meetings and festivals, as deemed appropriate. Education and awareness activities about child protection needs may also be incorporated into the traditional celebrations through plays, folklore, and dances.

In addition to child protection, the issues of stigmatization of PLHIV may be addressed through folk plays and dances. To implement this form of public awareness, social workers may collaborate with youth groups on how folklore, plays, and dances can be utilized in creating awareness of available services, and the fostering of positive attitudes toward PLHIV: These are critical parameters stipulated in the National Policy on HIV (NACA, 2010).

Given the belief that traditional rulers are revered and are seen as the representatives of the gods people take what they say seriously. This belief may be a helpful measure in the summoning of communities for village meetings outside of festivals to address social protection needs, as well as a supportive factor, for social workers collaborating with community leaders in the facilitation of public awareness meeting. Usually, if there is a serious issue to be discussed, the entire village or town will be summoned by the traditional rulers through the town criers. When entire villages are brought together, issues identified, such as child protection deficits, can be addressed. This meeting would support the inclusion of villagers as stakeholders in the discussion and development of prevention measures and steps to sanction offenders.

Caution about harmful cultural practices

Recognizing ISC as a social protection complementary measure is culturally sensitive, and has the potential to enable comprehensive effective social initiatives on a governmental level. Social workers committed to the inclusion of ISC practices must be charged to recognize and address culturally induced tendencies to marginalize or exclude some members of the community, as well as cultural practices and beliefs that may be detrimental to the overall well-being of the community. Individuals in the context of family systems are negatively impacted by beliefs which support customs such as early marriage, child witchcraft, devaluation of the girl child, and other forms of gender discriminatory practices (Jones et al., 2012). There is also the existence of child labor in child fostering relationships, as well as physical abuse in form of child discipline. Though some of these practices have been intended to serve positive purposes, children are often exploited. Indigenous practices have also undergirded the marginalization or exclusion of some community members, relegating them to the life of an outcast. Amongst the Igbo people of Nigeria, an *Osu* in Ibo land is an outcast, not because of any offense he/she has committed but because of the social status of his or her progenitor. Their forefathers are believed to be slaves to their local deity, a status that cannot be changed by time or education. In places where this belief is still in practice, a free man is not permitted to freely associate with an *Osu*. Marriage between a free person and an *Osu* is forbidden.

It is imperative that sustainable and transformative social protection approaches in Nigeria engage with cultural beliefs, practices, and structures. Understanding and accepting the values and customs which interface with ISC, advocacy for indigenous practices must also be sensitive to the detrimental aspects of cultural beliefs and practices, which may undermine the efficacy of ISC. Revisiting and celebrating the virtues of ISC must be intentional in eradicating detrimental practices, while promoting social protection and care that is free of discrimination.

Conclusion

Focusing on social protection in Nigeria in the context of other current challenges such as terrorism and religious intolerance is imperative. Child-sensitive social protection deficits such as child trafficking, labor, and abuse weaken the overall sense of safety of the nation, despite the government's struggle to meet the challenges through legislations and programs. Such policies and programs are the Child's Rights Act, National HIV Policy, Care of Persons in Need (COPE), and Family Nutrition and Support Program (FNSP). It was observed that these laudable governmental interventions are fraught with enforcement issues, inadequate funding, fragmentation, and poor coordination. Thus, governmental social protection initiatives are in need of formal and informal complementary care systems. ISC was identified as a complementary care system with practices, beliefs, and structures that are native to Nigerian communities. ISC practices are undergirded by strong African beliefs in supernatural forces, deities, and collectivist beliefs and customs. Such ISC practices as kinship care, traditional cash transfer programs, festivals and ceremonies, youth vigilante groups, and traditional power structures promote well-being. It was proposed that ISC practices are affirmed by stakeholders such as governmental organizations, NGOs, civil societies, religious organizations, and international social services entities, and supported through funding and collaborations, to strengthen social protection of children and persons affected by HIV/AIDS in Nigeria.

References

A bill for an act to provide and protect the right of the Nigerian child and other related matters, 2003. (2003). Retrieved from www.nigeriarights.gov.ng/files/download/40.

Agbu, O. (2008). *Re-visiting corruption and human trafficking in Nigeria: Any progress?* Retrieved from www.ungift.org/docs/ungift/pdf/vf/backgroundpapers/OsitaAgbu_1.pdf.

Akinola, O. (2014). *Graduation and social protection in Nigeria: A critical analysis of the COPE CCT program.* Paper presented at the International Conference on Graduation and Social Protection. Kigali, Rwanda. Retrieved from www.ids.ac.uk/files/dmfile/Graduationconferencepaper-Akinola.pdf.

Amanyeiwe, U., Hatt, L., Arur, A., Taye, A., Mehta-Steffen, M., De Valdenebro, M.C., Ogungbemi, K., & Kombe, G. (2008). *Nigeria HIV/AIDS service provision assessment* (Health Systems 20/20 Project). Retrieved from http://catalog.ihsn.org/index.php/catalog/3333/download/48506.

Amao, I., & Akinlade, R. (2014) *Child labor in horticultural households in Bauchi State: A gender perspective.* Retrieved from https://mpra.ub.unimuenchen.de/55708/1/MPRA_paper_55708.pdf.

Asian Development Bank (ADB). (2003). *Social protection strategy: Our framework and strategies.* Retrieved from www.adb.org/sites/default/files/institutional-document/32100/social-protection.pdf.

Atolagbe, M.O.B. (1989). *Principles and practice of social welfare.* Paper presented at the External Studies Programs Series University of Ibadan, Nigeria.

Avert. (2012). *HIV & AIDS in Nigeria.* Retrieved from www.avert.org/hiv-aids-nigeria.htm.

Barrientos, A. (2007). *Introducing basic social protection in low-income countries: Lessons from existing programs* (BWPI Working Paper 6). Retrieved from www.bwpi.manchester.ac.uk/medialibrary/publications/working_papers/bwpi-wp-0607.pdf.

Belgrave, F.Z., & Allison, K.W. (2006). *African American psychology from Africa to America.* Thousand Oaks: Sage Publications.

Central Intelligence Agency. (2013–2014). *The world factbook: Africa – Nigeria.* Retrieved from www.cia.gov/library/publications/the-world-factbook/geos/ni.html.

Department for International Development, United Kingdom (DFID UK), HelpAge International, Hope & Homes for Children, Institute of Development Studies, International Labour Organization, Overseas Development Institute, Save the Children UK, United Nations Children's Fund (UNICEF), United Nations Development Programme (UNDP) and the World Bank. (2009). *Advancing child sensitive social protection.* Retrieved from www.unicef.org/socialpolicy/files/CSSP_joint_statement_9.13.10.pdf.

Devereux, S., & Sabates-Wheeler, R. (2004). *Transformative social protection* (IDS Working Paper 232). Retrieved from www.ids.ac.uk/files/dmfile/Wp232.pdf.

Devex Impact. (2015). *The family nutrition support program (FNSP) in Nigeria.* Retrieved from www.devex.com/impact/partnerships/family-nutritional-support program-fnsp-in-nigeria-130.

Dioka, A. (2014). *Human development report 2014 makes a case for sustaining human progress by reducing vulnerabilities and building resilience.* Retrieved from www.ng. undp.org/content/nigeria/en/home/presscenter/pressreleases/2014/08/18/-human-development-report-2014-makes-a-case-for-sustaining-human-progress-by-reducing-vulnerabilities-and-building resilience-.html.

Eseadi, C., Achagh, W., Ikechukwu-Ilomuanya, A.B., & Ogbuabor, S.E. (2015). Prevalence of baby factory in Nigeria: An emergent form of child abuse, trafficking and molestation of women. *International Journal of Interdisciplinary Research Methods,* *2*(1), 1–12.

Fiszbein, A., & Schady, N. (2009). *Conditional cash transfers: Reducing present and future poverty.* Retrieved from http://siteresources.worldbank.org/INTCCT/Resources/ 5757608-1234228266004/PRR-CCT_web_noembargo.pdf.

Global AIDS Monitoring and Evaluation Team (GAMET). (2008). *World Bank global HIV/AIDS program report – West Africa HIV/AIDS epidemiology and response synthesis – Characterization of the HIV epidemic and response in West Africa: Implications for prevention.* Retrieved from http://siteresources.worldbank.org/INTHIVAIDS/ Resources/375798-1132695455908/WestAfricaSynthesisNov26.pdf.

Hagen-Zanker, J., & Holmes, R. (2012). Social protection in Nigeria (Synthesis Report). Retrieved from www.odi.org/sites/odi.org.uk/files/odi-assets/publications-opinion-files/7583.pdf.

Henry J. Kaiser Family Foundation. (2015). *Fact sheet: The global HIV/AIDS epidemic.* Retrieved from http://files.kff.org/attachment/fact-sheet-the-global-hivaids-epidemic.

Holmes, R., Samson, M., Magoronga, W., & Akinrimisi, B. (with Morgan, J.) (2012). *The potential for cash transfers in Nigeria.* Retrieved from www.odi.org/sites/odi.org. uk/files/odi-assets/publications-opinion-files/7578.pdf.

Huntley, S.S. (2013). *The phenomenon of baby factories in Nigeria as a new trend in human trafficking* (ICD Brief 3). Retrieved from www.internationalcrimesdatabase.org/ upload/documents/20140916T170728-ICD%20Brief%203%20-%20Huntley.pdf.

Ife, J. (2001). Local and global practice: Relocating social work as a human rights profession in the new global order. *European Journal of Social Work, 4,* 5–15.

Ifeadikanwa, C. (2013). *Homelessness in Nigeria.* United States: Xlibris Corporation.

Ikejiani, O. (2015). *Yam festival in Igboland: The origin of yam.* Retrieved from http:// kaleidoscope.igbonet.com/culture/yamfestival/oikejiani.html.

International Labor Office (ILO). (2005). National program on the elimination of child labor in Nigeria (Internal Evaluation Summaries). Retrieved from www.ilo.org/ wcmsp5/groups/public/--edmas/-eval/documents/publication/wcms_149868.pdf.

Jansson, B.S. (2001). *The reluctant welfare society: American social welfare policies – past, present, and future* (4th ed.). United States: Brooks/Cole Thomson Learning.

Jones, N., Presler-Marshall, E., Cooke, N., & Akinrimisi, B. (2012). *Promoting synergies between protection and social protection in Nigeria.* Retrieved from www.odi.org/sites/odi.org.uk/files/odi-assets/publications-opinion-files/7579.pdf.

Kay, R. (2011). (Un)caring communities: Processes of marginalization and access to formal and informal care and assistance in rural Russia. *Journal of Rural Studies, 27*(1), 45–53. Retrieved from http://eprints.gla.ac.uk/45365/1/45365.pdf.

Kazeem, K. (2011). An integrated approach to social work practice in Nigeria. *College Student Journal Publisher, 45*(1). Retrieved from www.freepatentsonline.com/article/College-Student-Journal/252632763.html.

Kidd, S., & Wylde, E. (with Tiba, Z., Daniel Stein, S., & Vanden, O.). (2011). *Targeting the poorest: An assessment of the proxy means test methodology.* Retrieved from www.unicef.org/socialpolicy/files/targeting-poorest.pdf.

Lladan, M.T. (2011). *Combating trafficking of children and women under international and Nigerian legal regimes.* Presented at United Nations System and Program Training Workshop. Lagos, Nigeria: Nigerian Institute of Advanced Legal Studies, Lagos.

McDonnell, J., & Melton, G. (2008). Toward a science of community intervention. *Family Community Health, 31*, 113–125.

McDowell, J. (2006). Indicator measurements in comprehensive community initiatives. In A.C. Michalos (Ed.), *Social indicators research series (Vol. 27). Indicators of children's well-being: Understanding their role, usage and policy influence* (pp. 33–93). Dordrecht: Springer.

National Agency for the Control of AIDS (NACA). (2010). *National HIV/AIDS strategic plan 2010–2015.* Retrieved from www.ilo.org/aids/legislation/WCMS_146389/lang--en/index.htm.

National Agency for the Control of AIDS (NACA). (2012). Federal republic of Nigeria global AIDS response country progress report. (Nigeria GARPR 2012). Retrieved from www.unaids.org/en/dataanalysis/knowyourresponse/countryprogressreports/2012count ries/Nigeria%202012%20GARPR%20Report%20Revised.pdf.

National Agency for the Prohibition of Trafficking in Persons and Other Related Maters (NAPTIP). (2007). *Fact sheet 4: Trends in human trafficking in Nigeria.* Retrieved from www.naptip.gov.ng/docs/FACTSHEET0001.pdf.

National Agency for the Prohibition of Trafficking in Persons (NAPTIP). (2015). *First quarter 2015 report.* Retrieved from www.naptip.gov.ng/docs/First%20quarter%20report.pdf.

National Association of Social Workers (NASW). (1973). *Standards for social service manpower.* [Monograph]. Washington, DC: NASW.

Ogunkan, D.V. (2011). Begging and almsgiving in Nigeria: The Islamic perspective. *International Journal of Sociology and Anthropology, 3*(4), 127–131.

Okpukpara, B.C. & Odurukwe, N. (2006). *Incidence and determinants of child labor in Nigeria: Implications for poverty alleviation* (African Economic Research Consortium [AERC] Research Paper Research Paper 156). Retrieved from www.sarpn.org/documents/d0002214/Child_labour_Nigeria_Jun2006.pdf.

Olagbegi, B.O. (2006). *Human trafficking in Nigeria: Root causes and recommendations* (Policy Paper Series Number14.2 [E]). Retrieved from http://unesdoc.unesco.org/images/0014/001478/147844e.pdf.

Olaore, A., & Drolet, J. (submitted). Indigenous knowledge, beliefs, and social care practices for children and families in Nigeria. *Journal of Ethnic and Cultural Diversity in Social Work.*

Oxford Business Group. (2013). *The report: Nigeria 2013.* Retrieved from www.oxfordbusinessgroup.com/nigeria-2013.

Pebley, A.R., & Sastry, N. (2003). *Neighborhoods, poverty, and children's well-being* (Draft). Retrieved from www.russellsage.org/sites/all/files/Pebley%26Sastry.pdf.

Samuels, F., Blake, C., & Akinrimisi, B. (2012). *HIV vulnerabilities and the potential for strengthening social protection responses in the context of HIV in Nigeria*. Retrieved from www.unicef.org/nigeria/HIV_sensitive_social_protection_the_case_of_Nigeria.pdf.

Sanubi, Franklins A. (2011). *Social protection as a residual safety net in democratic governance in Nigeria: A critical analysis of some current policy initiatives*. Retrieved from www.ids.ac.uk/files/dmfile/sanubi2011socialprotectionandgovernanceinnigeriac-spconferencedraft.pdf.

Uche, O.C.O., & Ogugua, P.I. (2013). Religion and African identity: A reflection on Nigerian situation. *Open Journal of Philosophy*, *3*, 248–254.

Uko, C. (2015). Community partnerships for care of orphans and vulnerable children: Sagamu community centre, Sagamu local government & Olabisi Onabanjo teaching hospital: A child welfare collaborative (Internship Report).

United Nations (UN). (1989). *Convention on the rights of the child*. Retrieved from www.ohchr.org/Documents/ProfessionalInterest/crc.pdf.

United Nations (UN). (2008). *Millennium development goals indicators: Official list of MDG indicators*. Retrieved from http://mdgs.un.org/unsd/mdg/host.aspx? Content=indicators/officiallist.htm.

United Nations (UN). (2015). *The millennium development goals report 2015*. Retrieved from www.un.org/millenniumgoals/2015_MDG_Report/pdf/MDG%202015%20rev%20%28July%201%29.pdf.

United Nations International Children's Fund (UNICEF). (2007a). *Child trafficking* (Information Sheet). Retrieved from www.unicef.org/wcaro/WCARO_Nigeria_Factsheets_ChildTrafficking.pdf.

United Nations International Children's Fund (UNICEF). (2007b). *The child's rights act* (Information Sheet). Retrieved from www.unicef.org/wcaro/WCARO_Nigeria_Factsheets_CRA.pdf.

United Nations International Children's Fund (UNICEF). (2006). *Child labor – UNICEF Nigeria 2006* (Information Sheet). Retrieved from www.unicef.org/wcaro/WCARO_Nigeria_Factsheets_ChildLabour.pdf.

United Nations International Children's Fund (UNICEF). (2015). *UNICEF social inclusion, policy and budgeting*. Retrieved from www.unicef.org/socialpolicy/index_social-protection.html.

United Nations Development Programs (UNDP). (2014). *Sustaining human progress: Reducing vulnerabilities and building resilience explanatory note on the 2014 human development report composite indices: Nigeria: HDI values and rank changes in the 2014*. Retrieved from http://hdr.undp.org/sites/all/themes/hdr_theme/country-notes/NGA.pdf.

US Advisory Board on Child Abuse and Neglect. (1993). *Neighbors helping neighbors: A new national strategy for the protection of children* (Fourth Report). Retrieved from www.clemson.edu/centers-institutes/ifnl/documents/neighbors_helping_neighbors.pdf.

Vaughan, O. (1995). Assessing grassroots politics and community development in Nigeria. *African Affairs*, *94*(377), 501–518.

World Bank. (2011). *Safety nets and transfers: CCT program country profile – Nigeria*. Retrieved from http://web.worldbank.org/WBSITE/EXTERNAL/TOPICS/EXTSO-CIALPROTECTION/EXTSAFETYNETSANDTRANSFERS/0,,contentMDK:220636 21~pagePK:148956~piPK:216618~theSitePK:282761~isCURL:Y,00.html.

World Population Review. (2015). World population review countries: Nigeria population 2014. Retrieved from http://worldpopulationreview.com/countries/nigeria-population/.

13 Social protection, disaster risk reduction and community resilience

Evidence from rural areas in Indonesia

Saut Sagala, Dodon Yamin, Alpian A. Pratama and Elisabeth Rianawati

Introduction

Social protection includes a number of measures or schemes in developed and developing countries to alleviate the burden faced by the poor in society. Social protection (SP) has various means and functions. One of the important functions is the role of SP in fostering disaster risk reduction (DRR), and climate change adaptation (CCA), which came to be defined and understood as adaptive social protection (ASP). Davies et al. (2009) admit that there is a high relevance of SP for reducing vulnerability in society. The similar characteristics among the goals, target groups and tools of SP and DRR make it promising for sharing opportunity in achieving community resilience (Davies et al., 2009; Heltberg et al., 2008). A valid question that remains is: What is the role of SP in promoting long-term community resilience in disaster contexts?

Twigg (2007) defines community resilience as a community that has capacities "to absorb stress or destructive forces through resistance or adaptation; to manage, or maintain certain basic functions and structures, during disastrous events; and to recover after an event" (p. 6). Resilience is a state where people can adapt to environmental changes (Adger, 2000, p. 1). In order to achieve community resilience, several initiatives are integrating SP, DRR and CCA approaches in disaster-affected areas. For instance, the Reducing Vulnerability to Climate Change (RVCC) project in Bangladesh distributed assets such as ducks to rear, in order to provide alternative livelihoods to the local community affected by climate change related disasters (Mallik, 2006, in Davies et al., 2009). Another form of social protection is the National Rural Employment Guarantee Act (NREGA) in India that guarantees 100 days of employment in a year to rural populations in public work programs such as de-silting irrigation and strengthening embankments (Davies et al., 2009). This chapter focuses on Indonesian social protection schemes in reducing community risks from disasters. In 2015, the Indonesian population reached 255.4 million people and about less than half of the population are living in rural areas and mostly are supported by agriculture (BPS, 2015). In Indonesia, poverty is found more in the rural areas rather than in the urban population, with poverty rates of 14.3% and 8.4% respectively in 2012 (OECD, 2015, p. 24).

In addition to poverty, a large number of rural areas in Indonesia are prone to disaster risks due to their geographic location in disaster prone areas. By the definition set in the disaster management regulation in Indonesia (No. 24/2007), the disaster prone area is "territory for a certain period of time are not able to reduce the adverse effects of a hazard (geological, hydrological, biological, climatological, geographical, social, cultural, political, economic, and technological)," such as along the coasts, high slopes areas and active seismic faults and volcanoes. Within the past decade (2004–2014), a large number of rural areas in Indonesia were hit by catastrophic natural hazards, such as tsunamis, earthquakes and volcanoes that claimed lives of nearly 200,000 people and resulted in about 10 million people injured (BNPB, 2015).

Slow onset disasters also plague Indonesia, particularly in the eastern parts of the country. For example, West Timor has been impacted by sea level rise and drought that deteriorated agriculture and fishery production, which consequently complicated the livelihood of the community in the long term. This situation has forced some people to be temporarily or permanently displaced within the country. For example, members of villages in the South of Sikka District, NTT Province in Indonesia had to move further into the mainland since their communities have been inundated by increasing sea levels.

In general, there are at least two generations of social protection programs in Indonesia (Sumarto & Bazzi, 2011). The first generation of social protection was initiated in 1998 and covered five major sectors of food security, education, health, provision of employment and community empowerment. The second generation was started in 2000 and was based on two national laws: National Law 40/2004 on national social protection system and National Law 24/2011 on national protection administered body. Under Law No. 40/2004, Indonesia has several social protection schemes including health protection, accidents at work protection, old age pension and death protection. Apart from nationally administered social protection, there are other measures implemented by the Indonesian government such as a direct cash transfer program or cash for work program.

In the second generation, the social protection programs were clustered into three divisions. The first division comprised of major social programs such as rice for the poor (Raskin), Unconditional Cash Transfer (UCT), Conditional Cash Transfer (CCT), Health Insurance for the Poor (Askeskin) and scholarship programs. The second division consists of National Program for Community Empowerment (PNPM), which was established in 2008. The third division focused on expanding the small-scale enterprises (SME) by providing microcredit (Sumarto & Bazzi, 2011).

The PNPM is a large-scale program that assists rural and urban poor communities to improve their living conditions through community infrastructure development and provides cash to the workforces involved in the program. It covered 200 million people in over 70,000 villages by 2011 (Sumarto & Bazzi,

2011). In some disaster prone areas, some of the works include the strengthening of water channels and establishing evacuation routes.

This chapter will discuss the role of PNPM in disaster risk reduction in Indonesia and its contribution to community resilience. The concepts related to social protection in reducing disaster risk and promoting long-term community resilience are explored by considering the role of SP in Indonesia. This chapter further discusses these concepts by considering several key questions as follows:

1   What is the role of SP initiatives in supporting disaster risk reduction in Indonesia?
2   What prerequisite conditions are needed to extend the role of SP in achieving community resilience?
3   How do social workers enhance community resilience?

The chapter presents a case study developed from research findings on the role of SP in promoting community resilience in Indonesia. Finally, the chapter considers how SP schemes have contributed towards reducing disaster risks and the contribution of social workers in enhancing community resilience in the study areas.

Literature

SP is defined by the International Labour Organization (ILO) as:

> a set of public measures that a society provides for its members to protect them against economic and social distress that would be caused by the absence or a substantial reduction of income from work as a result of various contingencies (sickness, maternity, employment injury, unemployment, invalidity, old age, and death of the breadwinner); the provision of health care; and, the provision of benefits for families with children.
>
> (ILO, 2003, p. 13)

The concept of SP is not static and evolves as societies change. The basic objective of SP is to cover the risks associated with being too poor. Different actors such as governments, local authorities and charitable organizations provided the earliest forms of public assistance.

Social protection in disaster risk management

Disaster risk reduction is the concept and practice of reducing disaster risks through systematic efforts to analyze and reduce the causal factors of disasters (UNISDR, 2014). According to the United Nations' Sendai Framework for Disaster Risk Reduction 2015–2030, disaster risk reduction needs to be based on an understanding of disaster risk in all its dimensions of vulnerability, capacity, exposure of persons and assets, hazard characteristics and the environment

(UNISDR, 2015, p. 14). While both social protection and disaster risk reduction are commonly designed for short-term programs, they have the potential to promote long-term community resilience. Enhancing capacity and reducing vulnerabilities is part of building resilience for society as stated in recent Sendai Framework (UNISDR, 2015). In the link between disaster risk management (DRM) and community resilience, SP can play a role to mediate and serve as a catalyst in the process toward community resilience. For example, the Stern Review (2007) states that SP could act as an important element of adaptation and that SP could give "additional resources required to tackle it, into planning and budgeting" (p. 425) of a comprehensive DRM. Moreover, social protection and disaster risk reduction have overlapping targets, such as to reduce the risks faced by vulnerable groups, to tackle the impacts of disaster, and to seek to build resilience in post-disaster contexts. Furthermore, when SP is introduced and added with the sustainable livelihood people have, it can be a resource not only to develop preparedness but also to sustain capacity toward resilience. This can be explained as follows. During the time of crisis, people become dependent on aid and external support to meet basic needs that cannot be met by the people themselves. This certainly cannot last long because sooner or later the short-term aid or relief will stop. Thus, the realization of sustainable livelihoods is needed. If the community in the disaster prone area is able to create sustainable livelihoods then they are able to implement the "living with risk" concept. This concept puts emphasis on a disaster risk reduction strategy rather than on humanitarian response and relief activities (UNISDR, 2004). Social protection aims to "help rural people not only to expand their assets, but to use them efficiently and adopt higher return activities" (Davies et al., 2009, p. 12); it could improve the overall resilience of the community and make them less vulnerable to disasters or climate change impacts.

Integration of social protection and disaster risk management

SP initiatives introduced in disaster prone areas to reduce the vulnerability of the people can be found in South Asia (Heltberg, 2007, in Davies et al., 2009; Béné et al., 2014), where India and Bangladesh have shown the most progressive advancement of SP and DRR integration (Davies et al., 2013). This is in line with recent attempts to shift DRR away from reactive, post-disaster coping strategies such as providing food aid toward more proactive and long-term disaster preparedness and management (Hellmuth et al., 2011; Heltberg, 2007). SP programs are also used in the absence of effective risk reduction and mitigation measures, or after these have failed or have been exhausted (Devereux et al., 2012). Examples include cash transfer programs developed in response to a disaster that offers direct assistance in the form of cash to the target group (Vishwanath & Yu, 2008). The cash transfer program or what is commonly known as cash for work (CFW) is often designed for a temporary period until economic activities pick up and generate employment opportunities. CFW programs have been implemented after floods in Bangladesh, in conflict-affected regions like

Afghanistan and the Democratic Republic of the Congo, and, most recently, in the tsunami-affected regions of Indonesia and Sri Lanka. In Indonesia the CFW program was a public work program involved 18,000 participants in 60 villages after the 2004 Asian tsunami (Doocy et al., 2006, p. 279). Public work programs in post-disaster contexts serve to create or restore much-needed infrastructure in the disaster-affected areas, through debris removal, repair of community water supply and sanitation, repair or construction of public buildings, and minor road repairs.

A number of comprehensive initiatives are presented by Davies et al. (2009), who examined 124 programs in South Asia that show full integration of SP, CCA and DRR approaches into adaptive social protection (ASP). They found the practice is relatively limited, although combining SP with DRR has become more common in the last 10 years. In the case of SP–DRR projects, a number of new and innovative approaches to vulnerability reduction can be observed. Of particular interest is the use of vulnerability mapping in food security and DRR projects where social and natural science disciplines focusing on risks and poverty assessment are brought together. This suggests that there has been some movement within the DRR community toward acknowledging and integrating the underlying social dimensions of vulnerability that people face.

Social work perspective for increasing community resilience

Miller et al. (2011) pointed out that social work is committed to responding to marginalized individuals, families and communities for achieving social justice. Furthermore, social workers contribute to building community awareness about social protection schemes and facilitating commnunity participation, and integrating community perspectives in the implementation process. In this manner social workers contribute to building community resilience. Without supports from social workers, social protection schemes have limitations to achieve wider community impacts, particularly with those who have limited access due to education, awareness and power. It is important to consider the roles of social workers in the implementation of social protection schemes. In developing countries, where governments have limitations, social workers are engaged in social programs offered by non-governmental organizations (NGOs) working on economic and social development issues (Tierney, 2012), and this is the case in Indonesia (Lassa et al., 2013). The next section describes social protection measures in Indonesia.

Social protection in Indonesia

President Susilo Bambang Yudhoyono launched PNPM Mandiri in 2007. This program was created to scale up poverty reduction programs from previous eras. PNPM Mandiri was designed to coordinate tens of poverty reduction programs administered by various departments that existed at that time. It adopted the use of community development as an operational approach. Several national ministries are involved in SP including the Ministry of Social Welfare, Coordinating Ministry for Citizen Welfare, Ministry of Education, Ministry of Health, Coordinating Ministry for Economy. PNPM was delivered in block grants to selected districts to rebuild community infrastructure at the village level in urban and rural areas. The districts were selected based on the severity of poverty and the magnitude of the poor population. The amount of block grant ranged from IDR1–3.5 billion or US$110,000–365,000 (Voss, 2012, p. 6).

Before PNPM Mandiri was launched in 2007, there were several poverty alleviation programs in Indonesia, which used the concept of community development for their program implementation. The earliest program was Inpres Desa Tertinggal (IDT), literally translated into "Presidential Instruction on Underdeveloped Villages," which began in 1993. The IDT program was implemented by providing funds of US$2,000 for every village each year. There were over 20,000 villages and the fund was provided for three years. The IDT program reached 28,376 villages with the total amount of grant of IDR1.5 trillion or US$110 million, and this is one of the largest social protection programs in Indonesian history (BAPPENAS, 2013, p. 14). In addition, the government provided technical support for rural communities in order to utilize the fund. The goal and targets of the program was to empower the poor in under-developed villages, such as laborers, forest dwellers, fishermen, peasants and young dropouts. Under-developed villages themselves are defined as "lagging behind in their development pace relative to the rest of the nation" (BAPPENAS, 1994, in Akita and Szeto, 2000).

Conceptually, the goal and the target recipient were as they should be. However, the IDT program was based on a biased database since the definition of poor people was determined by village meetings instead of by national definition or statistical database. Although this system reduced the potential local conflict, there was inequality of target recipients between villages, as the definition of poor people varied among villages. Moreover, since most of the under-developed villages were located in remote areas, the micro-enterprises arising from the IDT program in the villages were not supported by basic infrastructure like road and transportation and unavailability of receiving market (Sarman & Sajogyo, 2000, p. 27).

Learning from the strengths and weaknesses of IDT, the second generation of poverty alleviation programs was initiated, which included: Sub-district Development Program (KDP) carried out by the Department of the Interior in 1998, P2KP (Urban Poverty Programme) which was implemented the Department of Public Works in 1999, PEMP (Coastal Community Economic Empowerment) implemented by the Department of Marine and Fisheries, KUBE (Joint Group of Enterprise) carried out by the Ministry of Social Affairs, and others. These programs were run according to the policy and aim of each department, which were limited and sectoral (BAPPENAS, 2013).

In order to have an integrated poverty alleviation program, the Indonesian government launched the National Program for Community Empowerment (PNPM) in 2007. PNPM Mandiri program aimed to alleviate poverty using a "bottom-up" approach by providing mentoring and funds for the community to create their own projects related to basic infrastructures, small-scale enterprises and to provide funds for education purposes. Through a participatory development scheme, the program aims to promote critical awareness and self-reliance of the community.

PNPM Mandiri as social protection

The PNPM Mandiri was categorized in three areas: rural areas (Sub-district Development Program), urban areas (Urban Poverty Alleviation Program), and under-developed regions such as post-disaster or conflict areas (Accelerating Development of Underdeveloped Regions – Disadvantaged and Special District Program).

In 2008, the PNPM Mandiri program was integrated with the Regional Socio-Economic Development Infrastructure (RISE) to attach economic growth in rural areas with the economic growth in sub-district areas. PNPM Mandiri was reinforced with community development programs from various departments, sectors and local governments, whereas the priority was focused in poor villages.

The integration of pre-existing projects into the policy framework of PNPM Mandiri was done in order to have a more extended coverage of the poverty alleviation programs, particularly in remote and isolated areas. In addition, the effectiveness and efficiency of programs were expected to increase by eliminating overlapping programs. Given that the empowerment programs would take effect over 5–6 years, the PNPM Mandiri was projected to last until 2015, which is in line with targets for the Indonesian Millennium Development Goals (MDGs). The MDGS raised the prospect of women and children's well-being by reducing poverty, improving health and access to education. Moreover, Indonesia has achieved the first MDG goal to reduce extreme poverty ahead of 2015 due to strong per capita income growth and more efficient and well-targeted poverty reduction programs (OECD, 2015; UNICEF Indonesia, 2012). The government of Indonesia's success in strengthening economic recovery was accompanied by a series of social protection interventions such as health insurance for the poor, social assistance and community-based poverty reduction programs (UNICEF Indonesia, 2012, p. 6).

Research methodology and study areas

This chapter will share the results of research based on qualitative analysis of PNPM in two rural districts of Indramayu and Sleman in Indonesia. Indramayu is prone to floods and droughts, while Sleman is prone to volcanic eruptions. The data for this chapter is based on fieldwork surveys conducted by the authors. In Indramayu, the authors carried out field research such as observation and interviews, from 2011 to 2014, in disaster risk management studies and migration (Sagala & Sani, 2014; Sagala et al., 2012). In Sleman, the authors carried out field research from 2008 to 2013.

Rural areas in Indramayu

Indramayu District is located in West Java Province on the north coast of Java Island. Indramayu District is one of the poorest districts in the province of West Java Province. Many farmers do not own their land, and thus rent or borrow land from the landowners. It is reported that 11 of 31 sub-districts in Indramayu have high levels of poverty (BPS Indramayu, 2014, p. ii).

The district is mostly dominated by agriculture activities, and is the main source of national rice production. The impacts of climate change such as extreme weather, drought and floods have significantly hampered rice production. As a result, people's livelihoods have changed from agriculture-based sectors to business or commercial based sectors between 2005 and 2009.

Indramayu experiences floods due in part to the flat topography of the district, with the average slope of 0–2% and the altitude between 0–100 meters above mean sea level (Bappeda Indramayu, 2011, p. II–1). Both tidal floods and river floods contribute to the occurrence of floods in Indramayu District. In early 1990, flooding started to affect the eastern Indramayu District. Over the years, the flood area extended to the western part of the district. Indramayu's most recent flood map of 2008 shows that 20 of 31 sub-districts are prone to flooding. The potential flooding area has reached 40,000–50,000 hectares, covering residential areas and paddy fields (Ministry of Agriculture, 2010, p. 18).

Indramayu District is also a drought prone area. Since 1990, the drought-affected area was 171,071 hectares, which occurred on a large scale in 2003 and 2008, and reached about 102,000 hectares (BNPB, 2015). The crop failures due to the drought were equal to the loss of 65,000 tons of rice in 2008 alone (22,870 ha rice plantation failed to be harvested, 2008). The next section will describe the Sleman District.

Rural Sleman District

Sleman District is located in the northern part of Yogyakarta Province. The population of Sleman District in 2010 was 1,117,176 people, with the number of men as many as 555,070 (49.68%) and women as many as 562,106 (50.31%) (Bappeda Sleman, 2011, chapter II, pp. 12–13). Livelihoods in Sleman are mostly in the trading, hotels and restaurants (25%), in the service sector (24%), and in farming and agriculture (22%) (Bappeda Sleman, 2011, p. II-15). Sleman is the center of cow farming in Yogyakarta Province, accounting for 90% of the total livestock of cows (Yogyakarta Agricultural Bureau, 2011). A large portion of Sleman District is used for the agricultural sector, and this accounts for 63.5% of the total area, which is mainly used for rice plantation (44%) (Bappeda Sleman, 2011, p. II-10).

Overall, the geological condition in Sleman District is dominated by the presence of Mount Merapi. To date, there have been two major volcanic eruptions from Mount Merapi, the 2006 and 2010 eruptions. In 2010, Mount Merapi became active and released multiple eruptions between the months of September to November, in which two eruptions were notably enormous. The first one took place on October 26, 2010 and the second on November 11, 2010. Along with the massive damages to homes and local infrastructure, there were 2,347 fatalities reported and 500 people were injured (Sagala et al., 2012; The Secretariat of the JRF, 2012; Wimbardana et al., 2013, p. 2). An estimated 410,338 people were displaced and spread over about 640 different locations (Wimbardana et al., 2013, p. 2). The losses of livestock in Sleman District were estimated to be IDR48.2 billion (around US$5.4 million), whereas the impact to the agriculture sector amounted to IDR238.3 billion (around US$26.5 million) (Bappeda Sleman, 2011, p. II-5). Another impact of the eruption was the reduced dairy production by 50% to 70% (Priyanti and Ilham, 2011, p. 158). More significant losses were experienced in damaged settlements, which accounted for IDR580.8 billion (US$64.5 million) and in damaged infrastructure such as transportation, clean water networks, electricity, telecommunication, health and social services which in total accounted to IDR160 billion (US$18 million) (BAPPENAS & BNPB, 2011, p. i–ii). The next section discusses SP implementation and its role for community resilience in Indramayu District and Sleman District.

Social protection in rural Indonesia

Disaster risk reduction, SP measures and roles in achieving community resilience will be presented, and the role of social workers in each case study drawing upon the experiences of two rural districts.

Social protection program in Indramayu

The government of Indonesia and the Indramayu District government have launched various programs for poverty alleviation. Some of the social protection initiatives are as follows: Social Security Agency (BPJS), Aid for Low Income Students (BSM), PNPM Rural, Productive Economic Business (UEP) and the Women's Savings and Loans (SPP). Table 13.1 shows the various forms of social security in Indramayu District.

BPJS Program is a national program that integrates the social security and health insurance. BPJS is a statutory body established to administer social security programs such as health and employment. The program is aimed to Indonesian citizens in general, who are divided into two categories: recipients of health fund and non-recipients of health fund. The recipients of health fund are those who fall into poor and near-poor category; this category is exempted from monthly premiums, whereas the other category is required to pay monthly premiums. The premiums themselves are subsidized by the government of Indonesia. In 2014 the local government allocated US$3.6 million to support the national BPJS in Indramayu District, where BPJS was integrated with another health insurance known as Jamkesda (the regional health insurance). Currently, BPJS in Indramayu district was distributed to 75% of the population; some of the people who are not covered by BPJS are thousands of fishermen and

Table 13.1 Social protection programs in Indramayu District

Program	Abbreviation	Activity	Fund	Beneficiaries
Social Security Agency	BPJS	Health care insurance for Indonesian people, especially for the low income	US$3.6 million (National)	922,978 people
Low income Student Aid	BSM	Financial aid for education related fees	US$582,600	57,800 students
National Program for Rural Community Empowerment	PNPM Mandiri rural	Direct funds for the development of physical and economic infrastructure in the sub-district and village level	US$14.83 million	All sub-districts in Indramayu
Enterprise for Productive Economy	UEP	Empowerment of small and micro enterprises through micro-credit programs	US$544,600	2,253 groups
Women Saving and Loans	SPP	Funds for women	US$997,700	31,793 women

employees in around 175 private companies (Republika, 2015; Seruu, 2013). The people do not apply the BPJS due to their hesitancy to pay the monthly premium, even 22,000 of BPJS participants in Indramayu failed to pay a total amount of IDR5.6 billion (US$430,000) in 2015 (Barat, 2015).

The second poverty alleviation program in Indramayu is students aid (BSM), which is combined with the School Operational Assistance (BOS). BSM is distributed to poor and almost-poor students to cover their personal expenditure. BSM uses several approaches such as scholarships, cash transfer to students, contingent on enrollment, bursaries, among others. The BOS is transferred to secondary schools based on the number of poor students in each school. For each poor student, the school would receive IDR1.2 million (US$133) per year to cover the education fee. In 2014, the government of Indramayu allocated US$582,600 to fund 57,800 students. In 2015, the program was renamed as the "Program Indonesia Pintar" (PIP) or Smart Indonesia Program (OECD, 2015).

Poverty alleviation programs and the protection of the public in Indramayu District is focused on how to empower people who mostly work in the agricultural sector and fisheries. Health and education are generally administered by the local government of various national programs in the district of Indramayu. While the infrastructure and social sector are developed mainly through the PNPM rural scheme. The PNPM rural scheme in Indramayu consists of several programs such as: Savings and Loan for Women, cash transfers, micro-credit programs and Prospective Family programs. Each program will be discussed in the next section.

Program Keluarga Harapan or Prospective Family program is a cash transfer based program, which targets the very poor household. The short-term goal of the program is to alleviate the economic burden of the very poor household, whereas the long-term goal is to break the chain of intergenerational poverty, so the next generation can come out of the poverty trap (TNP2K, 2015). In this program, the very poor family should be represented by the female family members in receiving the cash transfer. The cash transfer received for a family ranged from IDR1,300,000–2,800,000 (US$100–215), which varied according to the size of the family, the number of school-aged members of the family and the maternal condition of the mother (TNP2K, 2015). In Indramayu, around 10,000 very poor families received the PKH grant in 2014, whereas the total budget for the whole Indramayu District is IDR10 billion per year (US$770,000) (Republika, 2014).

Kredit Usaha Rakyat (KUR), literally translated into "credit for people's enterprise," provides grants from IDR5–500 million (US$385–385,000) which aims to enable the development of small or medium enterprises in the local community (TNP2K, 2015). The grants were distributed through banks that have partnerships with the government of Indonesia for the KUR program. The initial scheme from the government was to provide grants without collateral, when the amount is below IDR20 million (US$1,540), nonetheless as the procedure of KUR is handed over to the bank, in some cases the bank requires the people to provide collateral to obtain the credit (Kustiasih, 2011). As a result, out of

52,000 recipients of KUR in four districts of West Java Province – including Indramayu District – only 17% or 8,840 recipients are farmers and fishermen (Kustiasih, 2011).

The saving and loan program for women is a form of social empowerment program in the economic sector. The program focuses on providing assistance to women's groups covering various social, economic and cultural aspects. The aim of the program is to develop a normative paradigm of entrepreneurship for women in order to inspire home business or house production activities. Empowering women in entrepreneurship is considered to be a strategic approach as the structure of production and business in Indonesia is dominated by micro, and small and medium enterprises (SMEs), which account for 55.2 million units (99.98%) (Ministry of Cooperatives and Small and Medium Enterprise, 2012, p. 3). Interestingly, 60% of SMEs are run by women (Ministry Women's Empowerment and Child Protection, 2012, p. 2). Nonetheless, in spite of the considerable number of women entrepreneurs, the patriarchy norms in Indonesia impede the growth of women SMEs, particularly in rural areas (UN-ESCAP, 2013). One of the biggest challenges faced by women is obtaining external financial support and funding for their SMEs. For example, some women are required to produce the co-signature of a male family member when applying for credit. In other cases, women have to compete with the male to obtain credit schemes, which may be deemed to be more reliable by financial institutions, due to sociocultural reasons, such as patriarchy norms (UN-ESCAP, 2013). It is estimated that 41% of women entrepreneurs fund their own SMEs, in comparison to 29% who obtain commercial credit (UN-ESCAP, 2013, p. 26). In 2014, the Ministry of Home Affairs and the local government allocated a budget of US$997,700, which was given to 31,793 women in Indramayu District through small loans. Another economic empowerment program in rural Indramayu was a scheme called Productive and Economic Enterprise (UEP), which aimed to enhance the creative economy. Under this scheme in 2014, the local government allocated a fund of US$544,600 which was given to 2,253 groups of people in Indramayu District. These small groups of enterprise were the targets of empowerment so that the budding enterprises would be more resilient to economic hazards.

Cash transfers are provided in order to meet basic needs as a result of rising fuel prices and to improve community resilience. For example, the Rural Agribusiness Development (PUAP) is an organization formed by the Ministry of Agriculture and operates in rural areas. PUAP comprises a local farmers' union, known as GAPOKTAN in Indramayu, and its supervising agency, Mitra Tani. Through PUAP, the government distributes the funds to the farmers' union, and monitors its implementation through the supervising agency. In addition to economic empowerment in Indramayu District, PNPM Self-Supported Rural also initiated community empowerment by involving them in the development of rural infrastructure such as the construction of roads, drainage, sanitation facilities and schools. The budget for the development of infrastructure was the biggest allocation noted to date, which amounted to US$14.83 million for building the facilities in villages and sub-district of Indramayu. However, in the implementation the rural PNPM faced several challenges and constraints such as capital or loans granted by PNPM Mandiri program were not sufficient to meet the needs of the community. The loans were provided in small amounts and led to the under-developed community businesses. Other challenges that were found in the implementation of PNPM in Indramayu are:

1   the lack of community participation in the conception and development of projects;
2   the lack of coordination in target village selection, which have resulted in several conflicts between villages; and
3   the high dependency of villagers toward the capital given from PNPM program (Katiman, 2012).

Social protection programs in Sleman

The government of Indonesia provided emergency disaster assistance using the PNPM to distribute disaster recovery management support. In November 2010, during the Coordination Meeting for Merapi Disaster Management, the Vice President of Indonesia, Mr. Boediono, instructed immediate assistance for livelihood projects to commence, between the emergency response phase and the rehabilitation and reconstruction phase. One of the most prominent examples of a livelihood project was volcano-based tourism, which generated temporary income for the community (Sagala et al., 2012; Wijayanti & Sagala, 2012) and which was used for the recovery and revitalization of the affected communities (Kemenko Kesra, 2011). In addition, the cash for work program was launched so that the community could have an alternative source of livelihood to support recovery and to restore prior cattle ownership jobs and feeding grass affected by the Mount Merapi eruption.

Cash for work in Sleman was implemented under PNPM Urban and PNPM Rural schemes (Coordinating Ministry for People's Welfare of the Republic Indonesia and PNPM Support Facility (PSF), 2011). Cash for work activities were a strategic initiative during the transition from emergency to the recovery phase. The cash for work activities enabled communities to earn some income from simple works. The program helped the affected community members to revive and recover from the impacts of the Merapi eruption shocks. The assistance enabled affected community members to strengthen coping strategies and build adaptive capacity, and contributes to disaster risk reduction by protecting the most vulnerable through livelihood diversification (Davies et al., 2008).

In addition, cash for work activity in Sleman covered both temporary and permanent settlement, infrastructures and public facilities, such as cleaning up tourist attractions such as the Mbah Maridjan Tomb.

The PNPM Support Facility committee established the Disaster Management Support project in 2011 (Choi & Tomlinson, 2013). The project supports the community through three main programs such as PNPM Urban, Community-based Settlement Rehabilitation and Reconstruction (Rekompak) program, and PNPM Rural. The cash for work program ended in December 2011 (BAPPENAS and BNPB, 2011). The grant for the second stage came from the governments of Australia, Denmark, Netherlands, United Kingdom, United States, and the European Union, which was managed by the World Bank through the PNPM Support Facility program with funding of US$4.3 million (Choi & Tomlinson, 2013).

The target groups were selected by interviewing the village leader to get information on the poorest households in the community, workers' database, and a collection based on the Family Register and National Identity Card by local neighborhood leaders. The cash for work program was divided into two phases. The funding source of the first phase (2011–2012) was allocated from Emergency Response Fund managed by the National Board for Disaster Management (BNPB). The second phase started from January until December 2012. The first phase cash for work activity involved around 14,000 workers from local neighborhoods and 195,936 for the second phase. The standard wage ranged from US$3–7 per day per worker depending on the worker's skill level (Kemenko Kesra, 2011). In some locations, cash for work activities were in synergy with activities of other agencies that were using heavy equipment. Thus, cash for work made an even wider impact on the welfare of the surrounding communities.

Residents who were affected by the Mount Merapi eruption were evacuated to some fixed residential locations. The fixed residential places were located outside the hazardous area based on maps established by the government. The development of fixed residences was funded by the Java Reconstruction Fund (JRF) and carried out with the help of Rekompak. To build this permanent housing, each family received funding of IDR30 million (US$2,500) for the house construction. However, the amount was not sufficient to build a house. Therefore, the community collectively built their homes and a local committee coordinated the construction.

To improve the condition of the local community after the disaster, the government provided support by distributing resources (Tobin & Whiteford, 2002). The Indonesian government distributed cows in Sleman to indemnify livestock that died from heat clouds. Compensation was divided based on the age of cattle that died: US$850 for one adult cow, US$550 for one young cow, and US$350 for a calf (Wimbardana et al., 2013, p. 11).

In some locations, cash for work activities were in synergy with activities of other agencies that were using heavy equipment. Thus, cash for work made an even wider impact on the welfare of the surrounding communities. For instance, a cash for work project was designed to build a bridge between the villages of Umbulharjo and Kepuharjo, as well as building the main hall of Kepuharjo village. Further, the National Team for the Acceleration of Poverty Reduction (TNP2K) worked closely with Community-Based Settlements Rehabilitation and Reconstruction Project (PNPM/Rekompak) to reduce poverty.

To date, the PNPM Support Facility (PSF) has disbursed over US$6 million mostly in cash for work activities in two provinces of Daerah Istimewa Yogyakarta (DIY) and Central Java. Over 750,000 employment days have been generated to first clean-up Merapi-affected villages (January–June 2011) and then to reconstruct their basic infrastructure (July–December 2011). While the cash for work program is now closed, the remaining funds will finance sub-projects selected through the PNPM process.

ASP in Sleman shows its benefit for affected communities in short-term recovery. In the long-term, however, it should be related with the community's own livelihood sources. For this, it is important to integrate the program with the economic recovery process after the volcano eruption (Sagala et al., 2012).

Disaster risk reduction, social protection and community resilience in Indonesia

The results of these studies show how the community proposes the use of community empowerment funds to support the reconstruction of physical infrastructure in order to contribute to community disaster preparedness and to mitigate risks. While the program was initially designed on a short-term basis, the impacts of the physical infrastructure protect livelihoods that foster community resilience. This chapter suggests community resilience from SP programs relies on the high involvement and participation of community members in the design of programs. There is a need to consider some of the strategies adopted in the implementation of SP to support community resilience. Social workers, such as PNPM facilitators, are important to enhance the awareness and involvement of communities in the utilization of SP programs. These facilitators work to explain how PNPM works to the communities. As discussed in Indramayu, social workers in the PNPM program contribute to shaping and stimulating the discussions among stakeholders and the direction of the programs. Similarly, in Sleman, social workers facilitate the PNPM program to integrate with the recovery process after the eruption of Mount Merapi in Sleman.

ASP can serve as means to reduce disaster risk, to recover from disaster, and ultimately, to contribute to community resilience. SP has limitations because it needs to tap into a community's own resources. In West Sumatra (Indonesia), Vanhoebroek and Sagala (2010) found that the recovery process following the 2009 earthquake was partly supported by the social capital that people have. Since the funding for housing reconstruction should be integrated from several sources and involve several stakeholders, the role of facilitators from universities and local NGOs is very important. Social workers in the Sapayuang Community Organization assisted in the process through meetings, raising awareness, and coordinating and stimulating collaboration among communities and different actors. Social workers bring their expertise in community development and community organizing. The social work facilitators involved stakeholders in the process to identify problems and potential solutions. This also included formal and informal processes in the affected communities. Thus, acceptance of all stakeholders was achieved through the steps supported by social work facilitators.

A study of four earthquake-affected areas in Indonesia observed the recovery process particularly on housing reconstruction (Pribadi et al., 2014). The four affected areas are Aceh (by earthquake and tsunami in 2004), Yogyakarta (by earthquake in 2006), West Sumatra and West Java (by earthquake in 2009). It was found that norms and social networks determined the shape and speed of housing reconstruction (Pribadi et al., 2014, p. 219). The housing reconstruction in Yogyakarta, Central Java (2006) was considerably more successful, due to the fact that the government of Indonesia distributed the housing fund directly to the beneficiaries through their bank accounts instead of distributing it through agencies, which were more complicated in Aceh (2004). In addition, in order to prevent overlapping of aid disbursement, the community applied a "community group" program to manage resources to reconstruct their housing or used local materials to minimize the cost of transportation. A combination of natural resources, social capital of the community (e.g., norms and social networks) and social workers sped up the recovery process.

Figure 13.1 summarizes the process from disaster risk reduction to community resilience through the the PNPM and social work facilitators. Social workers facilitate the process of achieving resilience by integrating PNPM to enhance the disaster risk reduction measures. For example, PNPM has provided road infrastructures that helped increase livelihood sources for the communities. The infrastructure provides a means for commuting, and engaging in economic activity or evacuation in disaster events. Although the amount of funding received is relatively small, PNPM can stimulate collective action in order to build community resilience.

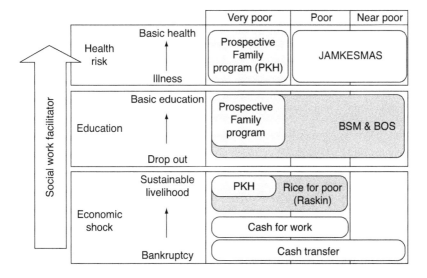

Figure 13.1 National strategies in social protection programs (TNP2K, 2011).

Conclusion

This chapter demonstrates the linkages between disaster risk reduction, social protection and community resilience, taking into account case studies from two districts in Indonesia. The similar characteristics among the goals, target groups and tools of SP and DRR make it promising for sharing opportunities in achieveing community resilience. Social protection has been utilized in developing countries to alleviate the burden faced by those with low incomes in society. In this chapter two case studies are presented to demonstrate how adaptive social protection through PNPM program can facilitate disaster risk reduction in disaster prone areas. ASP shows its benefit for affected communities in short-term recovery. In the long-term, however, it should be related with the community's own livelihood sources.

SP provides temporary or short-term benefits but also contributes in the long term to strengthen community capacities. Communities affected by climate change and disasters can access SP initiatives and funding to redevelop infrastructure that will further increase community preparedness and mitigate risks. ASP can serve as means to reduce disaster risk, to recover from disasters and extreme weather events, and ultimately, to achieve community resilience. The results of the studies presented in this chapter discuss the role of social work facilitators in terms of their practice in shaping social protection. By taking into consideration the needs to address disaster risk reduction and resilience, social workers can increase community awareness and build supports from other stakeholders.

To achieve community resilience, SP initiatives msut consider the local community context, including the community's own natural and social resources (social capital). This is promoted through the integration of community resources and their networks. The high involvement of community is required to integrate SP and DRR, which is enhanced by social workers in their practice.

References

22.870 ha rice plantation failed to be harvested (2008, August 1). *News @ Kompas.com*. Retrieved from http://nasional.kompas.com/read/2008/08/01/01264192/22.870.Ha. Tanaman.Padi.Puso.

Adger, W. (2000). Social and ecological resilience: Are they related? *Progress in Human Geography, 24*(3), 347–364.

Akita, T., & Szeto, J.K. (2000). Inpres Desa Tertinggal (IDT) program and Indonesian regional inequality. *Asian Economic Journal, 14*(2), 167–186.

Bappeda Indramayu. (2011). *Medium term development plant of Indramayu district 2011–2015*. Retrieved from www.bapeda.indramayukab.go.id/data/rpjmd/BAB-II-RPJMD.pdf.

Bappeda Indramayu. (2014). Medium term development plant of Indramayu district.

Bappeda Sleman. (2011). Medium term development plant of Sleman district. Retrieved from http://bappeda.slemankab.go.id/wp-content/uploads/2014/09/Bab-2-GAMBARAN-UMUM.pdf.

BAPPENAS (National Development Planning Agency). (1994). *IDT program implementation guidance*. BAPPENAS, Jakarta.

BAPPENAS. (2013) *Evaluation of PNPM Mandiri*. Directorate of Sectoral Development Performance Evaluation (BAPPENAS).

BAPPENAS & BNPB. (2011). Action plan for the rehabilitation and reconstruction eruption of Mount Merapi, DIY and Central Java Province in 2011–2013. Retrieved from http://perpustakaan.bappenas.go.id/lontar/file?file=digital/112720-%5B_Konten_%5D-Konten%20C7527.pdf.

Barat, J. (2015, August 24). *22.199 peserta menunggak, BPJS Rugi Rp 5,6 Miliar*. Retrieved from www.pikiran-rakyat.com/jawa-barat/2015/08/24/339644/22199-peserta-menunggak-bpjs-rugi-rp-56-miliar.

Béné, C., Cannon, T., Davies, M., Newsham, A., & Tanner, T. (2014). *Social protection and climate change*. OECD Development Co-operation Working Papers. Retrieved from www.keepeek.com/Digital-Asset-Management/oecd/development/social-protection-and-climate-change_5jz2qc8wc1s5-en#page1.

BNPB. (2015). *Database of disasters in Indonesia* (DIBI). Retrieved from http://dibi.bnpb.go.id/DesInventar/simple_data.jsp.

BPS. (2015). *Indonesia in numbers*. Retrieved from www.bps.go.id/linkTabelStatis/view/id/1274..

BPS Indramayu (2014). *Statistic of Indramayu District in 2014*. The Statistical Bireou of Indramayu District (BPS). Retrieved from http://indramayukab.bps.go.id/index.php/publikasi/128.

Choi, N., & Tomlinson, K. (2013). *2013 PSF progress report*. Jakarta: PSF Secretariat.

Coordinating Ministry for People's Welfare of the Republic Indonesia & PNPM Support Facility (PSF). (2011). *Where there is a will, there is a way: Cash for work in early recovery post Merapi eruption*. Office of the Coordinating Ministry for People's Welfare, Jakarta. Retrieved from http://psflibrary.org/catalog/repository/MERAPI%20BOOK%20lowres.pdf.

CRED. (2015). *EM-DAT database*. Retrieved from www.emdat.be/publications.

Davies, M., Guenther, B., Leavy, J., Mitchell, T., & Tanner, T. (2009). Climate change adaptation, disaster risk reduction and social protection: Complementary roles in agriculture and rural growth? *IDS Working Papers*, *2009*(320), 1–37.

Davies, M., Guenther, B., Leavy, J., Mitchell, T., & Tanner, T. (2008). "Adaptive social protection": Synergies for poverty reduction. *IDS Bulletin*, *39*(4), 105–112.

Davies, M., Béné, C., Arnall, A., Tanner, T., Newsham, A., & Coirolo, C. (2013). Promoting resilient livelihoods through adaptive social protection: Lessons from 124 programmes in South Asia. *Development Policy Review*, *31*(1), 27–58.

Devereux, S., Eide, W.B., Hoddinott, J., Lustig, N., & Subbarao, K. (2012). Social protection for food security. High Level Panel of Experts on Food Security and Nutrition, a zero draft consultation paper, March 19, 2012. Retrieved from www.fao.org/cfs/cfs-hlpe.

Doocy, S., Gabriel, M., Collins, S., Robinson, C., & Stevenson, P. (2006). Implementing cash for work programmes in post-tsunami Aceh: Experiences and lessons learned. *Disasters*, *30*(3), 277–296.

Hellmuth, M.E., Mason, S.J., Vaughan, C., van Aalst, M.K., & Choularton, R. (Eds.). (2011). A better climate for disaster risk management. International Research Institute for Climate and Society (IRI), Columbia University, New York, USA.

Heltberg, R. (2007). Helping South Asia cope better with natural disasters: The role of social protection. *Development Policy Review*, *25*(6), 681–698.

Heltberg, R., Jorgensen, S.L., & Siegel, P.B. (2008). *Climate change, human vulnerability, and social risk management.* Washington, DC: World Bank.

ILO. (2003). *Report of the Director-General: Working out of poverty.* International Labour Conference, 91st Session, Geneva.

Katiman. (2012). *PNPM Mandiri implementation in poverty reduction (Case study: PNPM rural and urban in district Lohbener and Kandanghaur, Indramayu district, West Java Province)* (Master's Thesis). University of Gadjah Mada, Yogyakarta.

Kemenko Kesra. (2011). Where there is a will there is a way. *Cash for work in early recovery post Merapi Eruption PNPM Mandiri.* Jakarta: Coordinating Ministry for People's Welfare of the Republic of Indonesia and PNPM Support Facility (PSF).

Kustiasih, R. (2011, August 2). KUR is not complicated. *Financial Business Kompas.* Retrieved on October 5, 2015, from http://bisniskeuangan.kompas.com/read/2011/08/02/0507305/KUR.Bukan.Kredit.Usaha.Rumit.

Lassa, J.A., Li, D.E., Rohi, R., & Sura, Y.B. (2013). Civil society roles in governing disaster reduction at national and local levels. IRGSC, Working Paper No. 6. June 2013.

Miller, C., Tsoka, M., & Reichert, K. (2011). Impacts on children of cash transfers in Malawi. In S. Handa, S. Devereux, & D. Webb (Eds.), *Social protection for Africa's children.* London: Routledge.

Miller, W.R., & Rollnick, S. (2012). *Motivational interviewing: Helping people change.* New York: Guilford Press.

Ministry of Agriculture. (2010). *Road map of agriculture strategy.* Retrieved from www.google.co.id/url?sa=t&rct=j&q=&esrc=s&source=web&cd=6&cad=rja&uact=8&ved=0CEUQFjAFahUKEwiozbD6n43IAhWFJpQKHVrfANc&url=http%3A%2F%2Fwww.pertanian.go.id%2Fdpi%2Fdownlot.php%3Ffile%3Droad_map_strategi_sektor_pertanian.pdf&usg=AFQjCNHPZgwJh9Au8Ol1Fte66UdZ6MD-yA&sig2=tZ4IrEDQFUh2_mfnca1oLQ&bvm=bv.103388427,d.dGo.

Ministry of Cooperatives and Small and Medium Enterprise. (2012). *Strategic plan, Ministry of Cooperatives and Small and Medium Enterprise 2012–2014.* Ministry of Cooperatives and Small and Medium Enterprise, Jakarta.

Ministry Women's Empowerment and Child Protection. (2012). *Policy and strategy: Increasing the productivity of women economy (PPEP).* Ministry Women's Empowerment and Child Protection, Jakarta.

National Planning Agency. (2011). Action plan for the rehabilitation and reconstruction of Mount Merapi eruption Yogyakarta and Central Java Province year 2011–2013. BAPPENAS and BNPB, June 2011.

OECD. (2015). *OECD economic surveys.* Indonesia.

Pribadi, K., Kusumastuti, D., Sagala, S., & Wimbardana, R (2014). Post-disaster housing reconstruction in Indonesia: Review and lessons from Aceh (2004), Yogyakarta (2006), West Java (2009) and West Sumatra (2009) earthquakes. In R. Shaw (Ed.), *Disaster recovery: Used or mis-used opportunities.*

Priyanti, A., & Ilham, N. (2011). Impact Mount Merapi eruption to farm economy. *Wartazoa, 21*(4), 153–160.

Republika. (2014, April 28). *Thousands of very poor family have not accepted pkh.* Retrieved from http://nasional.republika.co.id/berita/nasional/jawa-barat-nasional/14/04/28/n4qlao-ribuan-keluarga-sangat-miskin-belum-terima-pkh.

Republika. (2015, August 26). *175 companies in indramayu have not registered their employees to BPJS health.* Retrieved from http://nasional.republika.co.id/berita/nasional/daerah/15/08/26/ntnfjo280-175-perusahaan-di-indramayu-belum-daftarkan-pekerjanya-ke-bpjs-kesehatan.

Sagala, S., & Sani, I.R. (2014). *Livelihood adjustments to climate changes and foreign migrant worker*. Working Paper of RDI 9/2014.

Sagala, S., Rosyidie, A., Wimbardana, R., Pratama, A.A., & Ratna, A. (2012). *Promoting tourism in hazard zone area for local economic development: Case study of tourism in Cangkringan, Mt. Merapi*. Paper presented at the International Conference on Sustainable Built Environment Yogyakarta, July 10–12, 2012.

Sagala, S., Alpian A. Pratama, Teti Argo, & Asirin. (2012). The role of migrant worker remittances to reduce flood due to sea level rise risks in Indramayu. Journal of Tata Loka, University of Diponegoro, Indonesia.

Sarman, M. & Sajogyo. (2000). *Problem in poverty alleviation: Reflection from the east part of Indonesia*. Jakarta.

Sarman, M.D.S. (2000). *Reflection of poverty alleviation program from East Region of Indonesia*. Depok: Puspa Swara.

The Secretariat of the JRF (Java Reconstruction Fund). (2012). *Java reconstruction fund final report 2012. Disaster response & preparedness: From innovations to good practice.*

Seruu (2013, November 26). *Thousands of fishermen in Indramayu are not insured.* Retrieved from http://city.seruu.com/read/2013/11/26/192718/ribuan-nelayan-di-indramayu-belum-dapat-asuransi.

Stern, N.H. (2007). *The economics of climate change: The Stern review*. Cambridge University Press.

Sumarto, S., & Bazzi, S. (2011). Social protection in Indonesia: Past experiences and lessons for the future. *MPRA Paper No. 57893*. Retrieved from https://mpra.ub.uni-muenchen.de/id/eprint/57893.

Tierney, K. (2012). Disaster governance: Social, political, and economic dimensions. *Annual Review of Environment and Resources, 37*, 341–363.

TNP2K. (2015). *Program Keluarga Harapan (PKH)*. Retrieved from www.tnp2k.go.id/id/tanya-jawab/klaster-i/program-keluarga-harapan-pkh/

Tobin, G.A., & Whiteford, L.M. (2002). Community resilience and volcano hazard: The eruption of Tungurahua and evacuation of the Faldas in Ecuador. *Disasters, 26*(1), 28–48.

Triyoga, L.S. (2010). *Merapi dan Orang Jawa: Persepsi dan Sistem Kepercayaan* [The Javanese people and Merapi volcano: Perceptions and system of belief]. Jakarta: Grasindo.

Twigg, J. (2007). Characteristics of a disaster resilient community: A guidance note. DFID DRRICG.

UN-ESCAP. (2013). *Enabling entrepreneurship for women's economic empowerment in Asia and the Pacific*. Retrieved from www.unescap.org/sites/default/files/SDD_PUB-Executive-Summary-Enabling-entrepreneurship-for-women%27s-empowerment.pdf.

UNICEF Indonesia (2012). *MDGs and equity for children in Indonesia: An overview*. Retrieved from www.unicef.org/indonesia/A1-_E_Issue_Brief_MDG_REV.pdf

UNISDR. (2004). *Living with risk: A global review of disaster reduction initiatives*. Retrieved from www.unisdr.org/files/657_lwr1.pdf.

UNISDR. (2014). UNISDR annual report 2014. Retrieved from www.unisdr.org/we/inform/publications/42667.

UNISDR. (2015). *Sendai framework for disaster risk reduction 2015–2030*. Switzerland: UNISDR.

Vanhoebroek, P., & Sagala, S. (2010). *Not so helpless victims: Social capital roles in the 2009 West Sumatra earthquake recovery*. Indonesia: Research Report of International Federation of Red Cross and Red Crescent (IFRC).

Vishwanath, T., & Yu, X. (2008). *Providing social protection and livelihood support during post-earthquake recovery*. Washington, DC: World Bank.

Voss, J. (2012). *Rural PNPM, impact evaluation. April, 2010.* Jakarta: PNPM Support Facility.

Wijayanti, A.R., & Sagala, S. (2012). Bounce back after volcano disaster: The assessment of community's capacity in restoring livelihood destruction. PlanoCosmo International Conference, 2012, Bandung, Indonesia. School of Architecture, Planning, and Policy Development, V-55–V-68.

Wimbardana, R., Sagala, S., Pratama, A., & Rosyidie, A. (2013). Assessing community's socio-economic enhancement in post disaster recovery: Case study of Mount Merapi. The 2nd Planocosmo International Conference, 2013 Bandung. School of Architecture, Planning, and Policy Development, Institute of Technology Bandung.

Yogyakarta Agricultural Bureau. (2011). *The statistics of Yogyakarta Province livestock year 2006–2010.* Yogyakarta Province.

14 Conclusion

Julie Drolet

Introduction

The chapters in this book demonstrate a renewed and growing importance given to social protection as a human right and as a precondition for economic and social development. The ILO Recommendation No. 202 on the implementation of national floors of social protection (SPF) was adopted in 2012 by 185 ILO member states. Social protection floors guarantee universal access to health services and income security through the life cycle for children, unemployed and poor, older and disabled persons. Internationally, there are rights-based national social protection floors or measures of it that have been successfully implemented in many countries. The case studies in this book serve to present diverse social protection initiatives, and share successful and emerging experiences among stakeholders on promising practices and areas for future development. Building critical knowledge and innovative practices in social protection is of interest to social workers and students who are seeking to develop a new understanding and to implement actions in support of the right to social protection. Social protection floors contribute to the realization of the human right to social security and to social services, founded in the Universal Declaration of Human Rights, the Convention on the Rights of the Child, and other international legal instruments. There is an urgent need to work toward the goal of establishing social protection floors, and the future role of social workers in this process. In the literature reviewed in this book there is growing evidence that social protection floors are ambitious but feasible, affordable and effective in the reduction of extreme poverty. The post-2015 global development agenda incorporates social protection as a key component to reduce inequalities, to eradicate extreme poverty, and to support a number of sustainable development goals such as promoting gender equality, decent work, climate adaptation and universal health coverage.

Social work and social development perspectives

This book adopts a social work and social development perspective to understand social protection initiatives. Social workers aim to promote human rights and social justice in national and international contexts, and promote social development. Social development is a developmental perspective that is concerned with people's well-being and progressive social change. The interconnections between economic policy and social policy are captured in a social development approach that calls for a holistic and transformative approach to eradicate poverty and to promote social inclusion. Rather than focus on the economy per se, a social work and social development perspective recognizes the important social and human dimensions that must be considered. A critical social work approach demonstrates how the daily lives of individuals are linked to wider political, social, cultural and/or economic structures and systems. Social injustices such as poverty, social exclusion, inequalities, discrimination, oppression, abuse and exploitation are a key concern for social workers. A social work and social development perspective is people-centered, and requires a multifaceted approach and a variety of strategies to design and implement policies and programs to meet people's needs, to promote people's aspirations, and to uphold people's dignity. Further, given the complex environmental challenges due to climate change and related natural disasters, the role of the natural environment is considered in this volume with adaptive social protection that integrates the social, economic and environment dimensions.

The book explores the term "social protection" and its main components using a social development perspective and approaches in policies, programs and initiatives. The origins of the term "sustainable development" that linked economic, social and environmental dimensions in international policy and initiatives are presented, and the newly adopted Sustainable Development Goals in the post-2015 development framework. The concept of livelihoods, and related approaches and strategies, is highlighted, as well as the term "sustainable livelihoods" given the need for people to earn a living in sustainable manner. A gender perspective that considers gender equality, gender equity and gender inequality is necessary for transformative social protection. Varied definitions and understandings of poverty relevant to social protection initiatives are presented, including a multidimensional approach to eradicating poverty.

Learning from the regions

Chapters 1 to 7 of this book explore the key concepts and definitions relevant to social protection from a social work and social development perspective. Chapters 8 to 13 present case studies based on social protection initiatives in Asia (India, Indonesia), Africa (Ghana, Nigeria, South Africa) and Latin America (Brazil). The authors in this book share a concern about poverty, inequality and new forms of insecurity for individuals, families, communities and public sector institutions. Social workers are concerned with the social impacts of the economic crisis and the lived human experience. Each chapter discusses the role of social work in the development and promotion of social protection initiatives, and the implications for the social work profession to build on promising practices, key challenges, contributions to international cooperation and priorities for action.

Implications for social work policy and practice

The International Federation of Social Workers (IFSW) strongly supports the implementation of social protection floors as they offer an integrated approach addressing multidimensional vulnerabilities. Social protection floors with the guarantees for health services and basic income throughout the life cycle will stabilize and better the life of many clients of social work. Given the role of social workers in the implementation of social protection policies through key social service programs and service, it is necessary to consider the actual, potential and future roles of social workers in achieving national social protection floors around the world.

The Global Agenda for Social Work and Social Development, a joint commitment to action of the three global organizations of professionals (IFSW) and educators (IASSW) in social work and social development activists (ICSW) adopted in 2012 explicitly supports social protection floors. With the adoption of social protection initiatives governments are assuming their responsibility for the well-being of people living within their geographical boundaries and for the provision of appropriate social services. Social workers and their international social work organizations are willing to assume their role to contribute to the implementation and functioning of social protection floors as members of civil society and as professionals in public or private social services.

The topic of social protection is increasingly gaining international interest and attention. The 2012 Social Work and Social Development Conference held in Stockholm featured several keynote presentations and workshop sessions on social protection floors, and the idea for this book emerged from a session at this conference, which indicates a high level of interest in social protection as a social work research and professional activity. It is unknown at this time how social protection is covered in academic courses, but it is anticipated that it will be increasingly integrated in cross-national, national and international social policy, and social and economic development courses taught across the disciplines.

Social workers bring knowledge and expertise to contribute to the development of social protection floors that meet the needs and cultural traditions of marginalized, at-risk and vulnerable people with whom they work. Social workers are positioned to make the voice of their clients heard, advocate with them and empower them to claim their rights. With the expected proliferation of social protection systems it is important that social workers prepare themselves to participate in this task and understand the active role they can play in the conception, implementation, managing, delivering and monitoring of social protection floors.

The role of social work will vary in relation to different benefits and provision schemes depending on the organizational and administrative structures, on division of labor, on the acquired status of the profession, and on cultural and traditional ways of support for and by families and communities in varying contexts. The social work profession works to meet the need for integrated social services, to promote social protection floor inclusion for all, and to advocate for the inclusion of social workers. Consistent with the social development para-digm, social workers offer a range of skills, strategies, principles and activities at the individual, family, community and policy levels. Social work education and training plays an important role in building capacity of the profession in coun-tries where there are not enough qualified social workers to develop social pol-icies and to deliver social services. Social work and human service professionals facilitate access to health services, unemployment benefits, social insurance pro-grams, assistance for older people (pensions and basic allowances), child protec-tion, family allowances, welfare and social services, cash and in-kind transfers, temporary subsidies for utilities and staple foods, employment programs and skills development, and work to meet the needs of poor, vulnerable and disad-vantaged families. It is important to recognize and respect the role of social workers in the implementation of national social protection systems, and inter-national development practitioners can learn from them.

Future of social protection

Social protection initiatives can enhance human resilience, and need to take into account people's vulnerabilities and capacities across the life cycle. In an increasingly interconnected world what was once local is now global, as people experience direct change in their lives due to international economic, social and environmental forces. Social workers are particularly concerned with the needs and rights of the marginalized, at-risk, vulnerable and excluded. The post-2015 development agenda and Sustainable Development Goals provide an opportunity for the international community to reduce poverty and vulnerability, and build resilience. This is particularly important with the increase in natural and (hu) man-made disasters.

"Universal access to basic social services – education, health care, water supply and sanitation, and public safety – enhances resilience" (UNDP, 2014, p. 5). There is an urgent need to expand social protection to meet the needs of more people around the world. For developing countries faced with the chal-lenges of underemployment, labour market policies are not enough, considering that most jobs are in the informal economy (UNDP, 2014). Many people employed in the informal sector, as well as the working poor, the self-employed and the unemployed have no social protection or social security coverage and no access to safety nets. Many migrant workers also lack access to social protection because they have crossed borders that define eligibility and accessibility to pro-grams and services. This needs to change. And it will change because we must do better.

Social protection is an important topic in the Social Sciences, Humanities, Social Policy, Management, International Development Studies, Social Work and Human Service. This book provides examples of how social workers can get involved in realizing the right to social protection. The conceptual chapters and case studies are of interest to a wide range of individuals, including international academics, researchers, practitioners, and students in the social sciences, humanities, and health fields such as demographers, population geographers, social workers, sociologists, health researchers, economists, engineers, population health, nurses, anthropologists, political scientists, social policy analysts, planners, and others working in the broad field of international cooperation.

Innovative social protection policies and initiative will be designed and developed in the coming decade, and social workers will play an important role in their implementation. This is necessary for a human-centered and sustainable social development.

Reference

UNDP. (2014). *Human development report 2014: Sustaining human progress – reducing vulnerabilities and building resilience*. Retrieved on October 26, 2015 from http://hdr.undp.org/en/2014-report.

Index

Page numbers in *italics* denote tables, those in **bold** denote figures.

For Product Safety Concerns and Information please contact our EU
representative GPSR@taylorandfrancis.com
Taylor & Francis Verlag GmbH, Kaufingerstraße 24, 80331 München, Germany